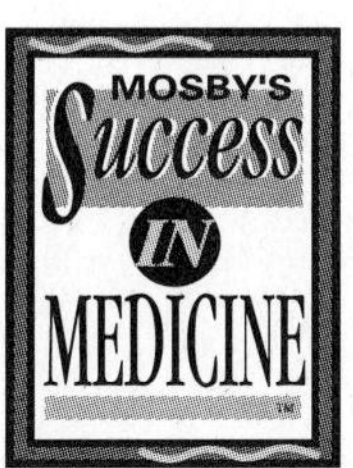

Histology & Cell Biology

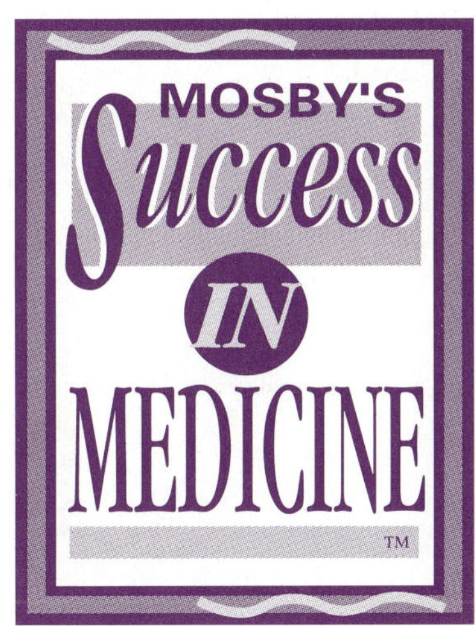

Histology & Cell Biology

E. Robert Burns, Ph.D.

Course Director, Microscopic Anatomy,
Professor of Anatomy,
Department of Anatomy,
College of Medicine,
University of Arkansas for Medical Sciences,
Little Rock, Arkansas

M. Donald Cave, Ph.D.

Professor of Anatomy,
Department of Anatomy,
College of Medicine,
University of Arkansas for Medical Sciences,
Little Rock, Arkansas

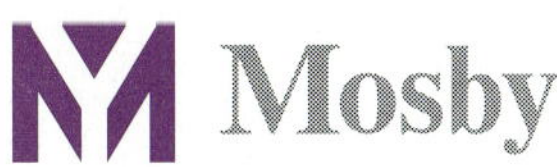 Mosby

St. Louis Baltimore Boston Carlsbad Chicago Naples New York Philadelphia Portland
London Madrid Mexico City Singapore Sydney Tokyo Toronto Wiesbaden

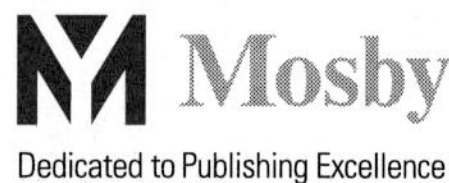

Dedicated to Publishing Excellence

A Times Mirror
Company

Vice-President and Publisher *Anne S. Patterson*
Editor *Emma D. Underdown*
Developmental Editor *Christy Wells*
Project Manager *Dana Peick*
Production Editor *Jeffrey Patterson*
Manufacturing Supervisor *Tony McAllister*
Book Designer *Amy Buxton*
Cover Design *Stacy Lanier/AKA Design*

Printed in the United States of America
Composition by Graphic World, Inc.
Printing/binding by R. R. Donnelly

Mosby–Year Book, Inc.
11830 Westline Industrial Drive
St. Louis, Missouri 63146

Published in the United States as Ace the Boards

Library of Congress Cataloging-in-Publication Data

Burns, E. Robert.
    Mosby's USMLE step 1 reviews—histology & cell biology/E. Robert Burns, M. Donald Cave.
        p.   cm.—(Ace the boards)
    Includes index.
    1. Histology—Examinations, questions, etc.   2. Cytology—Examinations, questions, etc.   3. Pathology, Cellular—Examinations, questions, etc.   I. Cave, M. Donald.   II. Title.   III. Series.
    [DNLM: 1. Histology—examination questions.   2. Cytology—examination questions. QS 518.2 B967m 1996]
    QM554.B85   1996
    DNLM/DLC
    for Library of Congress   95-52478
                                                                    CIP

        ISBN 0-8151-8927-3   (IBM)
        ISBN 0-8151-8928-1   (MAC)

96 97 98 99 00 / 9 8 7 6 5 4 3 2 1

PREFACE

ACE The Boards: Histology and Cell Biology is a complete review of the topics contained in a modern, medical Microscopic Anatomy course (i.e. cell biology, basic tissues, histology, and organology). Wherever possible we have presented a cell biology approach to histology and organology. A unique feature of this book is the attention given to cell proliferation and cell cycle kinetics of the tissues and organs.

Structure and function correlation is the basic theme of this book. Structure separated from function exists in an isolated, relatively uninteresting setting. Structure correlated with function is more meaningful and therefore easier to learn. A natural extension of learning normal structure and function is to begin the process of thinking about some abnormal structure and function relationships. This book contains many clinical or histopathologic correlations, which bridge the gap between what is normal and what is pathologic.

Each of us has been teaching freshmen medical students for 25 years. This book has gradually evolved from written materials provided to students during that time. We have constantly revised, reworked, and reconfigured this information in response to advice, suggestions, and criticism from our students.

Pedagogical Features

Concise, bottom line information is presented in *outline style format.* Tables, charts, lists, and diagrams summarize material for ease in integrating. Open layout and special design allow room for notetaking.

Each chapter contains a sampling of *multiple-choice* or *matching review questions* useful for preparing for the USMLE and other exams. *Perforated answer sheets* in the back of the book allow you to tear out the scoring sheets and have the answers right at your fingertips.

A computer *diskette* with over *500 categorized questions* provides immediate feedback on answers and allows you to pinpoint exactly the areas you want to study.

The crisp *illustrations* enhance understanding through the use of color.

Marginal icons can be used to locate key information quickly.

ACKNOWLEDGMENTS

We thank Emma Underdown at Mosby for finding us and providing leadership and advice throughout the project. Emma's staff is to be commended for keeping us on track.

Without the input of literally thousands of freshmen medical students over the duration of our teaching careers, we would have command of the subject but not necessarily be able to make it understandable to medical students. We owe a significant amount of appreciation and thanks to our former, current, and future students. We especially thank Anna Monias for her thoughtful, detailed review of the entire manuscript.

Several people have played instrumental roles, which have enabled us to undertake this task. They include our parents, our mentors (Edith K. MacRae, PhD–MDC; S. Meryl Rose, PhD–ERB), and our colleagues.

Donna Cave (MDC) and Mary Lindsey (ERB) have helped us complete this work in a variety of immeasurable ways from typing, to editing, to good old fashioned partnership support. They may never know the extent or the impact of their support to us.

E. Robert Burns, Ph.D.
M. Donald Cave, Ph.D.

Test-Taking Strategies

Suzanne F. Kiewit, M.Ed.

Standardized national exams are a part of the medical education process in many countries. To perform well on standardized exams, it is imperative that you begin with a **plan.** Be as efficient and effective as possible by planning well.

MONTHS AHEAD OF THE EXAM

- Sit down with a blank calendar and block in your commitments: classes, final exams, scheduled events.
- Include time for activities of daily life: eating, sleeping, exercising, socializing, banking, maintaining your home, and so forth.
- The remaining time is available for study/review.
- Determine an orderly approach to the material you need to cover that fits your particular set of needs (e.g., subject-by-subject approach, systems approach, pathologic state approach).
- Assign the remaining time to content areas. This is done in various ways: material covered last year first, easiest material first, least comfortable material first, detailed subjects last, whatever. Your plan should reflect your goal: to maximize your score.
- Establish a warm-up, which may consist of breaking the tension in major muscle groups (neck rolls, shoulder rolls, etc.), a quick visualization of you performing successfully, or a brief meditation. Practicing this warm-up routine before each of your study sessions will make it a familiar activity that helps you learn effectively, as well as take exams effectively.
- Designate time at the end of your study period for overall review. Depending on your needs, that might be a week or just several days before the exam.
- Plan for feedback on your efforts. Schedule time for answering questions on the material you are reviewing and for taking at least one mock comprehensive exam.
- Do the comprehensive exam midway through your study period so that you can refine your efforts to reflect the degree of your performance.

DAYS AHEAD OF THE EXAM

- Divide each day into thirds: morning block, afternoon block, and evening block.
- Consider the time of day that is most productive for you and do the most difficult or least favorite material at that time.
- Assign more blocks of study to those areas requiring the most review to reach a comfortable knowledge level.
- A popular way to use blocks is to pair subjects or materials. For instance, pair strong content with weaker content so that you are not always in the position of not knowing material (which would invite negative feelings or ineffectiveness). Or pair a conceptual subject with a detail subject, such as physiology with anatomy, so that you are not always doing the same kind of thinking (this invites positive effort).
- Use your most productive blocks of time for actual study/review. Use the nonpeak times for reinforcement of material covered or feedback by answering questions on material that you have covered.

Planning the Blocks

- Once you determine time allocations for each content area and an orderly approach that fits your needs and goals, you want to specify what you plan to do during each block.
- Be specific as to content area, material to study, and task; for example, MICRO: review chart on viruses; PHYS: answer questions on renal; and so forth.
- Each study block will last approximately 3 to 4 hours. To be most efficient and effective, plan to take a 5- or 10-minute break every hour. If you are having difficulty getting into the study mode, plan to study for 25 minutes, then take a 5-minute break. Reserve longer breaks for switches between subjects. Get up and move around on breaks.

BEFORE THE EXAM

You can maximize your exam performance by taking control. Adults tend to perform better when they feel that they have a measure of control. With comprehensive exams, it is easy to feel out of control. You are told what time to arrive, where to go, what writing instrument to use, and so on. You want to assume control of as many aspects as possible to maximize your performance:

STUDY   Follow the wise advice of planning your work and working your plan to maintain satisfactory preparation with regard to study.

SLEEP   Get a good night's rest. Sleep needs vary, but 6 hours is usually minimum. Try to get the appropriate amount of sleep that you require.

NUTRITION   Maintain proper nutrition during both study time and exam time. Eat breakfast. Choose foods that help keep you on an even energy level. Eat light lunches on exam days. If you have a favorite food and can take it with you, treat yourself.

MEDICATION   It may be cold, flu, or allergy season. Take no medications that may make you drowsy.

CLOTHING   Heating and cooling systems are rarely balanced enough to suit everyone. Wear articles of clothing that can be added or removed as necessary. Strive for personal comfort.

READINESS   Develop physical, mental, emotional, and psychologic readiness for the exam. Keep your thoughts about the exam and your preparation efforts positive. You must believe that *you can do this!*

ARRIVAL   Plan to arrive as close to the designated time as possible and still allow yourself sufficient time to check in. Keep to yourself so that other people's anxieties will not affect you. Find your seat.

ACCLIMATION   Settle in and get comfortable. Take several deep breaths . . . RELAX. A relaxed mind thinks better than a tense one. Do your warm-up routine.

ATTENTION   Pay attention to the proctor. Complete all identification material as required. Read all instructions carefully. Ask for clarification as needed. Do not open your test until told to do so. Once you begin, quickly glance through the whole test to see how it is set up and how questions are organized. Again, you want to take control of the situation. A quick review eliminates surprises and allows you to develop a plan.

DURING THE EXAM

Plan Your Approach

There are numerous approaches to answering questions. Answer questions in the order that appeals to you. Doing the easier ones first may give a psychologic boost; however, the ones you skip may stay on your mind and cloud your thinking.

Another approach is to answer each question in sequence. Start with the first one in the section with which you begin and fill in an answer for each question. Do not leave any blanks! The theory behind this is that if you spend any time at all on an item, you should mark your best response at that time and go on. If you are not certain of your choice, mark "R" on the test for review and return to it later as you have time.

There are various formats to questions. The most popular is the one-best-answer multiple choice item. These typically pose a question and ask you to choose between five options. Another popular question type is the matching sets. These may include short leading lists or long leading lists of up to 26 items from which to choose.

Some students plan to do the matching items first. If you prefer matching items, this is a reasonable plan because it helps you get started with items about which you feel confident. It is also reasonable because matching items are not good items on which to guess if you run short of time. **You** must decide the order in which you want to do the questions.

Complete the Answer Sheet Carefully

There are two schools of thought on this matter. One is to fill in the answer sheet **item by item** as you go. This method minimizes transcription errors. The other method is **block transfer.** Complete a logical chuck of questions in the test (one or two pages) and then transfer responses to the answer sheet. Be sure that the last question number on the page is the last numeral you blacken. This method saves time and offers a mini–mental break at the end of each block. Such minibreaks help decrease fatigue during a long exam. Choose the method that will work for you and *practice* it as you take prep questions.

Budget Your Time

Know how much time is allotted and check the number of questions. A quick calculation will give you the average number of seconds or minutes you can spend on each item and still complete the exam. Obviously, some questions may go more quickly and balance out the ones that take longer. To keep track, you need a pacing strategy. A good strategy is to establish checkpoints at 30-minute intervals. When you overview the exam, circle the numerals corresponding to where you should be at 30 minutes, 60, 90, 120, and so on. For example, if you have 200 questions on a 3-hour exam, you should be at question number 33 at 30 minutes. As you complete the exam, check your time at the circled items. This technique keeps you from watching the clock too much, yet permits multiple opportunities to adjust your pacing.

If you find yourself spending too much time on any one question, select your best choice at that time, mark an answer, and "R" it for later review. The point is to keep going. Laboring too long on one question limits you from responding to other items you may know well. Remember, controlling your time helps you maximize your points.

ANSWERING THE QUESTIONS

- **Read and *understand* the stems and alternatives.**

  The most frequent error made on exams is misreading or misinterpreting the various aspects of a question. The **stem** is the introductory question or statement. The **alternatives** are the options from which you select the one best response. To encourage reading and understanding, use a process.

- **Follow a process to answer questions.**
  1. Quickly read the stem.
  2. Quickly read the options. (Combined, the first two steps create a preview of the item.)
  3. Carefully read, underline, and mark the stem in a timely fashion.
     - Selectively underline key words and phrases.
     - Pay attention to nouns, verbs, and modifiers.
     - Circle age and gender.
     - Note data in telescopic form (e.g., $\uparrow$ BP).
     - Graphically represent material if it helps you to understand (e.g., diagram the renal tubule to answer a question about reabsorption).
  4. Carefully read each alternative. Mark as appropriate.

- **Consider each alternative as one in a series of true, false, or not sure (?) statements.**

  Read each alternative. Rather than slashing out the ones you eliminate, work with each one and designate it as **true, false,** or varying degrees of **true/false/?.** This marking strategy requires you to make judicious decisions about alternatives relative to the stem. It also provides a record of your original thinking, which will save you rethinking time if you need to reconsider a question. Practice this strategy on preparation questions so it becomes second nature.

- **Avoid premature closure.**

  Sometimes you may read a question and anticipate a response. Such a reaction helps focus your

attention. However, be sure to read *all* the options so that you are selecting the *best* response. In one-best-answer multiple choice questions, there is one *best* and several *likely* responses. Avoid being misled; consider all the alternatives.

- **Be leery of negative stems.**

  Negative stems require shifting to a negative thinking mode to determine which alternatives are not correct. You can avoid this shift by using this strategy:
  - Circle such words as *except, least, false, incorrect, not true* to raise your awareness of them.
  - Cross out the negative and read the stem as though it were a positive.
  - Mark each option as T/F/?. The F option will then be the appropriate choice.

- **Keep your original answers.**

  To change or not to change answers is a difficult decision. The answer depends on a person's previous history. If you are the kind of student who, if you change answers, changes them from wrong to right, then selectively changing answers may be worthwhile. If, on the other hand, your past experience has been to change right answers to wrong answers, selectively changing answers is probably not a good idea. Good performers change answers, but only if they have reason, such as acquired insight or discovery of misreading or misinterpretation.

- **Stay calm and focused.**

  If a question upsets you, calm yourself. Take several deep breaths. Tell yourself, "I can do this!" Give yourself a mental or physical break. Pay special attention to the next two or three questions after a bout of emotional uneasiness. It is possible to miss items when attention is diffused.

THINKING THROUGH QUESTIONS

- **Use logical reasoning and sound thinking.**
  - Read the item carefully. After careful reading, ask "What is this question really asking?" Restate it so that you know what is being asked.
  - Engage in a mental dialogue with the question. Talk to yourself about what you do know. Always start with what **you** know. Verbalize your thinking.
  - If a diagram or graphic representation is included, orient yourself to it **first** so that the options do not lead your thinking.

- **Use information found within the questions themselves to help you answer others.**

There will not be obvious answers on a nationally standardized exam. However, there may be items or graphics that trigger remembrances.

- **Create a diagram, chart, map, or graphic representation of given information.**
  Material that is visually presented usually helps clarify thinking. Use selective, quick sketching as warranted.

- **Reason through information like a detective.**
  - Sift through the details (preview).
  - Determine the relevant information (selectively mark).
  - Put the clues together as in solving a puzzle (reason).

- **Read carefully and note key descriptors.**
  - Note words such as *chronic, acute, greater than, less than, adult, child.*
  - Attend to prefixes such as *hyper-, hypo-, non-, un-, pre-, post-.*

- **Analyze base words and affixes.**
  Studying a question at the word level may help you remember salient information. Look for base words or related words. Determine Latin or Greek word parts and use their meanings to assist you.

- **Consider similar options equally.**
  If you mark one alternative as "false" for a particular reason and you think another option is false for the same reason, it's probably "false" as well.

- **Trust the questions.**
  The questions are designed to determine if you have a working knowledge of the material. They are not written to confuse you. You need to believe that your medical school curriculum and your study efforts prepared you for most of the questions.

- **Meet the challenge of clinical scenarios.**
  Longer scenarios challenge you to discern the relevant from the irrelevant material. In doing so, you are given multiple clues to consider. To effectively handle the scenario, follow this strategy:
  - Scan the stem and read the first several lines.
  - Skip to the end of the stem and read the last several lines.
  - Check the alternatives to narrow your focus.
  - Now that you know what the question is about, go back to the stem; read and mark what's important to your informed decision making.
  - Make good T/F/? decisions.

- **Reread your underlines and markings when you are down to two choices.**

By the time you work through a stem and numerous alternatives, it is easy to lose the focus of the question. Checking your focus by rereading only the underlines to ensure that you are answering the question being posed.

ANSWERING MATCHING ITEM SETS

Matching items are used to measure your ability to distinguish among closely related items. They require knowledge of specific sets of information. As you study, be alert to potential material that could be tested in this way.

Matching items can be formatted in two ways. **Short leading list matching** items include a set of five, lettered options followed by a lead-in statement and then several numbered stems. **Long leading list matching** items include a set of up to 26 lettered options, followed by a lead-in statement and then several numbered stems.

To efficiently deal with a short leading list item, consider it as an upside-down multiple choice item with the same repeated options. To handle it effectively, do the following:

- Scan the list; determine the topic.
- Read the lead-in statement; determine the focus.
- Quickly read the stem; then read and mark key words.
- In the left margin, create a grid with A, B, C, D, E at the top.
- Make good T/F/? decisions about each stem, marking them in the grid. In this way you can see the pattern of your responses. Similarly, a grid with the item numbers can be drawn beside the leading list and responses marked there.

Handling long leading list matching items effectively requires some modifications in the process. It is not efficient to make T/F/? decisions about each option, so follow this strategy:

- Scan the list; determine the topic.
- Read the lead-in; determine the focus.
- Read a stem and generate your own response.
- Narrow the focus. Put a check mark by those related options in the long list.
- Read and mark specifics in the stem to differentiate among those alternatives you marked.
- Make good T/F/? decisions.

For each stem, mark the narrowed-list options with a different symbol (star, dash, etc.). Items are listed in logical order, alphabetically or numerically. When looking for an option such as "xanthinuria," do not start at the beginning of the list. Looking in the appropriate place saves valuable seconds.

TEST PSYCHOLOGY

How a question is worded can often influence your response to it. Most clues about "test psychology" are a function of the way in which a question is worded—test constructors cannot rename body parts, drugs, diseases, and so forth. Being aware of the psychology behind the wording can often help you answer the test question.

Using techniques of test psychology to arrive at a correct answer has limited value on standardized exams because those who construct the exams are well aware of the use of these techniques. Nonetheless, being aware of these techniques of test psychology may add another point or two to your score, and they can also enhance your sense of control. Knowing these techniques provides additional strategies to employ should the question temporarily confuse you.

The best way to take any exam is to be totally prepared with a strong knowledge base and personal test confidence. The following techniques should be used only if you have exhausted your knowledge base, eliminated all distractors, and cannot come up with the answer even with logical thinking and sound reasoning. Such techniques are **not** a substitute for knowledge, nor are they foolproof.

- **Identify common ideas or themes within the options and between the stem and options.**
  - Circle repeated words in the options.
  - Select the option with the most repeated words or phrases.
  - Circle words repeated in both stem and options.
  - Select the option that contains key words or related words from the stem.
- **Beware of words that narrow the focus or are too extreme because they tend to be incorrect.**
  Circle such words as *all, always, every, exclusively, never, no, not, none.*
- **Options that are look-alikes are good candidates for exclusion.**
- **Note qualifiers that broaden the focus because they may be correct.**

Circle words such as *generally, probably, most, often, some, usually.*

- **Identify antonyms or two opposing statements as potentially correct options.**
  Test constructors may use pairs of opposites, so this tip may lose its effectiveness.
- **Select the most familiar-looking option.**
  Always go from what you know. Alternatives with unknown terms may be likely distractors.
- **Select the longest, most inclusive answer.**
  This would include "All of the above" as a strong potential response.
- **In numerical items, knock out the high and low alternatives and select one in the middle that seems most plausible.**
- **In negatively stemmed questions, categorize responses; the one that falls out of the category is a likely candidate.**
- **Mark the same alternative consistently throughout the test if you have no best guess and cannot eliminate distractors.**
  Before the test, decide which letter (A, B, C, D, E) will be your choice. In this way, if you have given a question your best effort and cannot decide, mark your favorite response and move to questions that cover more comfortable material.

AFTER THE EXAM

- **Between sessions and overnight:**
  - Take a well-deserved break. Eat nutritionally.
  - If you feel the urge to study, study material that is comfortable, from a source with which you are familiar (e.g., personally developed study cards or your annotated review book).
  - If you discovered a recurring "theme," you might desire to consult that set of information.
  - Do something pleasurable. Relax. Get a good night's rest.
- **After the final exam:**
  - Recognize that this exam is a measure of what you know on a given day for a given set of information at a given point in time. Keep a reasonable perspective.
- **Celebrate!**

References
Bushan V, Le T, Amin C: First aid for the USMLE Step 1, ed 5, Norwalk, Conn., 1995, Appleton & Lange.

CONTENTS

19 Endocrine System 199

20 Sense Organs 211

Answers and Explanations to Multiple Choice Review Questions 223

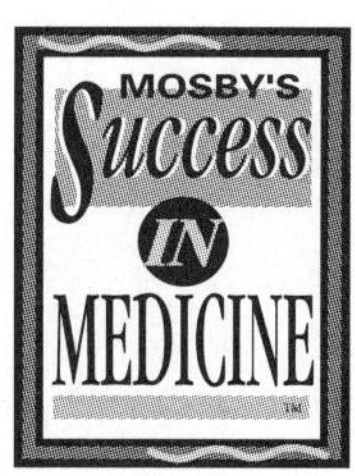

Histology & Cell Biology

Chapter 1

Introduction

The information covered in this book extends from the supramolecular organization of molecules in organelles, which can be envisioned by electron microscopy, to the organization of tissues in organs, which can be visualized with the naked eye. Table 1.1 summarizes this range in sizes.

The term Ångstrom (Å) is also used but less so nowadays. $1Å = 0.0001$ µm; $10,000$ Å $= 1$ µm; $1Å = 0.1$ nm.

- m = meter
- mm = millimeter
- µm = micrometer (micron)
- nm = nanometer

The *cell theory* first elaborated by Schleiden and Schwann in the nineteenth century has two major tenets:

- The cell is the fundamental structural and functional unit of biological systems.
- Cells arise only from preexisting cells.

The following are properties of cells that enable them to carry out the basic processes of life:

- Cells can harness and transform energy by extracting energy from foodstuff and converting it into a form that drives cellular reactions. This is largely a function of the enzymes in the cytosol and mitochondria.

Table 1.1   *Levels of Anatomic Organization*

DIMENSIONS	LEVELS	COURSE OF STUDY
1 m = 1000 mm	Organism ↑	Gross anatomy
	System ↑	
	Organ ↑	
1 µm = 0.001 mm	Tissue ↑	Cell biology and histology
1000 µm = 1 mm	Cell ↑	
	Organelle ↑	
1 nm = 0.001 µm	Molecule ↑	Biochemistry
1000 nm = 1 µm	Atom	

- Cells can control their own cellular environment by regulating what gets into them and what leaves them. This is largely a function of the plasma membrane.
- Cells replicate themselves and their constituents so that new cells arise from preexisting ones. This is largely a function of the replication and transcription of the DNA located in the chromosome.
- Cells differentiate and specialize enabling specific cells to carry out a specific function or functions.
- Cells interact to form larger units.

A *tissue* is a population of cells and their products that are specialized to perform a particular function or functions. There are four basic tissues:

- Epithelium
- Connective tissue
- Muscle tissue
- Nervous tissue

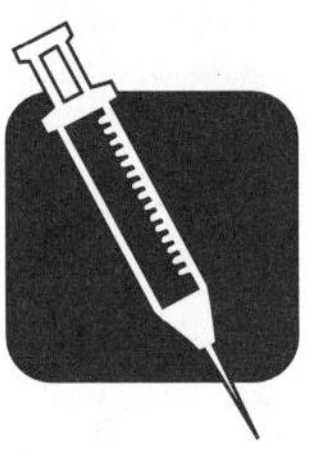

An *organ* is a group of tissues forming a structural unit and performing a specific function or functions. Most organs contain elements of all four tissues.

An *organ system* is a group of interconnected or interdependent organs that together perform aspecific function or functions.

An *organism* is a group of systems interacting in such a manner as to form a living economy.

Table 1.2   *Processing Tissues for LM and TEM*

Procedure	LM (Light Microscopy)	TEM (Transmission Electron Microscopy)	Purpose
1. Fixation	Formaldehyde solution	Glutaraldehyde and osmium tetroxide*	Preserves tissue morphology by coagulating protein, stops autolysis
2. Dehydration	Pass through graded ethanol series 35% → 100% EtOH		Removes water from cells and tissue
3. Clearing	Benzene (organic solvent)	Propylene oxide (organic solvent)	Enables cells and tissues to be penetrated with paraffin (LM) or plastic (TEM)
4. Embedding	Paraffin	Plastic (Epon)	Penetrates cells and intracellular spaces giving tissue rigidity for sectioning
5. Sectioning	5-10 μm on microtome	10-20 nm on ultramicrotome	Provides thin sections of cells and tissues
6. Mounting	Glass slide	Fine wire grid	Provides supporting medium for viewing and handling
7. Rehydration	Pass from benzene → 100% EtOH → 35% EtOH	Pass down 100% EtOH → 35% EtOH	Removes paraffin so that tissue can be stained with aqueous solution
8. Staining	Hematoxylin† and eosin‡	Uranyl acetate	Helps visualize tissue and cell components
9. Dehydration	Pass from 35% EtOH → 100% EtOH → benzene and mount under glass	Pass through 100% EtOH and air dry. Store in desiccant	Makes permanent

---

*Osmium tetroxide also stains lipid because osmium is electron dense and binds to lipid.

†Hematoxylin, a basic dye (positively charged at neutral pH), stains basophilic [acidic] components of the cell [e.g., nucleus].

‡Eosin, an acidic dye (negatively charged at neutral pH), stains acidophilic [basic] components of cell [e.g., cytoplasm].

Much of the information that we have gathered about cells and tissues has resulted from the applications of the light and electron microscopes. Because biological material is too thick to transmit light or electrons and because protoplasmic components are remarkably uniform in optical properties, it is usually necessary to cut thin sections of tissue (to transmit light or electrons) and stain them (to visualize components). To accomplish these ends the procedures shown in Table 1.2 are routinely utilized.

Fig. 1.1 shows an analogy between the light and electron microscopes. The *light microscope* (LM) and *transmission electron microscope* (TEM) have a similar arrangement of components.

The *illuminating system* serves to produce the required radiation (LM = visible light, TEM = electron beam) and direct it to the specimen.

The *source* emits radiation, which is used to form an image.

The *condensor lens* regulates the intensity of the illuminating beam on a specimen. Lenses for light microscopy are ground glass, which bends light rays, whereas lenses for electron microscopy are electromagnets, which control electrons.

The *specimen* is interposed between the illuminating and the imaging systems.

The *imaging* system is composed of the lenses, which produce a final magnified image.

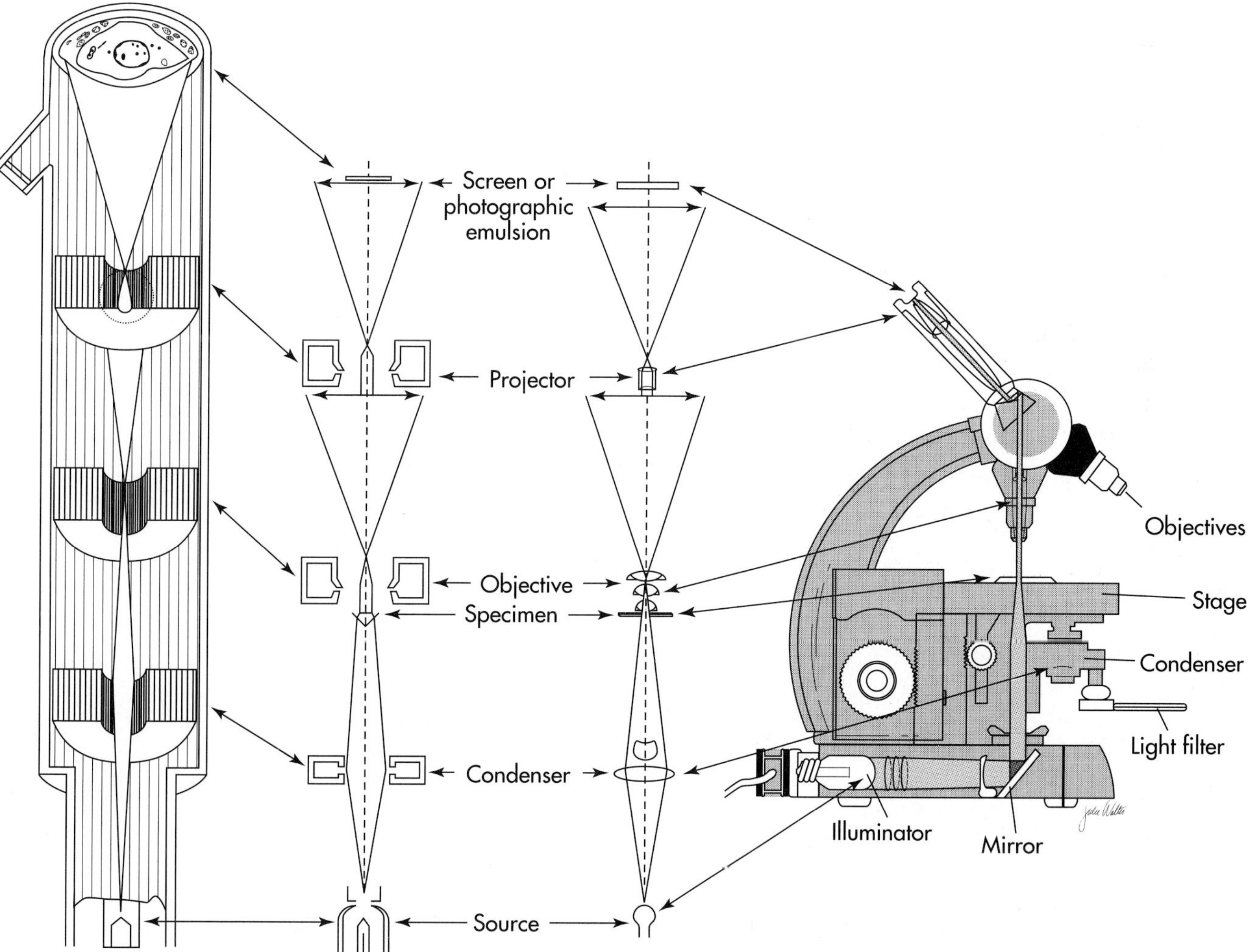

Fig. 1.1 Comparison of the light and electron microscopes. The light microscope utilizes optical lenses, and the electron microscope uses electromagnetic lenses to direct light rays or electrons. *(Modified from Junqueira LC, Carneiro J:* Basic histology, *ed 7, East Norwalk, Conn., 1992, Appleton & Lange.)*

The *objective* lens focuses the beam as it passes through a specimen to form a magnified intermediate image.

The *projection* lens (or ocular) magnifies a portion of the intermediate image to form the final image.

The image recording system consists of the eye (LM), the fluorescent screen viewed by the eye (TEM), and the photographic film (LM and TEM).

The critical factor in microscopy is resolution, which is the smallest distance at which two particles can be distinguished as separate objects. The highest resolution of the light microscope is 0.2 µm. Practically, bacteria and mitochondria, which measure 0.5 µm in thickness, are the smallest objects resolvable with the LM. In the TEM, resolutions of 1.0 nm are achieved.

Variants of light microscopy include *phase contrast microscopy* and *interference microscopy,* which enable visualization of cells and organelles without staining and therefore can be used to visualize living cells.

Scanning electron microscopy (SEM) is a variant of EM, which enables pseudo-three-dimensional views of the surfaces of cells, tissues, and organs. Whereas TEM uses electrons that have passed through a specimen or been diffracted by it to form an image, SEM uses electrons that are scattered or emitted from the specimen's surface. Resolution here is about 10 nm.

■ Some Special Procedures for Studying Cells

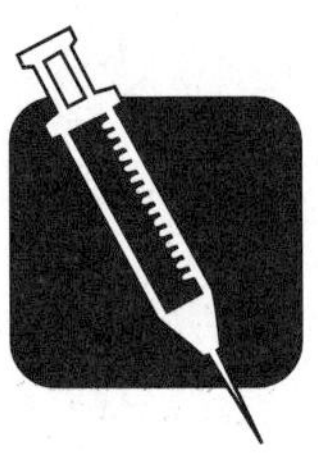

● **Autoradiography** Autoradiography (ARG) is a means for localizing radioactive compounds in cells and tissues. Living cells are provided with a radioactively labeled precursor (usually tritium or ^{3}H) to a cellular component. The precursor and its associated radioactivity are incorporated into the cell. The tissue is fixed and prepared for LM or TEM as described previously (Fig. 1.2). Tritium decays, emitting an electron. The electrons in the

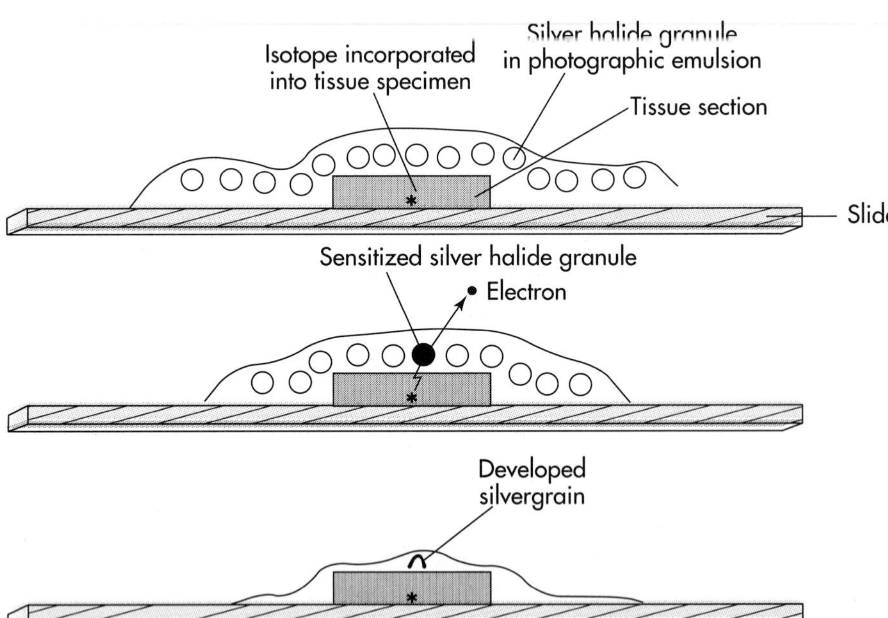

Fig. 1.2 Autoradiography. A fixed tissue section containing a macromolecule that has been labeled with a radioisotope is placed on a microscope slide or electron-microscopical grid and covered with melted photographic emulsion under darkroom conditions. The slide is exposed in the dark. The radioisotope decays emitting electrons that then sensitize some of the silver halide granules in the emulsion. On photographic development the sensitized silver halide granules are reduced to elemental silver causing a silver grain to overlie the portion of the section that contained the radioisotope.

tissue can be detected by a photographic emulsion, where silver halide microdetectors in the emulsion that are sensitized by the electrons produce black elemental silver grains on photographic development. It is therefore possible to coat a section (for LM or TEM) of a tissue exposed to the radioactive precursor with photographic emulsion and localize the radioactivity in the tissue by studying the distribution of silver grains.

Another application of ARG is in situ hybridization. This technique is based on the ability of nucleic acids to hybridize, or anneal, under conditions where the base sequence of a strand of nucleic acid (the *probe*) is complementary to the base sequence of a target. If the probe is labeled with ^{3}H and then hybridized with target nucleic acid (RNA or denatured DNA), after extensive washing to remove unhybridized probe, the hybrid molecules can be detected by ARG. In this manner, specific genes on chromosomes or messenger RNAs in the cytoplasm can be localized in cells or tissues.

● **Immunocytochemistry** Immunocytochemistry is a technique that allows localization of specific chemical components within cells and tissues. The chemical component must first be isolated and purified from the tissue. The isolated-purified component is then injected into an animal of another species (host) where it acts as an antigen. An *antigen* is a foreign substance that upon introduction into a host animal stimulates the production of specific *antibodies* (humoral) to the antigen.

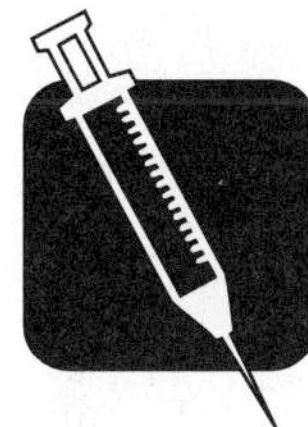

The B lymphocytes (plasma cells) of the host animal into which the isolated-purified component (antigen) is injected produces a specific antibody (humoral) to the antigen. An antibody (humoral) is a specific protein produced in response to the introduction of a specific antigen into an animal. The antibody combines and binds to the specific antigen molecules. The humoral antibodies are synthesized by the host. The immunoglobulins that contain the antibody are isolated from the host.

Alternatively, antibodies may be prepared by monoclonal antibody techniques (see below). With use of monoclonal methods, highly purified antibodies are produced in cell culture by cloned cells (hybridoma cells). The *immunoglobulins* that contain the specific antibody are coupled (covalently) with fluorescent compound (LM) or gold (LM and TEM) or are coupled to a histochemically detectable enzyme (horseradish peroxidase, HRP). (Fig. 1.3).

The fixed tissue that has been sectioned for LM or TEM as described above is placed in solution containing the fluorescent compound-, HRP-, or ferritin-coupled immunoglobulin. Subsequently the section is extensively washed to remove unbound immunoglobulin. The specific antibody to the isolated and purified chemical component (antigen) binds to that antigen in the section. The section is now viewed to note where the antibody, now bound to the antigen, is localized.

• LM—The specimen is viewed in the fluorescent microscope, which has a UV source and specific filters that transmit light of the wavelength that excites the fluorescent compound in the antibody causing it to fluoresce at a different wavelength. Fluorescent molecules absorb light at one wavelength and emit it at another. Fluorescein emits an intense green fluorescence when excited with blue light.

• TEM—The gold particles that are bound to the antibody are electron dense and have a characteristic appearance. They can be identified in the TEM or LM.

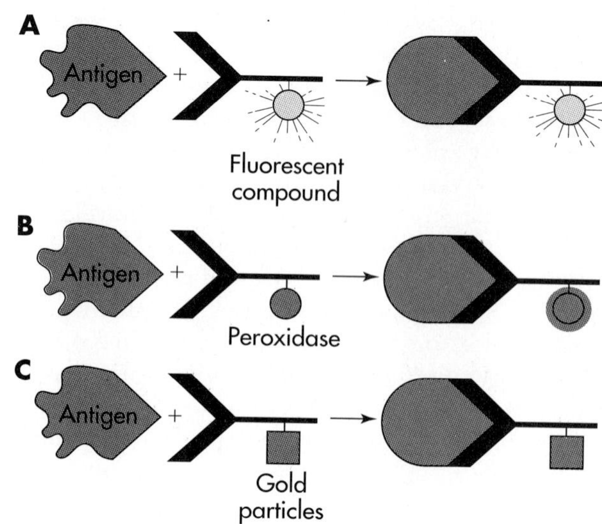

Fig. 1.3 Three methods for labeling and identifying specific proteins in sections by immunocytochemistry. **A,**The antibody is coupled to a fluorescent compound like fluoroscein isothiocyanate or rhodamine. After incubation of the section with labeled antibody it is examined in the fluorescent microscope. **B,**The antibody is coupled to horseradish peroxidase. After the antibody-antigen reaction the peroxidase is detected by a histochemical reaction for peroxidase and studied with the light microscope or electron microscope. **C,** The antibody is coupled to gold particles previously bound to protein A. Protein A reacts with the antibody labeling it. Preparations prepared in this way can be viewed by LM or EM. *(From Junqueira LC, Carneiro J:* Basic histology, *ed 7, East Norwalk, Conn., 1992, Appleton & Lange.)*

- The HRP can be localized for LM or TEM by enzyme histochemistry.

The localization of the compound in the section is thus identified. There are two variants of the immunocytochemical technique:

— *Direct method* Sections suspected of containing an antigen are incubated with a labeled antibody to that antigen, and the antibody-antigen complex is visualized.

— *Indirect method* Sections suspected of containing the antigen are incubated with an unlabeled antibody to the antigen. Then the antibody-antigen complex is detected by incubation of the tissue with a second labeled antibody directed against the first antibody. This second antibody is usually prepared in a species different from that used to produce the first antibody and is usually an antiimmunoglobulin. (It is an anti-antibody.)

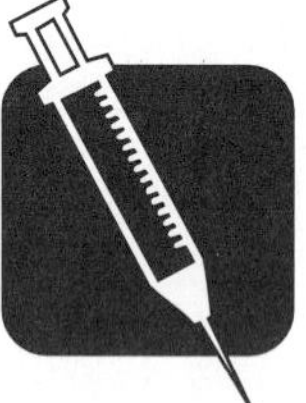

● **Cell and tissue culture** Cell and tissue culture is a technique for isolating cells and growing them outside of the body (in vitro methods). In vitro refers to cells grown 'in glass,' in contrast to in vivo, which is 'in a part of a living organism.' Cells in tissues are dispersed mechanically or with enzymes like trypsin or collagenase and are seeded onto a glass or plastic substrate where they adhere and frequently form single cell layers (monolayers) or can be maintained in suspension. Cells are grown in chemically defined media supplemented with growth factors, hormones, and serum components.

Most vertebrate cells die after a finite number of divisions in culture. It is believed that this limited life-span is related to the life-span of the animal from which the cells were originally derived, but some cells undergo a change that makes them effectively immortal. Such cells proliferate indefinitely, giving rise to a *cell line.*

The genetic uniformity of cells in culture can be improved by cell cloning in which a single cell is isolated and allowed to proliferate to form a large colony. A cell clone is a collection of cells that are descendants of a single ancestor cell.

When a suspension of cultured cells is treated with agents that cause cell fusion (polyethylene glycol, certain viruses), the plasma membranes of two cells fuse, and the fused cell with two separate nuclei is called a *heterokaryon.* Cells from different cell types or even different species of organisms can produce heterokaryons. Eventually heterokaryons will produce *hybrid cells* in which the two separate nuclear envelopes fuse and bring all chromosomes into one nucleus.

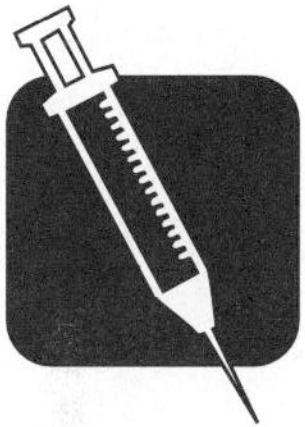

- *Organ culture* is the culture of whole organs or parts of them from their embryonic rudiments. The term refers to the culture of organs or organ fragments under conditions that keep the architecture of the organ intact.

- *Cell fractionation* is a process by which separate organelles and cellular components are separated usually by centrifugation to enable the study of that organelle in a relatively pure state in the absence of other cell components. Cells are disrupted in such a way that many of the organelles are left intact. The individual organelles are separated using differential centrifugation, velocity sedimentation, or equilibrium sedimentation, in a density gradient. These centrifugation techniques separate the organelles based on their mass, size, and shape, or buoyant density. Fractionated cell homogenates that maintain their biological functions are referred to as *cell-free extracts.*

- The *monoclonal antibody technique* greatly increases the specificity of antibodies and can be used in combination with immunochemistry (see above). Antibodies are produced simply by injection of an antigen into an animal of another species (e.g., a goat or rabbit). The antiserum contains a heterogeneous mixture of antibodies, each produced by a different antibody-secreting cell (B lymphocyte). Each antibody recognizes a different part of the antigen or even impurities in the antigen preparation. Such an antibody is referred to as *polyclonal* because it is the product of many B lymphocytes.

The problem of antibody heterogeneity is overcome by propagation of a clone of cells from a single antibody secreting B lymphocyte so that a homogeneous preparation of antibodies is obtained. To accomplish this, an antibody-producing B lymphocyte from an animal is fused with cells from an immortal "B" lymphocyte (or plasma cell) tumor (a myeloma). From the resulting heterogeneous mixture of cells, hybrids that have the ability to make a particular antibody are selected. These *hybridomas* are propagated as individual clones, each producing a single type of monoclonal antibody. This antibody will recognize a single antigenic site on an antigen.

MULTIPLE CHOICE
REVIEW QUESTIONS

1. Match the following:

    ________ 10,000 Å
    ________ 0.001 mm
    ________ 1000 nm
    ________ 0.1 nm
    ________ 0.1 mm

    a. 1 µm
    b. 0.001 nm
    c. 1 nm
    d. 1 Å
    e. 100 µm

2. Identify the smallest structure:

    a. Digestive system
    b. Red blood cell
    c. Connective tissue
    d. Mitochondrion
    e. Stomach

3. Which technique would be most appropriate to follow the movement of newly synthesized protein through a cell?

    a. Immunocytochemistry
    b. Autoradiography
    c. Staining with hematoxylin and eosin
    d. Staining with osmium tetroxide
    e. None of the above is correct

4. Match the following:

    ________ Mitochondrion
    ________ Heart
    ________ Stomach
    ________ Epithelium
    ________ Muscle

    a. Organelle
    b. Tissue
    c. Organ
    d. System
    e. Organism

5. Which technique would be most useful in demonstrating the localization of a specific protein like actin in a cell or tissue?

    a. Autoradiography
    b. Staining with hematoxylin and eosin
    c. Immunocytochemistry
    d. Uranyl acetate staining
    e. Freeze fracture microscopy

Chapter 2

Cell Biology: Cytoplasmic Organelles

THE CELL SURFACE

The **cell surface** encloses the cell, defining its boundaries and maintaining differences between the intracellular and extracellular environment. The cell surface is composed of the **plasma membrane** and the **cell coat (glycocalyx)**.

In transmission electron microscopy (TEM), the plasma membrane appears in section as two electron-dense lines, with the thickness of each measuring 3.5 nm. Between the two lines is a layer of less dense material measuring 3.0 nm in thickness. The total thickness of the tripartite structure is 9.5 nm. The membrane has an **external surface** and an internal **(protoplasmic) surface**.

Freeze fracture and **freeze etching** enable visualization of the faces of the membrane. This is accomplished by freezing cells in liquid nitrogen, fracturing the membrane with a razor blade, sublimating the H_2O, coating the membrane with carbon platinum, removing the tissue debris, and viewing the replica (made of carbon-platinum).

The cleavage, or fracture plane, occurs in the membrane in the center of the less dense layer. The cleavage plane reveals the membrane **faces** (Fig. 2.1).

- The **E face** (with the external surface) demonstrates few granules.
- The **P face** (with the protoplasmic surface) demonstrates many granules.

Scanning electron microscopy (SEM) indicates that the cell surface is an extremely dynamic structure, showing variation in surface contours indicative of movement.

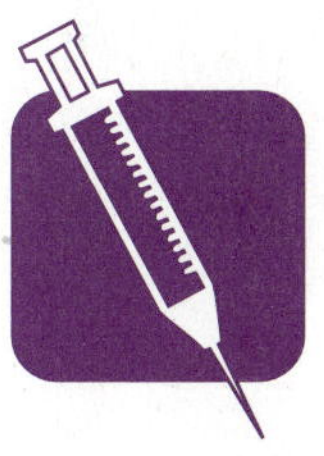

■ **Molecular Organization of Membranes** Membranes are composed of **lipids** and **proteins.** Much of the lipid is **phospholipid.** Phospholipids are amphipathic molecules. They have hydrophilic and hydrophobic ends (e.g., phosphatidylcholine, sphingomyelin, phosphotidylserine, phosphatidylethanolamine). The plasma membrane also contains cholesterol and glycolipids, which are amphipathic to some extent.

Associated with the lipids are proteins. The proteins function in the following different ways:

- Structural proteins
- Enzymes
- Pumps
- Channels
- Receptors

Lipid in the membrane is arranged as a **bimolecular layer.** The lipids are arranged in two layers, back to back. (Freeze fracture cleaves membranes between

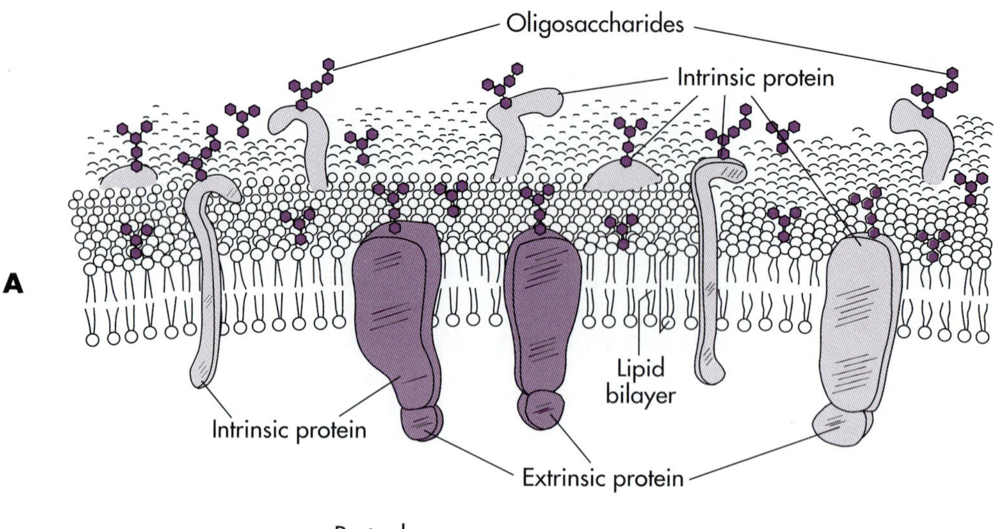

Fig. 2.1 The plasma membrane and glycocalyx. **A,** Organization of lipids in a bilayer that is penetrated by intrinsic membrane proteins. **B,** A plasma membrane that is cleaved according to the freeze-fracture technique to reveal the E and P faces of the membrane. *(Modified and redrawn from Fawcett DW: A textbook of histology, ed 11, Philadelphia, 1986, Saunders.)*

these two layers.) The hydrophilic heads of the lipids are directed toward the surfaces of the membrane (forming the dark lines of TEM). The hydrophobic tails of the lipids are directed toward the interior of the membrane (forming the less dense layer of TEM). Phospholipids in solution spontaneously form such a bimolecular structure.

Whereas the basic structure of the membrane is provided by lipids, most of the specific functions of the membrane are carried out by protein.

● **Extrinsic (or peripheral) membrane proteins** are those on the surfaces of membrane. They do not penetrate the lipid layer. Extrinsic membrane proteins have the following characteristics:

  • They are rich in hydrophilic amino acids.

  • They may be covalently bound to or held in place by noncovalent interactions with other membrane proteins, lipids, or oligosaccharides.

- They differ in distribution on the external and internal surfaces of the membrane.
- There are those proteins common to both surfaces. Some are found only on the internal surface, and some are found only on the external surface.

● **Intrinsic** (or **transmembrane**) **proteins** are those that penetrate the lipid layer of the membrane. These account for the granules apparent on the E and P faces revealed by the freeze-fracture technique. They are rich in hydrophobic amino acids (surrounded by lipid) and hydrophilic amino acids (on the cell surfaces). They differ in penetrance of the lipid layer.

— *Single-pass transmembrane proteins* The polypeptide chain crosses the membrane once.

— *Multipass transmembrane proteins* The polypeptide chain crosses the membrane many times.

There is no known example of a polypeptide that only partially penetrates the lipid membrane.

There is little if any exchange (flip-flop) of lipids or proteins between the inner and the outer layers of the bimolecular leaflet (except at the site of membrane assembly in the endoplasmic reticulum). Instead the lipids move laterally in their individual layers of membrane enabling the movement of proteins. When two cells are fused, it has been shown that the membrane proteins quickly (within seconds) distribute over the entire plasma membrane of the resulting heterokaryon cell demonstrating the fluidity of the plasma membrane and the proteins within it.

● **Uniformity of cellular membranes** The internal membranes of the cell (mitochondria, nuclear membranes, Golgi complex, lysosomes, endoplasmic reticulum) are similar in appearance to one another and to the plasma membrane (trilaminar appearance). They differ, however, in lipid composition and in protein composition (e.g., organelle-specific enzymes). The theory of membrane flow describes the ready exchange of membranes within cellular compartments.

- Plasma membrane → endocytotic vesicle membrane
- Membrane of secretion granule → plasma membrane
- S.E.R. → transfer vacuole → Golgi → condensing vacuole → secretory granule → plasma membrane
- Golgi membrane → lysosome membrane

Phospholipid molecules are synthesized in only one monolayer of the membrane, that being the cytosolic monolayer of the endoplasmic reticulum. Endoplasmic reticulum-bound **phospholipid translocators** catalyze a flip-flop exchange of specific phospholipids to the opposite monolayer.

■ **The Cell Coat or Glycocalyx** The majority of transmembrane proteins are glycosylated in the endoplasmic reticulum and Golgi complex and for this reason are always present on the noncytosolic surface of the endoplasmic reticulum membrane. They end up on the external surface of the plasma membrane (as per exocytosis) (Fig. 2.2).

Glycolipids, which have oligosaccharides attached to the polar ends of the

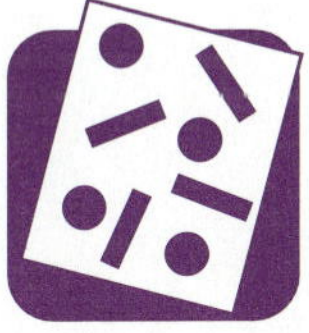

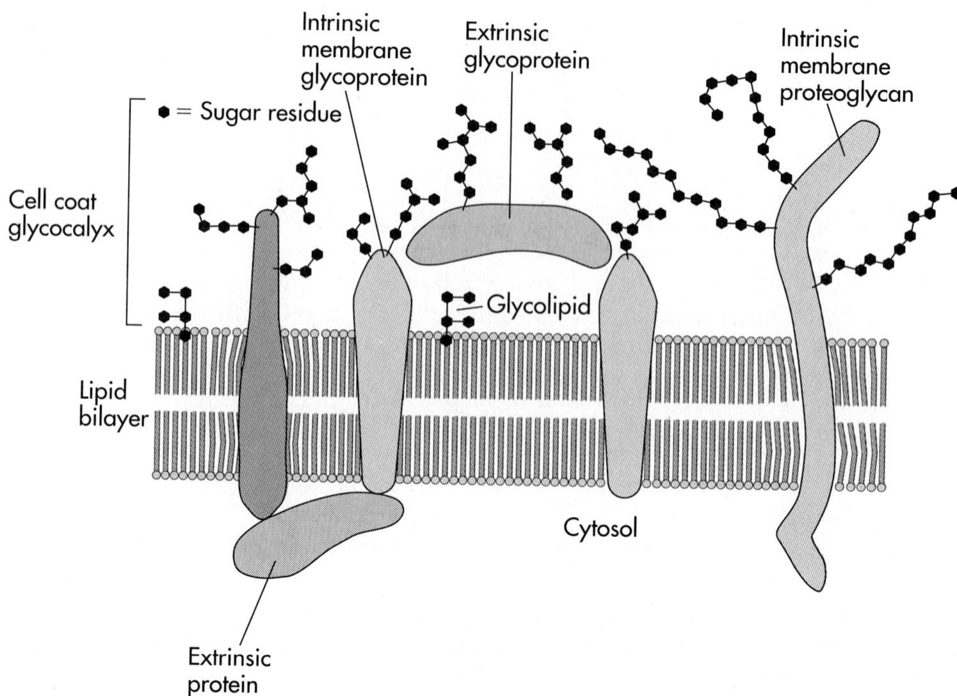

Fig. 2.2 The cell coat of glycocalyx. The glycocalyx is made up of the oligosaccharide side chains of glycolipids and intrinsic membrane glycoproteins and the polysaccharide chains on intrinsic membrane proteoglycans as well as extrinsic membrane glycoproteins and proteoglycans. The carbohydrate is on the external surface of the membrane. *(From Alberts B, Bray D, Lewis J, et al:* Molecular biology of the cell, *ed 3, New York, 1994, Garland Publishing.)*

phospholipids, are glycosylated in the endoplasmic reticulum, where they are found exclusively on the noncytosolic half of the lipid bilayer. These oligosaccharides also end up on the external surface of the plasma membrane and contribute to the cell coat.

The membrane glycoproteins and glycolipids are asymmetrically distributed so that their oligosaccharides are protruding from the noncytosolic surface of internal cell membranes (ER, Golgi, etc.) and the external surface of the plasma membrane.

The external cell surface is thus coated with oligosaccharides that make up the cell coat. Unlike the plasma membrane, which shows little morphological variation in different cell types (despite showing significant differences in lipid and protein components), the cell coat shows extensive morphological variation in different types of cells.

- It may be robust and strong.
- It may be extremely tenuous.
- It may be firmly attached by being covalently attached to proteins (intrinsic and extrinsic) or to lipids (glycolipids) of the cell membrane.
- The cell coat may be loosely attached or absorbed to the cell surface. Many of these components have been secreted by the cell and are a part of the extracellular matrix. They are glycoproteins and proteoglycans.

The functions of the cell coat are variable.

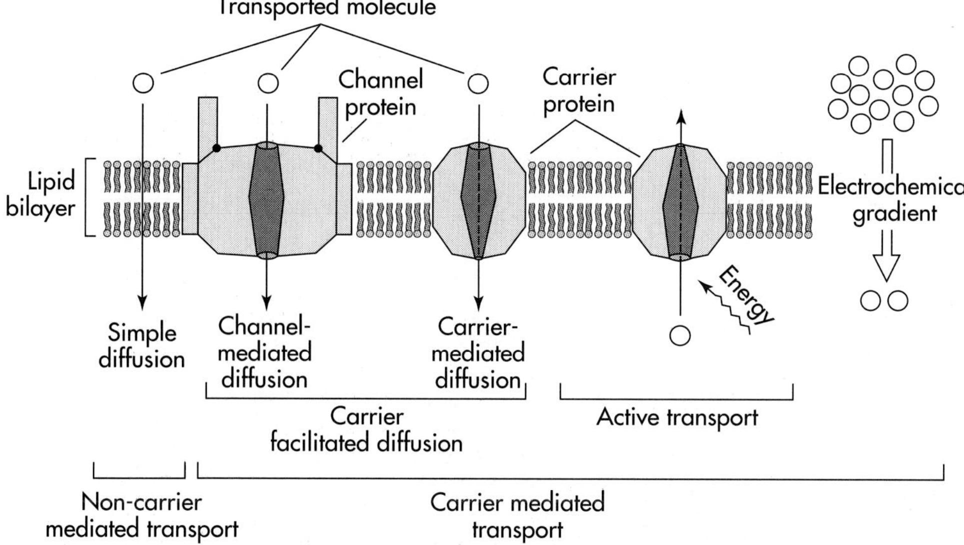

Fig. 2.3 Comparison of means of transport across the plasma membrane. Simple diffusion (non–carrier mediated transport) and facilitated diffusion occur spontaneously and can transport down an electrochemical gradient. Active transport requires an input of energy and can transport against an electrochemical gradient. *(Modified from Alberts B, Bray D, Lewis J, et al: Molecular biology of the cell, ed 3, New York, 1994, Garland Publishing.)*

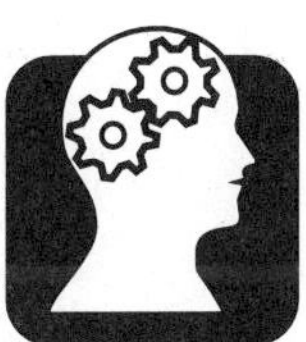

- It may act as a barrier, readily permeable to water and small molecules but not to large molecules.
- It aids in selective regulatory properties of plasma membranes (recognition sites).
- It may have a supporting function. Intercellular matrices are cell coats of adjacent cells that fuse, thus increasing the strength of the tissue.
- It may have a lubricative function.

Functions of Membranes There are several general functions common to the plasma membrane of most or all cells. Membranes are barriers to the movement of large molecules, allowing movement of small (nonpolar) material or of lipid-soluble material, or both types. The membrane is impermeable to charged molecules. The charge and high degree of hydration prevents them from entering the bilayer. This is largely a function of the lipid portion of the membrane. Membranes regulate movement into and out of cells (Fig. 2.3).

- **Non-carrier mediated transport** (diffusion) shows physical rather than chemical specificity. It is largely a function of the lipid in the membrane. Lipid-soluble material, small nonpolar, and small uncharged polar molecules like H_2O, CO_2, O_2, and EtOH readily diffuse through the membrane.

- **Carrier-mediated transport** demonstrates chemical specificity. This is largely a function of membrane proteins. The carriers are granules seen on the E and P faces as shown in Fig. 2.3.

  - **Carrier-facilitated diffusion** is not energy dependent. If the molecule is uncharged, its concentration drives transport. It moves down a concentration gradient. If the molecule is charged, its transport is driven by an electrochemical gradient. It moves down an electrochemical gradient.

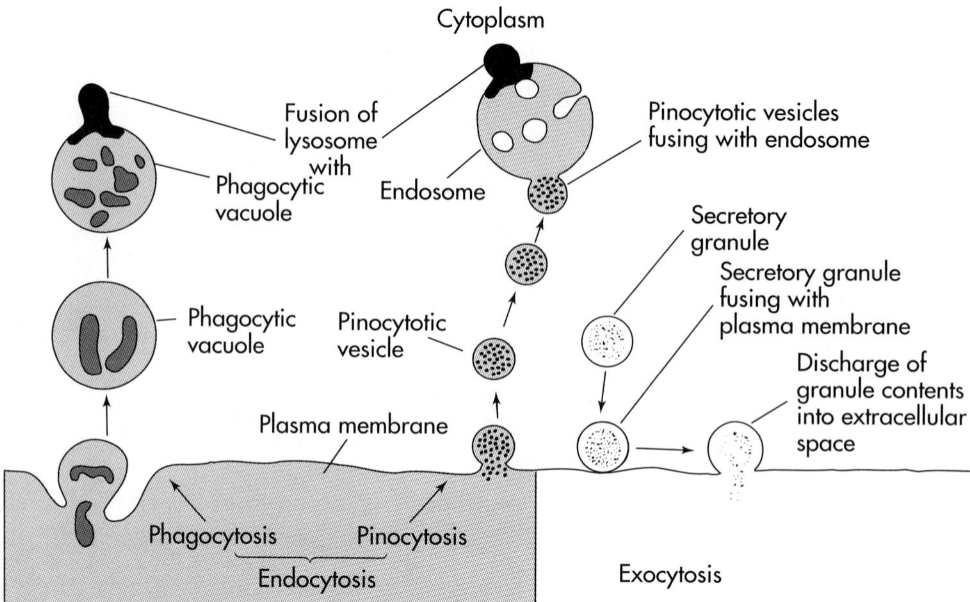

Fig. 2.4 Comparison of endocytosis and exocytosis. Two types of endocytosis are illustrated. Phagocytosis is the uptake in bulk of solid material. Pinocytosis is the uptake in bulk of fluid and dissolved material. Exocytosis is the release of material in bulk from vesicles in the cytoplasm. *(Modified from Ross RB, Reith EJ:* Histology: a text and atlas, *New York, 1985, Harper & Row.)*

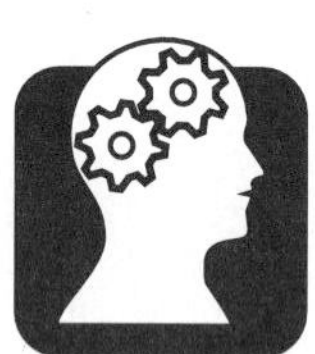

- **Active transport** requires energy. It goes uphill against an electrochemical gradient.

These processes are mediated by **membrane transport proteins.** All membrane proteins studied up to now are multipass transmembrane proteins. There are two classes of membrane transport proteins.

- **Carrier proteins** (carriers, permeases, and transporters) bind the solute and undergo a series of changes to transfer the bound solute across the membrane.

- **Channel proteins** need not bind solutes but form hydrophilic pores that extend across the membrane. When these pores are open, they allow specific solutes to flow through them.

Fig. 2.4 shows the mechanism by which cells take in or give out substances in bulk.

- **Exocytosis** is the mechanism by which large quantities of material are liberated in bulk from the cell. It involves fusion of the cytoplasmic surfaces of membranes.
- **Endocytosis** is the uptake in bulk of large amounts of material by cells. It involves fusion of external surfaces of membranes.
  - Phagocytosis is cellular eating (uptake of solids).
  - Pinocytosis is cellular drinking (uptake of fluids).
  - Receptor-mediated endocytosis enables a degree of specificity to be imparted to the endocytotic mechanism.
  - Specific molecules are bound by membrane receptors on the cell's surface. The receptor and bound molecules enters a coated pit.

(The coated pit has the protein clathrin on its cytosolic surface.) The pit forms a coated vesicle (still coated with clathrin). The vesicle sheds its clathrin coat to become an endosome. The pH of the endosome is such that it enables release of the receptor from the specific bound molecule, regenerating the receptor.

● **Specialized functions of cell membranes** Excitability (ability to transmit a nerve impulse or an action potential) is a special function of the neuron plasma membrane. Specialized cellular attachment areas are found in areas where cells are in close contact with one another. Their general functions are as follows:

- Stick cells together into mechanically coherent tissues (as the occludens and adherens junctions do).
- Provide a permeability seal so that tissue as a whole acts as a barrier to diffusion (as the zonula occludens does).
- Mediate direct communication between cells so that materials can move from the cytoplasm of one cell to the cytoplasm of an adjacent cell without passing through the extracellular space (as a nexus, or gap junction, does).

There are several specialized types of **cellular attachment sites,** as shown in Fig. 2.5.

1. There are attachment sites where there is direct membrane-to-membrane contact.

The **occludens junction** is also called the *tight junction.* The outer leaflets of the plasma membrane fuse, and so that the entire thickness is less than that of two membranes. Actually it is the matching ridges of the membranes that fuse. Freeze etching reveals fibers that run parallel with the ridge inside each cell membrane, actually believed to be rows of intrinsic membrane proteins.

There are several morphological types:

- **Zonula** (beltlike) **occludens** completely encircles the cell.
- **Fascia** (sheetlike) **occludens** forms broad areas of contact.
- **Macula** (disklike) **occludens** is like a "spot" weld on the cell surface.

Zonula occludens junctions form a permeability barrier between cells; that is, if a group of cells are joined by zonula occludens junctions (as they are in some simple epithelia), materials cannot pass between the cells. To pass through a group of cells so joined, the material must pass through the cell and to do that it must pass through the cell membrane.

The **nexus** is also called the *gap junction.* The membranes are actually separated by a 2 nm electron-lucent zone (gap). The gap is spanned by membrane subunits (called connexons). The plasma membrane internal organization is modified showing channel-like intrinsic membrane proteins. In the connexon there are multiple pores composed of the protein connexin. Nexi (nexuses) provide direct cell-to-cell communication, hydrophilic channels for passage of small ions from one cell to the next.

2. There are also cell attachment sites where membranes are separated by a 15 to 35 nm interspace. In **adherens junctions,** the adjacent cell membranes are attached by proteinaceous material in the interspace (glycocalyx) between cells. There are condensations of filamentous material composed of tonofibrils in the cytoplasm, and they attach to the cell membrane. The tonofibrils are made up of keratin-containing intermediate filaments.

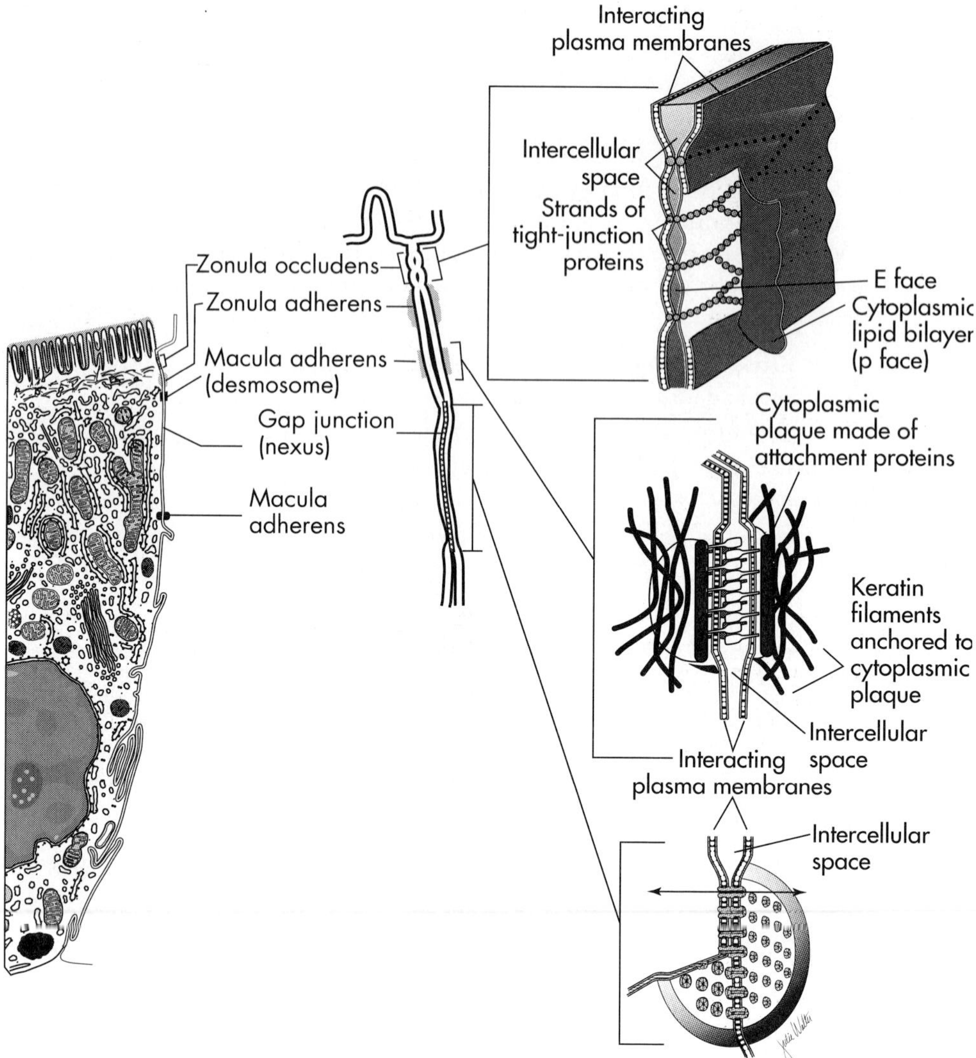

Fig. 2.5 The junctional complex of the absorptive simple columnar epithelial cell. This junctional complex consists of the zonula occludens, zonula adherens, and macula adherens. The cells also demonstrate nexi. In the occludens junction intrinsic membrane proteins arranged in rows in the adjacent cells provide membrane-to-membrane contact. In the adherens junction there is a space between the cells where elements of the glycocalyx hold the two cells together. In the nexus, intrinsic membrane proteins provide channels between the two cells. *(Modified from Lentz T: Cell fine structure, Philadelphia, 1971, Saunders.)*

There are several morphological types of adherens junctions.

- Zonula adherens
- Macula adherens (also called *desmosome*)

Interdigitations of the cell membrane can also act as cellular attachment sites. Such interdigitations function in the following ways:

- Increasing the surface area of contact between two cells, facilitating movement of material from one cell to the next.
- Increasing adherence of cells to one another in a mechanical way.

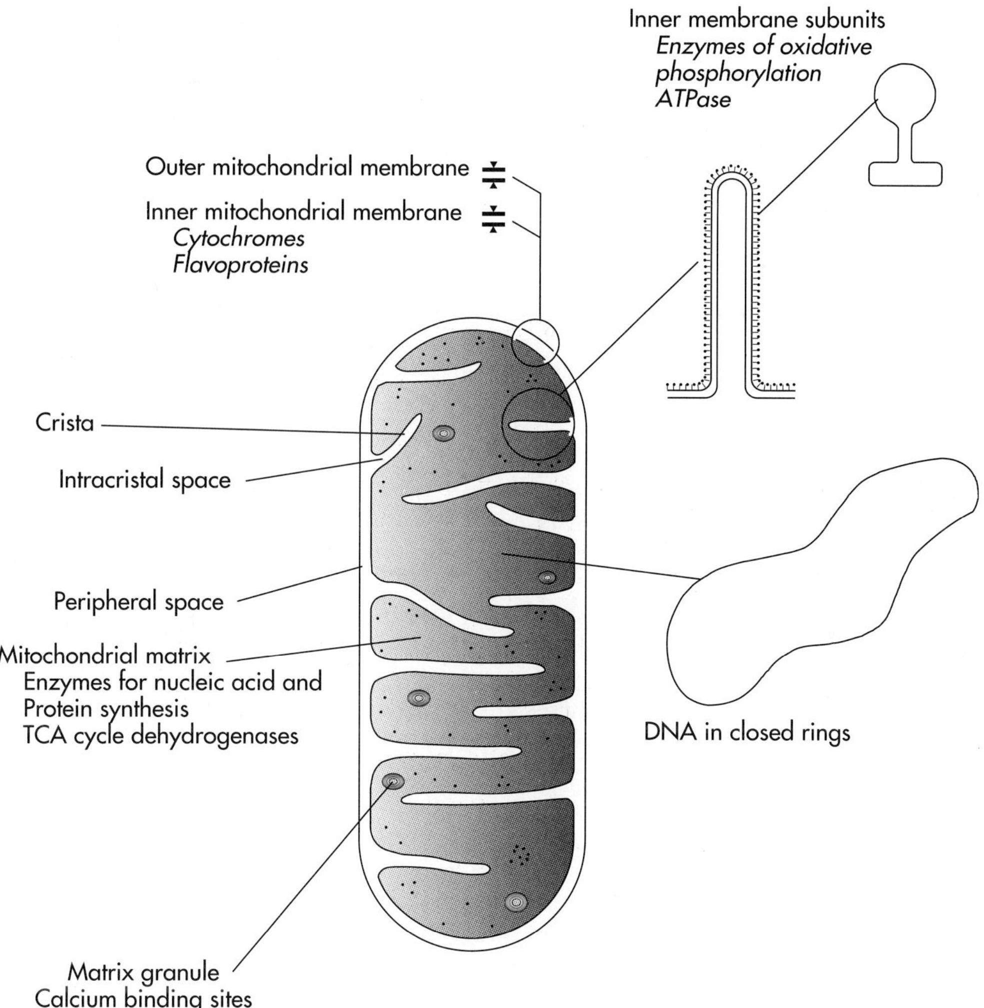

Fig. 2.6 The mitochondrion with some of its structural and functional components. *(Modified and redrawn from Fawcett DW: A textbook of histology, ed 11, Philadelphia, 1986, Saunders.)*

MITOCHONDRIA

Mitochondria are uniquely capable of carrying out for themselves the two basic properties of living matter (Fig. 2.6). They are partially responsible for their own reproduction (they contain mitochondrial DNA), and they generate a usable form of energy (they synthesize ATP).

■ **Structure of the Mitochondrion** Mitochondria are surrounded by two membranes. These membranes each have a tripartite structure like that of the plasma membrane, but the membrane is thinner. The protein and lipid composition of these membranes differ from one another and from the plasma membrane and other intracytoplasmic membranes.

The **outer mitochondrial membrane** is usually devoid of any special structure. It is freely permeable of molecules up to the size of simple sugars. The **inner mitochondrial membrane** is relatively impermeable. Negative staining shows that the inner membrane is studded with elementary particles. The particles measure 9 nm in diameter (with 10 nm center spacing) and are carried on stalks that attach to one side (the matrix side) of the inner mitochondrial membrane. **Mitochondrial cristae** can be free or be continuous with the inner membrane. They are covered with elementary particles. Cristae are more prominent in metabolically active cells than in quiescent cells.

The outer and inner mitochondrial membrane forms the bounds of several spaces. *Peripheral space* lies between the outer and inner mitochondrial membrane. The *intracristal space* is continuous with the peripheral space. Contained within the inner membrane is the mitochondrial matrix region, which contains the following:

- Soluble and insoluble protein
- Electron-dense granules of calcium phosphate
- Ribosomes
- DNA filaments

All mitochondria appear to have the following enzymatic equipment associated with the generation of ATP:

- **TCA cycle dehydrogenase enzymes** are localized in the inner membrane and in the matrix.
- Respiratory enzymes of the **electron transport system** are localized on the inner membrane.
- **Phosphorylating enzymes** are localized in the inner membrane in the elementary particles.

Mitochondria also contain

- Membrane transporting proteins (translocase and permease enzymes), which transport materials through the inner membrane. They are highly specific and localized in the inner membrane. (They are involved in carrier-mediated transport into and out of the mitochondrial matrix region.)
- Enzymes involved in the turnover of mitochondrial constituents

A disorder of mitochondria termed **mitochondrial cytopathy** is a defect in oxidative phosphorylation. There is an increase in the size and number of muscle mitochondria. This is associated with a high basal metabolic rate without hyperthyroidism.

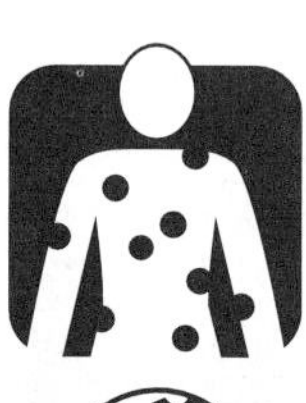
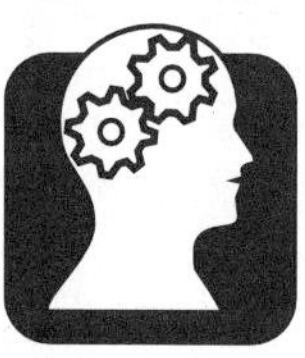

■ **Mitochondrial Reproduction** Mitochondria are partially self-replicating systems (i.e., they are not totally dependent on the nucleus for their genetic continuity). Mitochondria arise from preexisting mitochondria and are not completely new. They contain their independent genetic machinery.

Mitochondrial DNA is localized in the matrix region. It differs from nuclear DNA in the following ways:

- Its structural conformation is circular, measuring 4 to 6 μm in length. Each circle measures 15 kb (kilo–base pairs), which is enough to code for 5000 amino acids or about 25 average-sized proteins.
- Mitochondrial DNA is homogeneous. Each circular molecule appears to have the same genetic information as the others of that cell or in that organism.
- DNA is synthesized in situ in the mitochondrion.
- Mitochondrial DNA is synthesized throughout cell, and its synthesis is not limited to the S phase.

RNA is synthesized in the mitochondrion. This RNA is coded for by mitochondrial DNA. Ribosomes (differing from cytoplasmic type) are localized in the mitochondria.

Protein is also synthesized in the mitochondrion. Mitochondria contain all the components necessary for protein synthesis. Since the genome capacity of mitochondrial DNA is limited (about 25 proteins), not all proteins can be accounted for by mitochondrial DNA that has been sequenced. Mitochondrial DNA codes for

- a few subunits of the respiratory chain enzymes localized in the inner membrane
- mitochondrial ribosomal RNA
- 22 species of mitochondrial transfer RNA

Mitochondrial DNA does not appear to code for nonenzyme proteins of the outer membrane and matrix. Most (except for those mentioned above) mitochondrial enzymes are coded for by nuclear DNA rather than by mitochondrial DNA. Housekeeping enzymes (like RNA polymerase) are also nuclear coded.

It has been shown that mitochondrial reproduction involves the coordinated activity of the mitochondrial genome and the nuclear genome. Synthesis of nuclear encoded proteins on cytoplasmic ribosomes and transport into the mitochondria is coordinated with the synthesis of mitochondrial encoded proteins on mitochondrial ribosomes and results in the replication of the mitochondrion.

Several lines of evidence demonstrate similarities between the mitochondrial transcription/translation and that of prokaryotes, suggestive of a possible symbiont origin of mitochondria.

Mitochondria demonstrate maternal inheritance. The egg contributes all the mitochondrial DNA to the zygote. The sperm contributes none. Mitochondria show maternal genetics.

Lysosomes and Peroxisomes

Lysosomes are membrane-bound sacs within the cytoplasm that are filled with hydrolytic enzymes (Fig. 2.7). (Lysosomes are the digestive system of the cell.) Some of the enzymes of the lysosome are acid ribonuclease, acid deoxyribonuclease, acid phosphatase, cathepsins, and specific glycosidases and esterases. These enzymes are active at pH 5.0 and are of little consequence if released into the cytoplasm, which is at pH 7.2. A H^+ pump in the lysosomal membrane pumps H^+ into the lysosome maintaining the acid pH of the lumen.

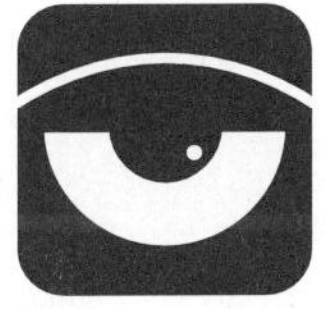

■ Modes of Lysosomal Activity

- **Heterophagic** activity is digestion of materials exogenous to the cell.
- **Autophagic** activity is digestion of the cell or cell components (arising intrinsically).
- **Autolysis** is self-destruction of entire cells.

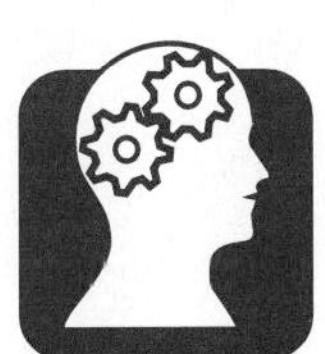

■ States of Lysosomal Activity

- **Endocytotic vesicles** arise by endocytosis (phagocytosis or pinocytosis).
- **Primary lysosomes** are filled with lysosomal enzymes but have not yet fused with an endosome and therefore have not begun digestion.
- **Secondary lysosomes** are lysosomes that have fused with an endosome, phagosome, or autophagosome, and demonstrate digestion. Several stages of secondary lysosomal activity are distinguished.

There are two types of digestive vacuoles.

- **Heterophagic vacuoles** contain material originating from outside of the cell (e.g., a bacterium).

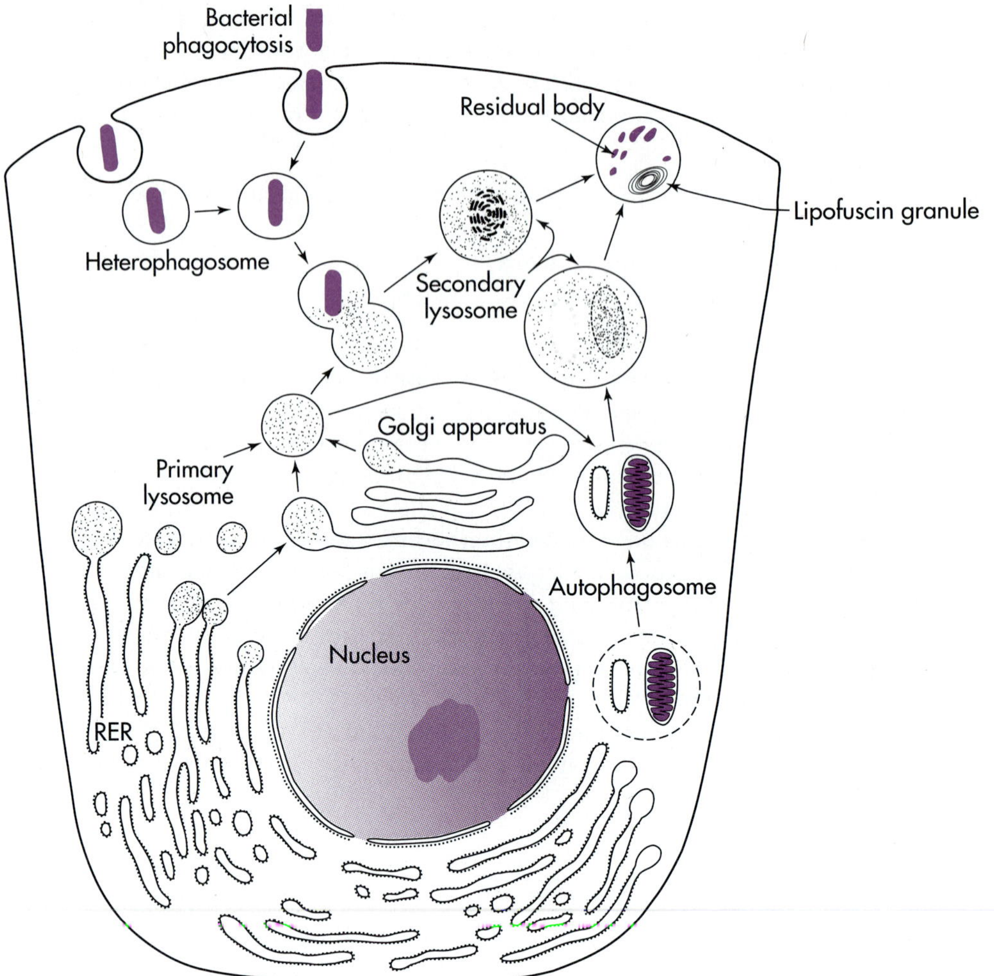

Fig. 2.7 Stages of lysosomal activity. Heterophagic activity *(upper left)* is initiated by the phagocytosis of a bacterium. Autophagic activity *(lower right)* is initiated with the sequestration of a cellular organelle within the membrane. *(Modified from Junqueira LC, Carneiro J: Basic histology, ed 7, East Norwalk, Conn., 1992, Appleton & Lange.)*

- **Autophagic vacuoles** contain material originating within the cell (e.g., mitochondria).

The **residual body** contains material that is the remains of heterophagic or autophagic activity. It is probably undigestible.

Lipofuscin granules are the final manifestation of lysosomal activity in long-lived cells that do not divide.

There is a whole catalog of genetic diseases that show abnormalities of the enzymatic machinery of lysosomes, examples of which are

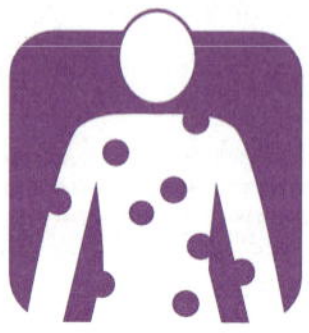

- **Glycogen storage disease type II** (Pompe's disease) is a disease of the liver. The lysosomes lack the enzyme glucosidase and can't adequately break down glycogen to glucose. Glycogen then segregates in vacuoles in hepatocytes and is not broken down.

- **Tay-Sachs disease** is an inherited recessive disorder with mental retardation and usually death by 5 years of age. Ganglioside G_{M2}, a normal lipid constituent of the plasma membrane, is continually synthesized and degraded in unaffected individuals. In Tay-Sachs, membranes of brain cells accumulate G_{M2} because of the absence of lysosomal hydrolase β-*N*-hexosaminidase A, which breaks down G_{M2}. Excess G_{M2} causes the symptoms.

In addition to these are industrial diseases in which the lysosomes become overloaded with indigestible material. The lysosomes of cells in the lung become filled with inert carbon particles causing **black-lung disease.** In the case of **silicosis,** the lysosomes of cells in the lung become filled with silica dust.

PEROXISOMES (MICROBODIES)

Peroxisomes (microbodies) are respiratory organelles involved in cell catabolism. They are membrane-lined organelles containing various oxidase enzymes (notably catalase). Their enzyme content differs in different cell types within a single organism. A common identifying characteristic of peroxisomes is the presence of catalase. Hydrogen peroxide accumulates in peroxisomes as a result of oxidative activity. Catalase breaks down hydrogen peroxide to yield water and oxygen. Peroxisomes are particularly prominent in cells involved in steroid synthesis. Like the lysosomes there is a whole catalog of diseases caused by enzymatic abnormalities of peroxisomes.

In one of these, Zellweger's syndrome, individuals afflicted have no peroxisomes. Their cells accumulate the waste products of catabolism. All major organ systems are affected as indicated by the description, cerebrohepatorenal syndrome.

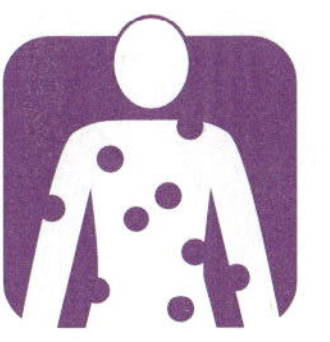

RIBOSOMES

Ribosomes behave like particles. Each ribosome is composed of

• The large 60S subunit, which contains 28S RNA and protein. The 28S RNA molecule measures 5 kb. The 60S subunit is composed of one 28S RNA molecule and 30 ribosomal protein molecules.

• The small 40S subunit contains 18S RNA and protein. The 18S RNA molecule measures 2 kb. The 40S subunit is composed of one 18S RNA molecule and 20 ribosomal protein molecules.

In the cytoplasm, the subunits behave as independent particles until they participate in the polysome formation at which time the 40S and 60S associate with messenger RNA to give rise to the functional 80S ribosome. The ribosome measures 15 nm in the section and 20 to 30 nm in negative gram-stained preparations.

In the EM it is seen to be composed of

• A long component (small subunit) (40S)
• Round component (large subunit) (60S)
• A cleft separates the large and small subunits and is where the RNA lies.

■ **Ribosome Function**   Functioning ribosomes act not as individual subunits but as aggregates attached to mRNA in polyribosomes (polysomes). These are extended arrays of ribosomes that are connected by a 1 nm wide strand of mRNA. The size of the polysome (length and number of ribosomes attached to it) is generally a reflection of the length of the mRNA (Fig. 2.8). Functioning ribosomes may exist as the following:

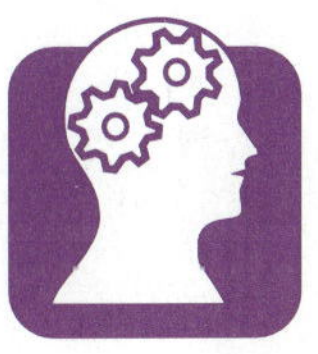

• Free polysomes in the cytoplasm, which are believed to be involved in the synthesis of proteins for intracellular use (i.e., cytosolic proteins).

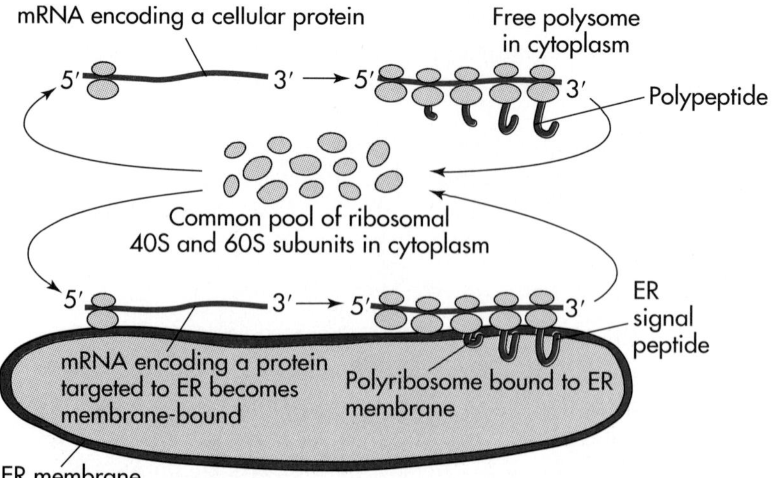

Fig. 2.8. Endoplasmic reticulum bound and free polysomes. A common pool of ribosomal subunits is used to synthesize proteins that remain in the cytoplasm and those that are transported into the endoplasmic reticulum. It is the signal peptide on the newly formed polypeptide that directs the ribosome to the endoplasmic reticulum. The messenger RNA molecule may remain permanently bound to the endoplasmic reticulum, whereas the ribosomes that move along it are recycled. *(Modified from Alberts B, et al:* Molecular biology of the cell, *ed 3, New York, 1994, Garland Publishing.)*

- Polysomes attached to membrane (RER), which are believed to be involved in the synthesis of proteins for extracellular use (as well as enzymes in lysosomes and proteins anchored in the membranes of the endoplasmic reticulum itself, the Golgi complex, and plasma membrane).

The polysome attaches to the endoplasmic reticulum in the following manner:

- There is a signal sequence in mRNA of proteins to be synthesized on RER.
- The translated product of this **signal sequence** (20 to 25 hydrophobic amino acids at the amino terminal end of the protein) interact with a cytosolic **signal-recognition particle (SRP).**
- The SRP-polyribosome complex binds to an **SRP receptor** in the RER. The SRP receptor is also called *docking protein.*
- **Ribophorins I** and **II** are intrinsic proteins of the RER (but not SER) that provide an attachment site for the large ribosomal subunit.
- There is vectorial discharge of the newly synthesized protein as it is translocated into the lumen of the RER.

Of the proteins synthesized on the RER, there are two basic outcomes.

- Water-soluble proteins that are translocated into the lumen of the endoplasmic reticulum to remain there or to be secreted from the cell, are released into the lumen. A **signal peptidase** cleaves the signal sequence, and the mature polypeptide is released from the membrane into the lumen of the RER.
- Proteins destined to become transmembrane proteins are only partly translocated across the membrane, and they become embedded in it. An addi-

tional hydrophobic segment in the polypeptide anchors the protein in the membrane, and so when the signal peptidase removes the signal peptide, the protein remains embedded in the membrane.

Many of the proteins synthesized on the RER are en route to other destinations (Golgi complex, lysosomes, plasma membrane). Proteins that are to remain in the ER contain an ER retention signal at their carboxyl terminus that retains them in the ER.

Proteins destined for other cellular membranes have different retention signals. This is referred to as a **default pathway** (*i.e.,* if the transmembrane protein does not have a signal to be retained by that organelle membrane, it is moved to the next [ER→Golgi→lysosome, etc.]).

There is also a **recovery pathway** to enable proteins that are not retained (but should have been) to be recovered.

ENDOPLASMIC RETICULUM (ER)

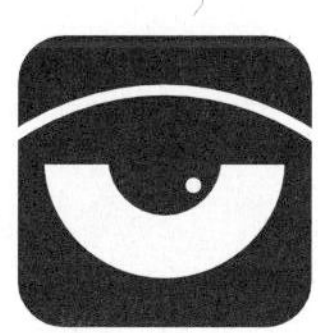

The endoplasmic reticulum is an anastomosing intracytoplasmic membrane system consisting of vesicular, tubular, and broad cisternal profiles often arranged in regular arrays. Two major elements are distinguished:

- Rough endoplasmic reticulum
- Smooth endoplasmic reticulum

Membranes of the endoplasmic reticulum measure approximately 5 nm in width and show a tripartite structure. They are continuous with the nuclear envelope, and they are pleomorphic.

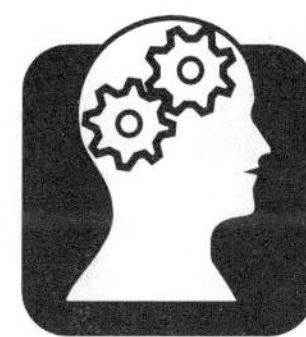

■ **Rough Endoplasmic Reticulum (RER)** Ribosomes are attached to the outer (cytosolic) surface of E.R., giving it a studded appearance. The smooth side faces the lumen. The ribosomes remain firmly attached during isolation procedures (**microsomal fraction**). The ribosomes are spaced about 15 nm apart. The large subunit faces the lumen.

Proteins synthesized on the ribosomes of the RER gain entrance to the lumen. The growing peptide is directed toward the lumen. (There is a canal through the center of the large subunit.) Discontinuities in the ER membrane allow the passage of the protein.

Proteins synthesized on the RER are primarily for extracellular use (secretion) or proteins in lysosomes and peroxisomes, as well as intrinsic membrane proteins.

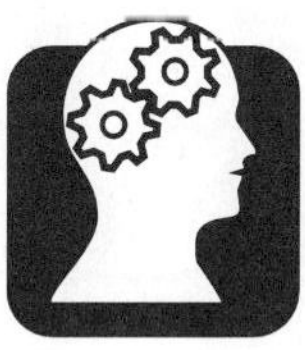

■ **Smooth Endoplasmic Reticulum (SER)** SER shows continuities with the RER. It is particularly well developed in cells with secretory or absorptive functions. When RER and SER are compared as to enzyme and polypeptide composition, they are very similar though not identical. Apparently most of the endoplasmic reticulum membrane components can diffuse between the RER and SER.

Functions of the smooth endoplasmic reticulum include the following:

● **Intracellular transport** Proteins synthesized on the RER are transported to the region of the Golgi complex by the SER. In cells that absorb lipid like intestinal epithelial cells, this lipid is either taken up by pinocytotic vesicles or resynthesized from absorbed fatty acids in the smooth ER. Transport or absorbed lipid is membrane bound.

● **Carbohydrate metabolism** Most of the proteins that are synthesized on the RER are glycoproteins. A preformed oligosaccharide (composed of *N*-acetylglucosamine, mannose, and glucose, and containing 14 sugars) is transferred en bloc to the proteins in the ER where it is linked to the side-chain amino group of asparagine. These oligosaccharides are referred to as **N-linked oligosaccharides.** Enzymes involved in synthesis of glycogen are localized in the smooth endoplasmic reticulum of hepatocytes.

● **Lipid metabolism** Enzymes involved in the synthesis of fatty acids and glycerol are localized in smooth ER. The SER plays an important role in phospholipid synthesis and membrane assembly. As indicated previously, phospholipids (and cholesterol) are incorporated into the cytosolic layer of the membrane, and then **phospholipid translocases** transfer some lipid to the luminal side of the membrane. Enzymes involved in the synthesis of steroid hormones are localized in the smooth ER. (Cholesterol is also an important membrane constituent.)

● **Detoxification** In hepatocytes, toxic substances are modified to form less harmful compounds by enzymes localized in the smooth ER. Detoxification is accomplished by enzymes that may carry out hydroxylation, demethylation, or glucuronizidation of the toxin.

GOLGI APPARATUS (GOLGI COMPLEX)

■ **General Organization of the Golgi Apparatus** In the light microscope, the Golgi apparatus is demonstrated by impregnation with osmium or silver. These deposit on a continuous network that shows a scale-like appearance. In the electron microscope, the Golgi apparatus is seen to have a very organized appearance. It appears as a group of cavities lined by membrane. Unlike the polymorphous smooth ER, it is very organized into stacks of flattened disk-like saccules. Around the surfaces of these saccules are many vesicles (20 to 100 nm diameter). There are transfer vesicles, associated with the immature face (*cis* face). There are also secretory vesicles associated with the mature face (*trans* face).

The Golgi apparatus is found in almost all eukaryotic cells. Its appearance is variable, and it shows a characteristic morphology and localization for a given cell type. For example, in the neuron, it surrounds the nucleus; in the secretory epithelial cell, it is near the apical end of the cell; in the plasma cell, it is localized at one end of the nucleus in the *hof.*

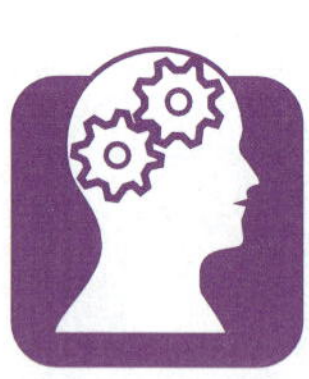

■ **Function of the Golgi Apparatus (Fig. 2.9)** Proteins processed by the Golgi apparatus are destined to be delivered to the following:

• Secretory granules→ exocytosis→ secretion
• Plasma membrane—intrinsic proteins
• Lysosomes—lysosomal enzymes

To perform these functions each vesicle must take up only appropriate proteins and fuse only with the appropriate target. A vesicle going to the plasma membrane must exclude proteins that stay in the Golgi and must fuse only with the plasma membrane, not other organelles.

The proteins processed by the Golgi are glycoproteins (they have N-linked polysaccharides attached to them). The oligosaccharides were added en bloc in

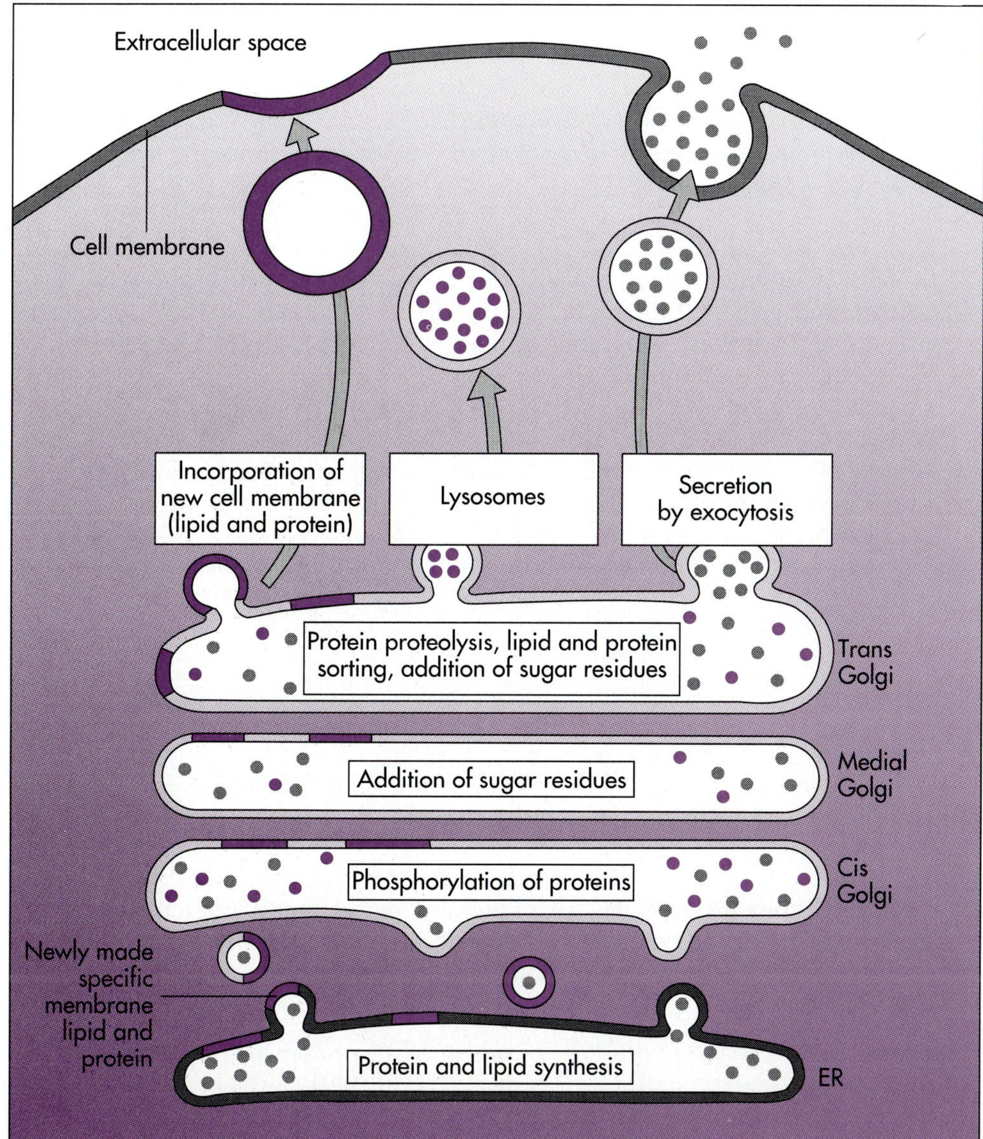

Fig. 2.9 The Golgi apparatus (or body) has three functional parts. The *cis* face, which receives transport vesicles from the smooth endoplasmic reticulum (SER) and phosphorylates some of the *n*-linked oligosaccharides associated with proteins that will be directed to the lysosome. The medial Golgi apparatus glycosylates lipids, proteins, and glycoproteins. The *trans* face glycosylates lipids, proteins, and glycoproteins and sorts different macromolecules into specific vesicles, which bud off the *trans* face. Membrane lipid, synthesized and assembled in the SER, is directed toward the plasma membrane by the Golgi apparatus. *(From Stevens A, Lowe JS:* Histology, *Brookfield, Vt., 1992, Gower Medical {London}.)*

the ER. These carbohydrate groups are modified in the Golgi (removal and addition of carbohydrate). Because the oligosaccharides are added on the luminal side of the ER and Golgi, their distribution is asymmetrical. As a result, the oligosaccharides of all membrane-associated glycoproteins and lipoproteins face the lumen of intracellular membranes whereas those of the plasma membrane (because of exocytosis) face the outside of the cell. Further modifications include

• Phosphorylation of mannose occurs in the *cis* cisternae and results in the lysosomal localization of these glycoproteins. The N-linked oligosaccharides of lysosomal proteins carry a unique mannose-6-phosphate marker (M6P). M6P receptors in the *trans* cisternae Golgi membrane identify these and package them in lysosomes.

• Glycosylation of N-linked oligosaccharides occurs in the medial and *trans* cisternae. Some of these proteins end up in the plasma membrane. Others end up in secretory granules.

Proteins for extracellular use, lysosomal enzymes, and some plasmalemma proteins are synthesized in the RER. Isotope tracer experiments show that labeled amino acids are processed as follows: RER → smooth ER → Golgi apparatus → Golgi vacuoles → secretion granules (lysosomes). The best evidence indicates that there are continuities between RER and SER, and that portions of smooth ER bud off and fuse with the Golgi apparatus. Secretion granules and lysosomes derive their membrane from the Golgi apparatus. The contribution to the Golgi of membrane from smooth ER provides for a loss of membrane from the Golgi to the secretion granules. Secretion granules form from Golgi saccules (presecretory granule → condensing vacuole → secretory granule) and are transported as membrane-bound vacuoles into the cytoplasm.

THE CYTOSKELETON

The **cytoskeleton** is made up of microtubules, microfilaments, and intermediate filaments. It is responsible for the cell's ability to adapt a variety of shapes and carry out coordinated movement (Fig. 2.10).

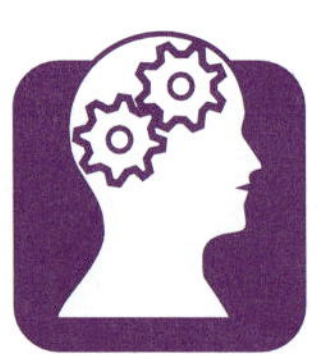

• **Microtubules** are slender tubular structures measuring 24 nm in diameter. They are variable in length and are composed of the protein tubulin. Alpha-tubulin and beta-tubulin ($50kD_a$ each) form tubulin dimers, which polymerize into microtubules.

In cross-section each microtubule is made up of 13 protofilaments, each composed of a linear array of tubulin dimers that run the length of the microtubule. Microtubules are polar structures with the following properties:

- The plus end is capable of rapid growth by adding tubulin dimers.
- The minus end loses subunits if it is not stabilized.
- Polymerization requires GTP (and GDP is incorporated into the microtubule).
- In most cells the minus end is stabilized when it is inserted into the microtubule-organizing center (MTOC), or centrosome.

Microtubules are stabilized when they bind microtubule-associated proteins (MAPS). Dyneins are MAPS that utilize ATP to move materials unidirectionally toward the minus ends of microtubules. Kinesins are MAPS that utilize ATP to move materials unidirectionally toward the positive ends of microtubules.

Microtubules are found in all cells. (They radiate from the centrosome.) They are particularly rich in the mitotic spindle, the cilia, the flagella, and the centriole.

The axoneme of cilia and flagella is a bundle of microtubules. The axoneme shows the characteristic central pair of singlet microtubules surrounded by a nine doublet array. Each doublet is one complete tubule and one partial microtubule fused to share a common wall. The microtubules in the axoneme are continuous. Dysmein side

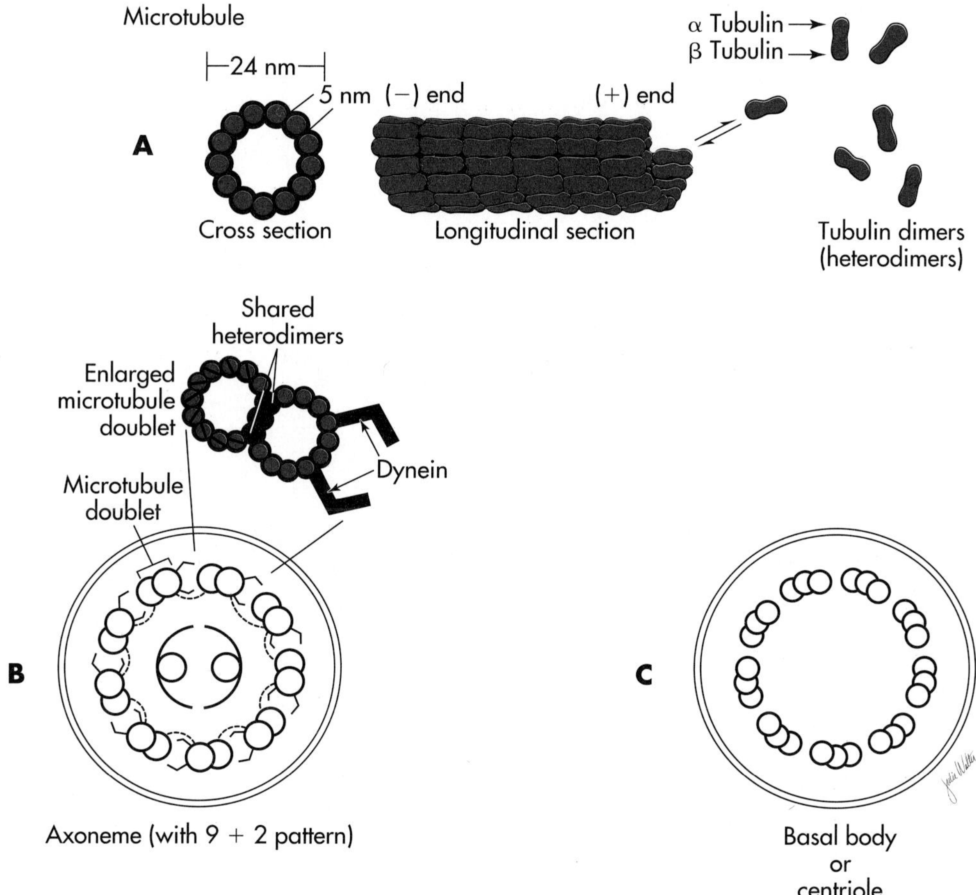

Fig. 2.10 Microtubules, cilia, flagella, and centrioles. **A,** A cross-section through a microtubule demonstrates a ring composed of 13 subunits of tubulin-containing protofilaments. **B,** A cross-section through a cilium or flagellum reveals a core of microtubules referred to as an *axoneme.* The axoneme is composed of two central singlet microtubules surrounded by nine doublet microtubules. **C,** A cross-section through the basal body of a cilium or flagellum or through the centriole reveals a ring composed of nine triplet microtubules. *(Modified from Junqueira LC, Carneiro J: Basic histology, ed 7, East Norwalk, Conn., 1992, Appleton & Lange.)*

arms extend between adjacent doublets and hydrolyze ATP to generate a sliding force between the doublets resulting in a bending movement that is responsible for beating. At the base of each axoneme is a basal body composed of nine triplet micro tubules. The basal body serves as a nucleation point for axoneme assembly. The centriole (located in the centrosome) is identical in structure to a basal body.

Functions of microtubules include

- support
- transport
- development of cell shape and polarity

■ **Microfilaments** **Microfilaments** are threadlike structures measuring 6 nm thick. They are composed of actin and proteins that interact with actin.

● **Actin-containing microfilaments** (Fig. 2.11) G-actin (globular actin) has a MW of 42 kDa. It spontaneously forms F-actin (fibrous actin). F-actin is

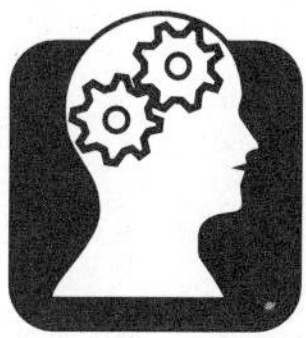

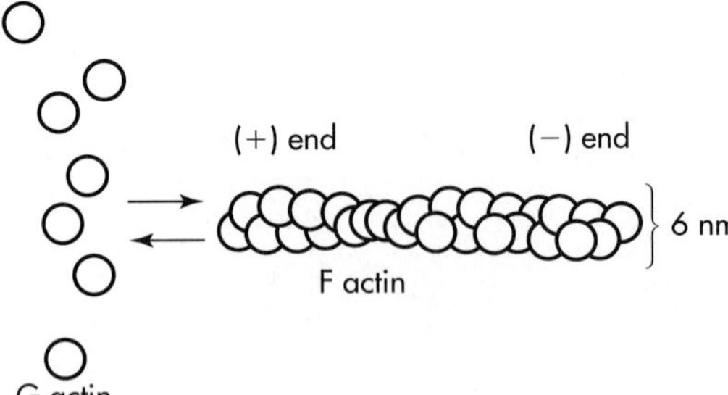

Fig. 2.11 Formation of microfilaments from G actin. Microfilaments are formed by the polymerization of G (globular) actin subunits into F (fibrous) actin containing microfilaments.

a double-stranded helical fiber composed of actin monomers. An F-actin filament has a positive end to which monomers are added rapidly. At the negative end of the filament, monomers are added more slowly. Polymerization requires ATP, and ADP is incorporated into the filament. Actin filaments can treadmill, continually adding to the positive end and removing from the negative end so that there is no net change in length.

■ **Proteins That Bind to F-actin and Modify It** **Profilin** and **thymosin** bind to G-actin monomers and prevent nucleation of filaments. Severing and capping proteins (like **gelsolin**) cut F-actin and prevent addition of G-actin monomers to F-actin. Gelsolin fragments microfilaments.

● **Cross-linking proteins**
- **Fimbrin** cross-links adjacent F-actin to form actin fibers.
- **Actinin** cross-links F-actin to form parallel arrays, or it binds to the membrane.
- **Filamin** cross-links F-actin to form a gel.
- **Tropomyosin** strengthens and stabilizes F-actin by forming parallel arrays on its surface.
- **Myosin** moves vesicles over the filaments and slides on the filaments.
- **Integrins** are intrinsic membrane proteins that bind to extracellular matrix components (like fibronectin) on the external surface of the membrane and bind to F-actin through vinculin and talin on the cytoplasmic side of the membrane.
- **Spectrin** and **ankyrin** are proteins that provide a supporting lattice on the cytosolic side of the red blood cell membrane. Spectrin is linked to the cytoplasmic tail of a transmembrane carrier protein by ankyrin bridges. The plasma membrane of the RBC is supported by a two-dimensional network of spectrin tetramers that are connected at their ends by actin filaments. Close relatives of spectrin (called fodrin) are found in the cortex of many vertebrate cells supporting the plasma membrane.

Microfilaments are found in virtually all types of cells (usually just beneath the plasma membrane). F-actin can form stable or labile microfilaments. *Stable microfilaments* are best known in muscle cells. *Labile microfilaments* are responsible for cell movements in nonmuscle cells.

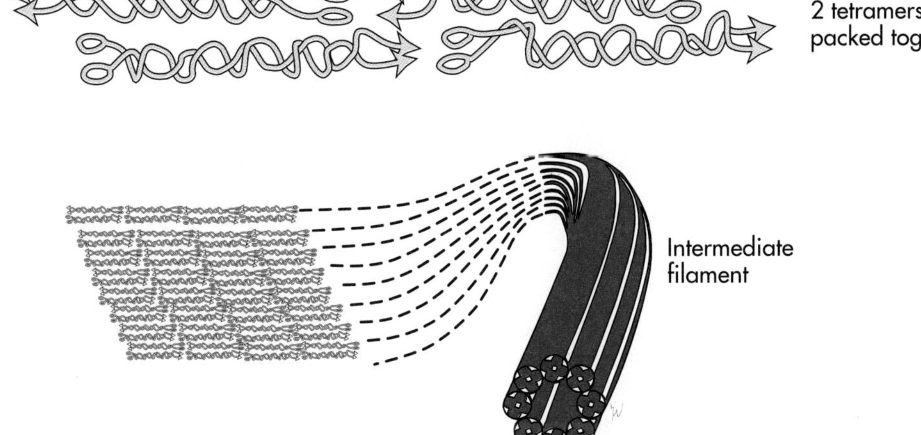

Fig. 2.12 A model of intermediate filament construction. A monomer coils with an identical monomer to form a dimer in which the central regions are wound together in a coiled coil. Two dimers then line up in an antiparallel tetramer. Within each tetramer the dimers are staggered allowing it to associate with another tetramer. In the final 10 nm intermediate filament the tetramers are packed together in a helical array. *(Modified from Alberts B, Bray D, Lewis J, et al: Molecular biology of the cell, ed 3, New York, 1994, Garland Publishing.)*

The following are functions of microfilaments:

- Movement (muscular system of cell)
- Gel formation (cell shape)
- Attachment

■ **Intermediate Filaments** measure 7 to 10 nm thick (Fig. 2.12). They show the most extensive cell and tissue diversity and are particularly prominent in cells subject to mechanical stress. Their function is support. (They are the skeletal system of the cell.)

- Desmin filaments are present in muscle cells.
- Vimentin filaments are present in mesenchymal cells.

- Keratin-like filaments are present in the epithelium (tonofilaments).
- Glial filaments are present in astrocytes.
- Neurofilaments are present in neurons.
- Lamins are a special class of intermediate filaments that form a meshwork that lines the inner nuclear membrane of all cells.

Unlike actin and tubulin, which are globular proteins, the various intermediate filaments are composed of elongate fibrous molecules that contain long tandem repeats forming coiled coil dimers. Two such dimers associate in a head-to-tail antiparallel manner to form a **nonpolarized** tetramer. The tetramers, which measure 48 nm in length, form filaments by associating in a staggered array. The monomers of different types of intermediate filaments differ in amino acid sequence and size but belong to a single gene family.

MULTIPLE CHOICE REVIEW QUESTIONS

1. Which of the following types of cellular association specializations most effectively provides a permeability seal in the space between cells?

   a. Nexus
   b. Zonula occludens
   c. Macula adherens
   d. Zonula adherens
   e. Macula occludens

2. Which of the following statements describes the P face of the plasma membrane?

   a. Covered with extrinsic membrane proteins
   b. Covered with polar heads of phospholipid molecules
   c. Covered with nonpolar tails of phospholipid molecules
   d. Covered with carbohydrate
   e. None of the above

3. Which of the following statements describes the cell coat?

   a. May act as a filter
   b. Rich in carbohydrate groups
   c. May be covalently linked to amino acids of intrinsic membrane proteins
   d. May be responsible for recognition sites on membrane
   e. All of the above are correct

4. Match the material with its method of transport:

   _____ Exocytosis
   _____ Pinocytosis
   _____ Non–carrier mediated transport
   _____ Active transport
   _____ Phagocytosis

   a. Uptake bacteria
   b. Uptake water droplets
   c. Secretion of enzymes
   d. Fatty acids
   e. Na$^+$ and K$^+$

5. Place in sequence from the outside of cell:

   _____ Polar heads of phospholipid molecules
   _____ P face
   __a__ Carbohydrate
   _____ E face
   _____ Nonpolar tails of phospholipid molecules

6. Which of the following would be considered autophagic activities of lysosomes?

   a. Digestion of bacteria
   b. Digestion of viruses
   c. Digestion of mitochondria
   d. Digestion of the contents of a phagocytotic vesicle
   e. All of the above

7. A cell is treated for 20 hours with chloramphenicol, an antibiotic that blocks mitochondrial protein synthesis but does not affect cytoplasmic protein synthesis. The synthesis of which proteins would you expect to be diminished?

   a. Proteins of the outer mitochondrial membrane
   b. Krebs cycle enzymes
   c. Cytoplasmic ribosomal proteins
   d. Lysosomal enzymes
   e. None of the above is correct

8. Treatment of cells with the antibiotic puromycin inhibits the attachment of messenger RNA to ribosomes. Ribosomes that have attached to messenger RNA before puromycin addition continue to move along messenger RNA. Treatment of a cell that is primarily synthesizing protein for intracellular use with puromycin for 5 hours would have what effects?

   a. Decrease the number of polysomes
   b. Decrease the protein synthesis
   c. Increase the number of free 40S and 60S subunits
   d. All of the above are correct
   e. None of the above is correct

9. Match the macromolecule with its site of synthesis:

   _____ Mitochondrial ribosomal RNA
   _____ Hydrolytic enzyme in lumen of intestine
   _____ Lysosomal DNAase
   _____ Hemoglobin in RBC
   _____ Succinic acid dehydrogenase (enzyme of TCA cycle)

   a. RER
   b. Metochondrial ribsomes
   c. Free polysomes
   d. Mitochondrial DNA
   e. Nuclear DNA

10. Place in proper sequence for synthesis of secretory protein:

    _____ Transfer vacuole
    _____ Secretory vacuole
    _____ RER
    _____ Golgi apparatus
    _____ Exocytosis

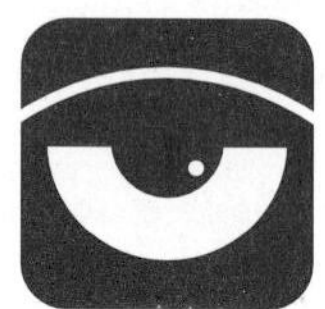

Chapter 3

Cell Biology: Nucleus and Cell Division

THE NUCLEAR ENVELOPE (FIG. 3.1)

The nucleus is surrounded by an **outer** and an **inner nuclear membrane.** Each membrane shows a tripartite structure. The membranes are separated by a space. Ribosomes cover the external surface of the outer nuclear membrane. The nuclear envelope is continuous with the RER. The **nuclear lamina** is composed of the intermediate filament lamin. Lamin lines the inner nuclear membrane. The nuclear envelope is incomplete. **Nuclear pores, or annuli,** are found where the inner and outer membranes fuse. The pores are incomplete openings (i.e., they are covered with a diaphragm composed of lamin).

CONTENTS OF THE NUCLEUS

- The **karyoplasm** is the fluid part of the nucleus.
- The **nuclear matrix** is the proteinaceous material that fills in the space between the chromatin. The nuclear matrix is continuous with the nuclear lamina.
- The **nucleolus** (see below)

Chromosomes contain the genetic "blueprint" of the cell (in DNA). Their appearance varies during different portions of the cell cycle. Chromosomes are most obvious at the time of cell division. In normal human cells, there are 23 pairs of chromosomes, with one member of each pair being derived from the maternal parent and one from the paternal parent. Each chromosome at metaphase is composed of two **chromatids.** The two chromatids at the site of the primary constriction are joined together by the **centromere,** which attaches to the mitotic spindle.

The chromosomes are composed principally of DNA and the basic protein **(histone);** more than 99% of the cellular DNA is localized in the chromosomes. Each chromosome has the following essential components:

- A **centromere,** which attaches it to the spindle and is responsible for its distribution to the daughter cell
- Several **origins of replication,** which enable it to replicate its DNA
- Two **telomeres** on the end of the chromosome

During cell division, chromosomes are inert genetically (i.e., they show little if any RNA synthesis). They are involved in the parceling out of DNA to daughter cells.

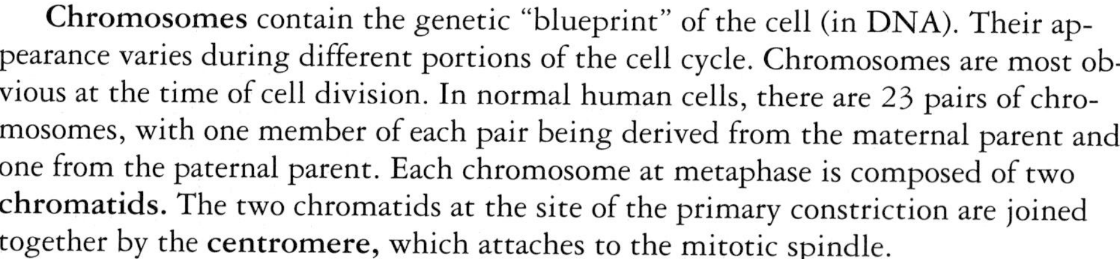

■ **Interphase Chromosomes = Chromatin** During interphase, chromosomes are not obvious; they are in an extended state. That chromosomes are present throughout interphase is demonstrated by cell-fusion experiments where interphase cells are fused with dividing cells; chromosomes can then be demonstrated in the interphase nucleus.

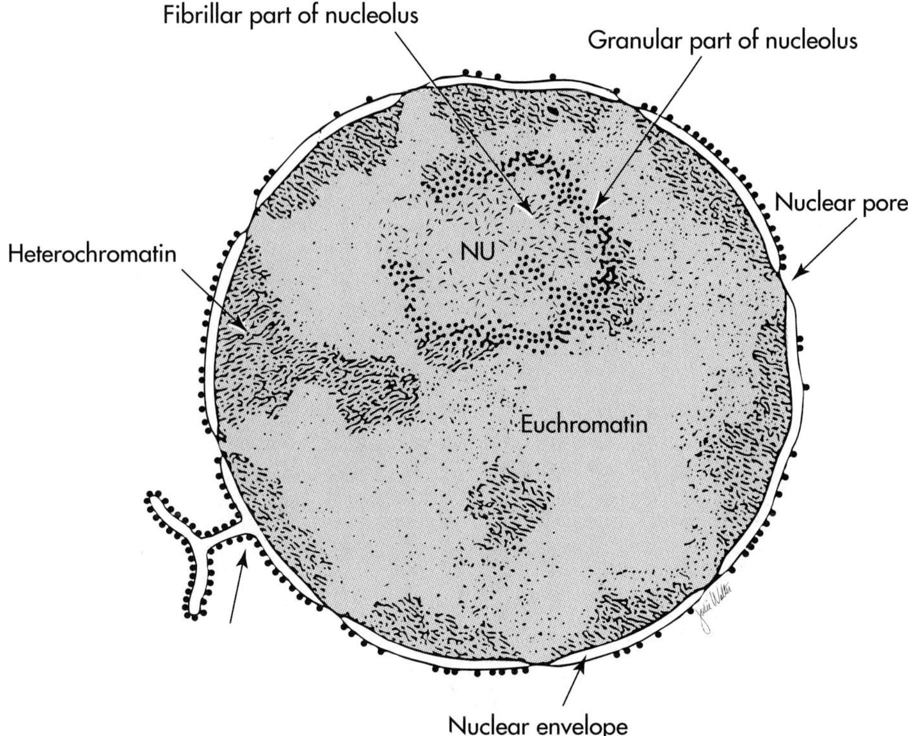

Fig. 3.1 The interphase nucleus. The interphase nucleus is bounded by the nuclear envelope. Two types of chromatin are evident: diffuse chromatin, or euchromatin, and dense chromatin, or heterochromatin. The nucleolus *(NU)* demonstrates a fibrillar and a granular area.

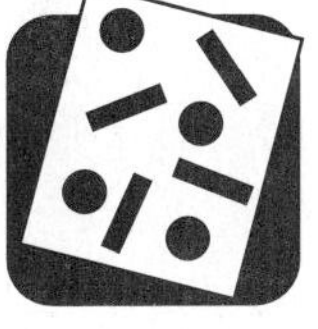

When chromatin is specially prepared for electron microscopy, it is visualized as beads on a string (Fig. 3.2). The beads are called *nucleosomes,* or "NU bodies," and measure approximately 8 to 10 nm in diameter. Each nucleosome contains approximately 150 base pairs of DNA. The DNA in the nucleosome is tightly coiled about and associated with histone protein. The core of each nucleosome contains eight tightly packed histone molecules, two molecules each of four histones (H2A, H2B, H3, and H4 histone).

Between the nucleosomes is a thread that measures 1.5 to 2 nm in thickness (which is approximately the thickness of DNA double helix). The thread contains approximately 50 base pairs of DNA. Another histone (H1 histone) associates with this DNA. Unlike the other histones, H1 histones show a lot of variation. Different tissues have different H1 histones. A chromatin fiber may approach 0.1 mm in length and is highly coiled in the nucleus.

There is good evidence to indicate that the DNA of each chromosome is represented by a single linear DNA double helix, which is organized into nucleosomes. The smallest chromosome contains approximately 50,000 kilo–base pairs of DNA. Such a molecule would measure approximately 2.0 cm in length. The DNA molecule undergoes several levels of coiling to form a structure that measures about 3 to 4 μm long at metaphase and fits into the interphase nucleus (about 10 μm in diameter). The chromatin is composed of the following:

- Nucleic acids [RNA (5%) DNA (35% to 40%)]
- Protein [Histone protein (about 35%) Nonhistone protein (about 10% to 20%)]

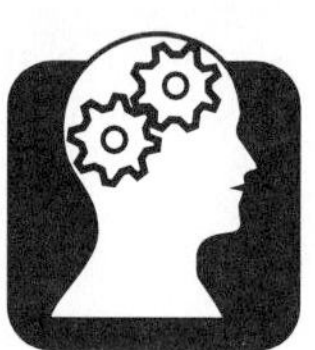

It is during interphase that chromosomes show their maximal activity (RNA synthesis).

— *States of chromatin activity* Euchromatin, or **diffuse chromatin,** is chromatin that is inactive in RNA synthesis. **Heterochromatin,** or **condensed chromatin,** is chromatin that is relatively inactive in RNA synthesis.

   • **Constitutive heterochromatin** is chromatin that is inactivated (heterochromatinized) for the developmental history of the organism from fertilization to death; i.e., it is never active. An example of this would be pericentric heterochromatin, which surrounds the centromeres and is never active in RNA synthesis.

   • **Facultative heterochromatin** may be inactivated (heterochromatinized) in one tissue and not another, or may be inactivated and activated during different periods of the cell cycle.

   Chromosomes function in several different ways.

   • They are repositories of genetic information (DNA) in all cell types.

   • They replicate DNA. The DNA is precisely replicated, duplicating the genome. In this manner an exact duplicate of the genome is provided to each daughter cell.

   • They transcribe DNA. When DNA is transcribed into RNA, genetic information is made available to the cell.

   Each region of the genome that encodes a functional RNA is a **gene.**

   • **Messenger RNA** (mRNA) encodes protein.

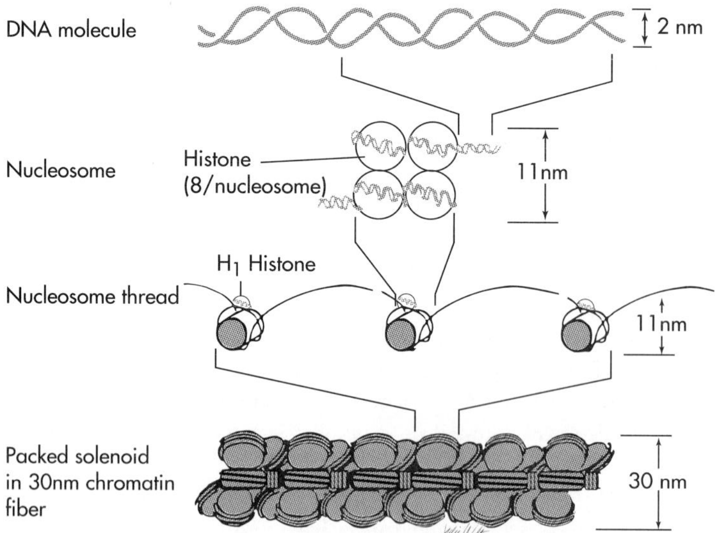

Fig. 3.2 Organization of DNA in chromatin. The DNA molecule coils twice around octamers of histone (each composed of 4 dimers of H2A, H2B, H3, and H4 histones) to form nucleosomes. Nucleosomes are linked by H1 histone, which aggregates to form the 30 nm chromatin fiber. *(Modified from Alberts B, Bray D, Lewis J, et al:* Molecular biology of the cell, *ed 3, New York, 1994, Garland Publishing.)*

- **Ribosomal RNA** (rRNA) forms part of ribosome the site of protein synthesis.
- **Transfer RNA** (tRNA) is involved in protein synthesis.

In regard to the transcriber function, not all genetic information is expressed by all cells (i.e., different cell types express different activities: erythrocytes, hemoglobin; plasma cells, antibody; etc.) Various mechanisms have been proposed in accounting for the control of differential gene expression. Histones and nonhistone proteins have been implicated in the regulation of genetic activity. There are no preferred histone-binding sites. Histones can occupy many positions on DNA.

Some sites on chromosomes appear to lack histones even though they are hundreds of nucleotides long. These sites can be detected with DNAase used at very low concentrations. **Nuclease-hypersensitive spots** are associated with sites of RNA synthesis. Different cell types show different hypersensitivity sites. Analysis of active chromatin reveals the following:

- H1 histone may be less tightly bound and perhaps different from H1 histones found in inactive chromatin.
- Other histones may be more acetylated than inactive chromatin.
- H2B histone may be more phosphorylated in inactive than in active chromatin.

■ The Nucleolus—Detailed Analysis of a Gene (or Genes) and Its Products

— *General organization of the nucleolus* The nucleolus is primarily composed of particulate elements (20 to 30 nm granules) and fibrillar elements. These may be intermingled or separated to form a **fibrillar core** and **granular cortex.**

The nucleolus undergoes changes during development and differentiation as a result of changes in cell metabolism and during different portions of the cell cycle (e.g., it disappears during cell division and reappears during interphase). The nucleoli disappear at late prophase. The sites where nucleoli were localized on the chromosome appear as secondary constrictions. The nucleolus is composed of

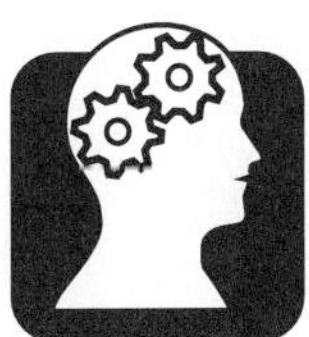

- protein, which is similar to the proteins in ribosomes
- DNA, i.e., nucleolar organizer DNA
- RNA that is a precursor of ribosomal 18S and 28S RNA

— *The role of the nucleolus in RNA synthesis* The genes that code for rRNA are localized in the nucleolus organizer. This can be demonstrated by in situ hybridization. DNA in chromosomes is made single stranded and hybridized with ^{3}H-labeled 18S and 28S RNA. The hybrid molecules are detected by means of autoradiography. The label appears exclusively over the nucleolus organizer (secondary constrictions). The data indicate that all the genes coding for rRNA are localized in the nucleolus organizer.

Moreover, in some lower forms it has been possible to isolate animals from which the nucleolar organizer is lost (by deletion). Such animals show no nucleoli and no secondary constrictions, and synthesize all other RNA forms except rRNA. Unlike other genes for which there is probably only one copy of the gene/haploid chromosome

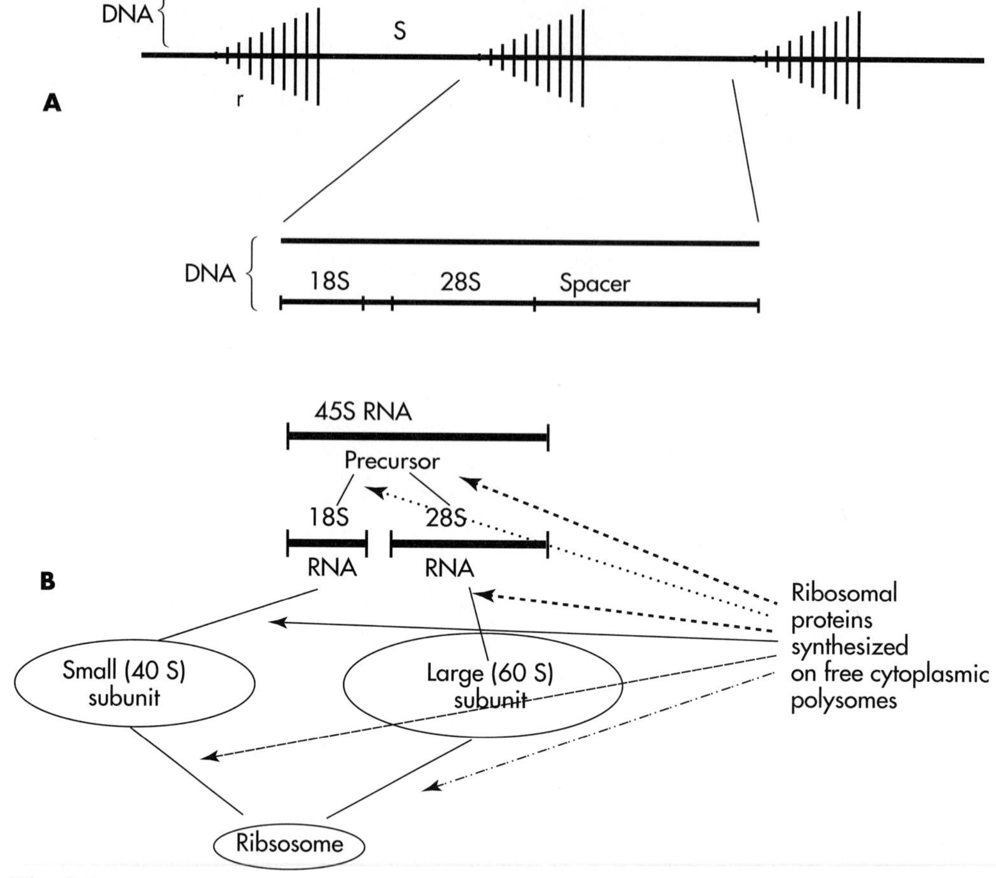

Fig. 3.3 Organization of the genes coding for ribosomal RNA and their transcription products. **A,** The genes coding for rRNA are localized in the chromosomal nucleolus organizer region. Each gene consists of a coding sequence that is transcribed into a ribosomal precursor RNA and a noncoding spacer sequence. The ribosomal genes are repeated many times in the nucleolus organizer and are arranged in a tandem array of coding and spacer sequences. **B,** Each gene is transcribed into a 45S RNA precursor molecule that is processed over several steps to give rise to the final 18S and 28S products. As they are synthesized and processed, the rRNA complexes with ribosomal proteins, which are synthesized on free cytoplasmic polysomes to form the large and small subunits of the ribosome.

complement, there are approximately 300 to 600 identical copies of the genes coding for 18S and 28S rRNA in human cells. The multiple copies of the genes coding for rRNA are arranged tandemly in the nucleolar organizer region. Separating each ribosomal gene that contains a segment coding for 18S and 28S RNA is a nontranscribed spacer DNA.

Ribosomal RNA is synthesized as a large (45S) precursor that is processed by means of several steps to give rise to the 18S and 28S products, which associate with ribosomal proteins to form the mature 40S an 60S particles (Fig. 3.3). The fibrous region of the nucleolus represents the 45S RNA precursor. The granular region of the nucleolus represents large and small ribosomal subunits.

— *Visualization of nucleolar genes and their products* If one treats nucleoli with distilled water, the nucleolar granules disperse and the

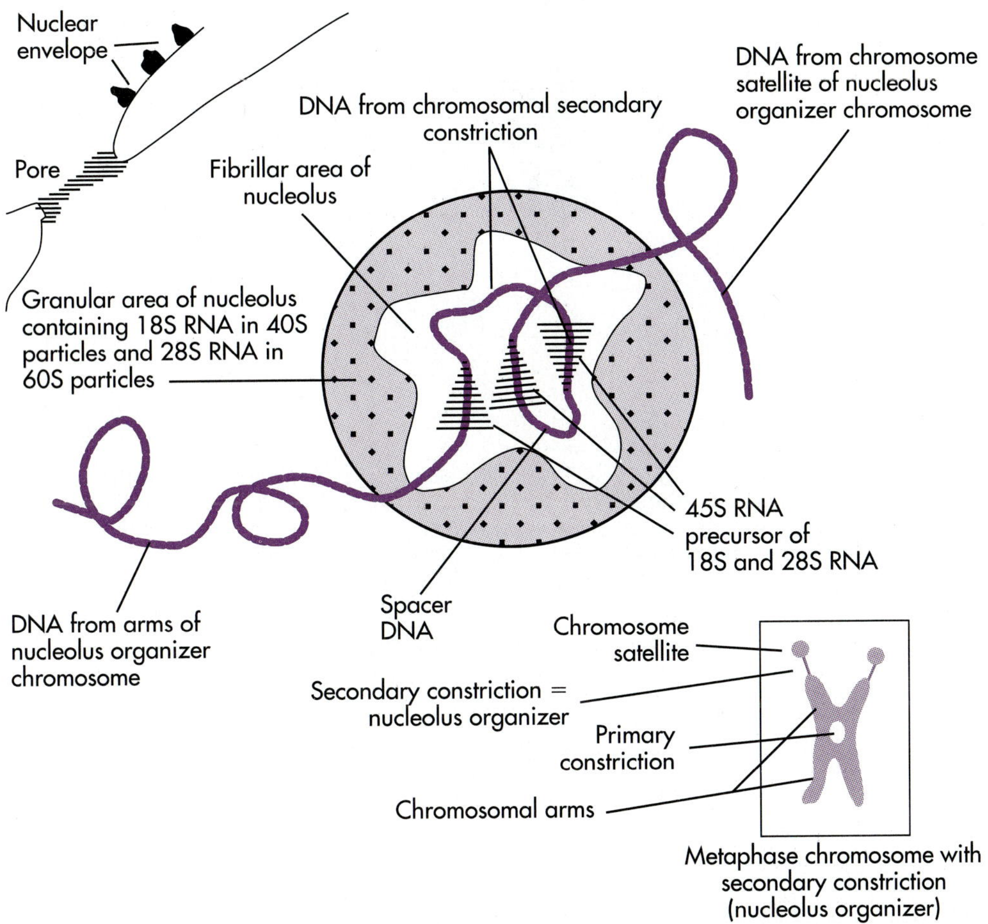

Fig. 3.4 Relationship of the chromosomal nucleolus organizer to the nucleolus. In the interphase nucleus the nucleolus organizer or organizers are localized in the granular area of the nucleolus where synthesis of the 45S precursor to rRNA takes place. As the 45S RNA is processed, it moves to the granular area of the nucleolus where the final 18S and 28S products are produced. The 18S and 28S products and associated ribosomal proteins are transported to the cytoplasm through nuclear pores where they provide for the small and large subunits of the ribosome.

fibrous regions become unraveled. Then the nucleolar contents are spread in a single layer, stained, and viewed in the EM. One visualizes a long thin axial thread with evenly distributed arrowhead-shaped fibrous matrix units separated by nonmatrix units (Fig. 3.4).

- The axial fiber is DNA.
- The fibrous side units are RNA.
- The length of an arrowhead-shaped matrix unit and its adjacent nonmatrix unit is equal to the length of the ribosomal gene and its nontranscribed spacer.
- The fibers in the matrix unit increase in length from one end to the other. This results from an increase in chain length as the RNA moves from the initiation site (shortest fiber) to the termination site (longest fiber).

In summary, the nucleolus contains the following products:

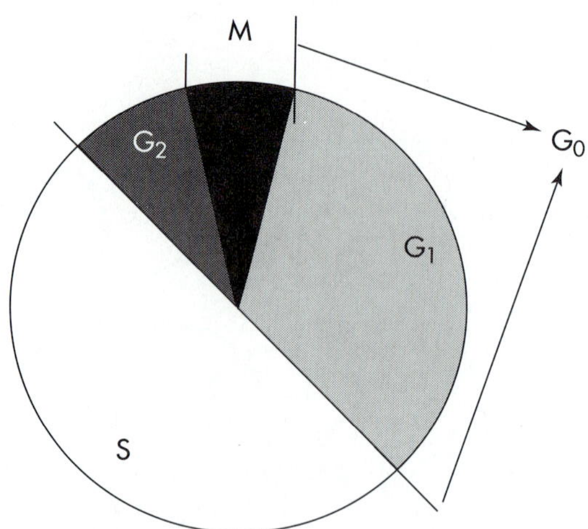

Fig. 3.5 The cell (intermitotic) cycle. The cell cycle consists of a non–DNA synthetic G_1 (gap 1) period followed by the S (synthesis) period in which DNA is synthesized, and that period is followed by another non–DNA synthetic G_2 (gap 2) period, which precedes cell division, or mitosis (M). Cells with a very long G_1 period are said to be in G_0.

- Nucleolar organizer DNA (location of the ribosomal RNA genes)
- Primary gene products (45S rRNA precursor)
- Derivatives of these products (ribosomal subunits)
- Enzymatic machinery for RNA synthesis

THE CELL CYCLE (FIG. 3.5)

In eukaryotic cells replication of DNA is limited toa specific portion of the cell cycle namely the S (synthesis) **period.** During the S period the cells incorporate labeled nucleotides (usually ^{3}H-thymidine) into DNA. The S phase is preceded by the non-DNA synthetic G_1 (gap 1) period, which follows cell division. (There is no thymidine incorporation in G_1-phase stage cells.) The S phase is followed by the non-DNA synthetic G_2 (gap 2) period, which precedes cell division. (There is no thymidine incorporation in G_2-phase cells.)

During the S phase the amount of DNA in the nucleus is precisely doubled (Fig. 3.6). The basic amount of DNA in a species is the amount of DNA found in the gamete. This is described as the "C" amount of DNA. This enables the amount of DNA to be described in a manner that is independent of the level of ploidy, which is described in terms of **n.** Since a new organism arises from fertilization involving two gametes, the minimum amount of DNA in somatic tissues is 2C.

Cell-fusion experiments have shown that if one takes cells in various interphase portions of the cell cycle and hybridizes them with dividing mitotic cells using Sendai virus the chromosomes can be visualized in the interphase cell. (Table 3.1)

- If a dividing cell is fused to a G_1-phase cell, the chromosomes of the G_1 cell demonstrate 1 chromatid per chromosome.
- If a dividing cell is fused to a S-phase cells, the chromosomes of the S-phase cell are fragmented into small pieces.
- If a dividing cell is fused to a G_2-phase cells, the chromosomes of the G_2 cell demonstrates 2 chromatids per chromosome.

This indicates that the replication of DNA is equivalent to duplication of the

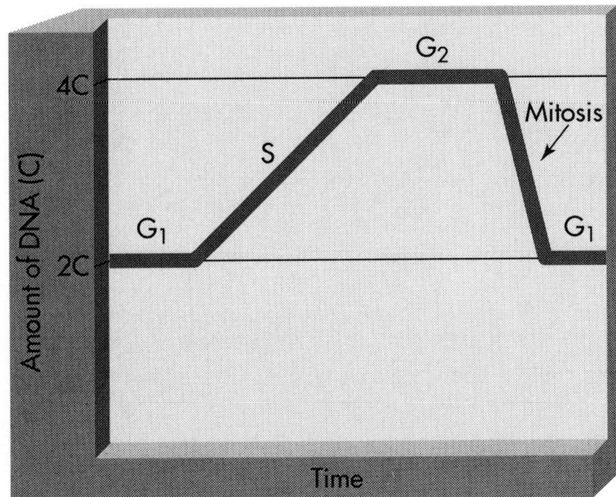

Fig. 3.6 Relationship of the cell cycle and mitosis to the amount of DNA in the nucleus. The amount of DNA in a haploid ($1n$) gamete nucleus is equal to C. The diploid ($2n$) G_1 nucleus contains 2C. During S phase this amount is precisely doubled. The diploid ($2n$) G_2 nucleus contains 4C. During mitosis this amount is halved to produce a diploid ($2n$) cell with 2C DNA.

Table 3.1

	G_1	S	G_2	M
Adrenal cortex	1863h*	7.5h	2h	1h
Intestinal crypts	3.5h	7.4h	2h	1h
Cultured fibroblast	16h	7.0h	2h	1h
Cultured cancer cell	8h	6h	3.5h	1h

*Cells with a long G_1 period are considered, by some investigators, to be in G_0.

chromosomes. Cells may differ in the relative duration of the cell cycle. Most of this variation is accounted for by differences in the duration of G_1.

Cell division is dependent on the cell having the G_2 amount of DNA. It cannot proceed unless DNA replication has occurred. The cell, however, does not need to replicate its DNA to stay alive.

The cell cycle control system is a set of interacting proteins that induce processes that duplicate and divide cells. The cycle can be stopped at two major checkpoints:

- The **G_1 checkpoint** is the point that S is initiated.
- The **G_2 checkpoint** is the point that mitosis is initiated.

The cell-cycle control system is based on two families of proteins. There are **cyclin-dependent protein kinases (Cdk)** that phosphorylate selected enzymes involved in the cell cycle activating them. **Cyclins** are proteins that activate Cdk by binding to it and control its ability to phosphorylate target proteins. **G_1 cyclins** bind to Cdk during G_1 and are required for entry into G_1. **Mitotic cyclins** bind to Cdk during G_2 and are required for entry in mitosis.

Certain drugs are known to specifically inhibit cells in various portions of the cell cycle.

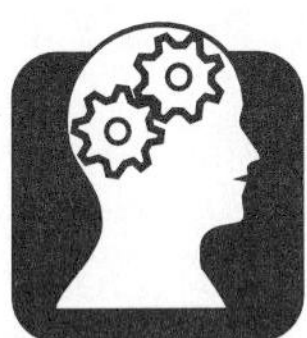

- Colchicine inhibits spindle formation and blocks cells in the metaphase of mitosis.
- 5-Fluorodeoxyuridine inhibits synthesis of enzymes that convert thymidine to deoxythymidylic acid and blocks cells at the G_1-S interface.
- Cytosine arabinoside and aminopterin also block cells at the G_1-S interface.
- Puromycin inhibits protein synthesis and blocks cells at the G_2-M interface.

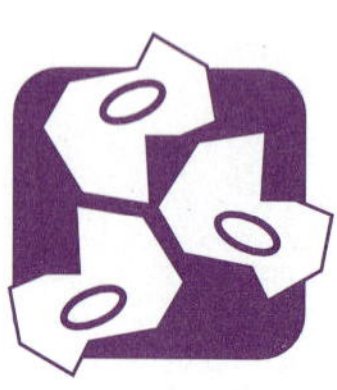

■ **The Cell Cycle in Societies of Cells** In the adult organism, there is specialization in regard to the frequency with which the cells undergo mitosis. Cells that can reproduce can be continuous or occasional replicator cells.

— *Continuous replicator cells are of two types:*

• **Vegetative intermitotic cells (VIM)** are undifferentiated cells. They have a short life-span, which begins at mitosis and ends at the next mitosis. They produce new cells to replace those lost or damaged. A cell in the basal layer of the epidermis is an example of a VIM cell.

• **Differentiating intermitotics (DIM)** are produced by vegetative intermitotics. They continue to divide as they differentiate and form specialized cells. They give rise to occasional and nonreplicating cells. A cell in the spinous layer of the epidermis is an example of a DIM cell.

— *Occasional replicators (reverting postmitotics)* (RPM) are cells that replicate only rarely or under special circumstances. These are specialized cells that may revert to divide. There are two classes of such cells.

• G_1 arrested (G_0) must pass through the S phase before dividing. (Most occasional replicators are of this sort.)
• G_2 arrested cells divide immediately without replicating DNA.

A hepatocyte is an example of a RPM cell.

— *Cells that do not reproduce* Nonreplicators (fixed postmitotics) **(FPM)** are highly specialized cells that no longer are capable of division. If damaged or killed, these cells will not be replaced unless they maintain a stem-cell population. An example of a nonreplicating cell is a cell found in the granulosum or corneum layer of the epidermis.

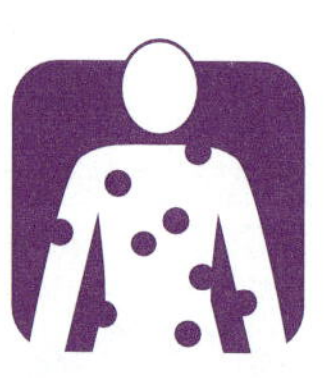

■ **Malfunctions of the Cell Cycle** Endoreduplication is failure of a cell to divide after passing through the cell cycle but to continue into the next cell cycle without dividing. This leads to polyploidy. In some cells this is normal. The megakaryocyte is a highly polyploid cell of the bone marrow that gives rise to platelets. In some cells this is abnormal. Many tumors contain highly polyploid cells.

There may be failure of an undifferentiated cell to differentiate. This occurs in the skin disease **psoriasis,** where the continuous replicating cells of the basal and spiny layers do not cease cycling and differentiate to form nonreplicating cells of the keratinized layer. The cells continue to pass through the cell cycle and thus form the erythematous plaque characteristic of psoriasis.

MEIOSIS AND MITOSIS

Instead of going through the individual stages of mitosis and meiosis, only the important most differentiating characteristics are mentioned.

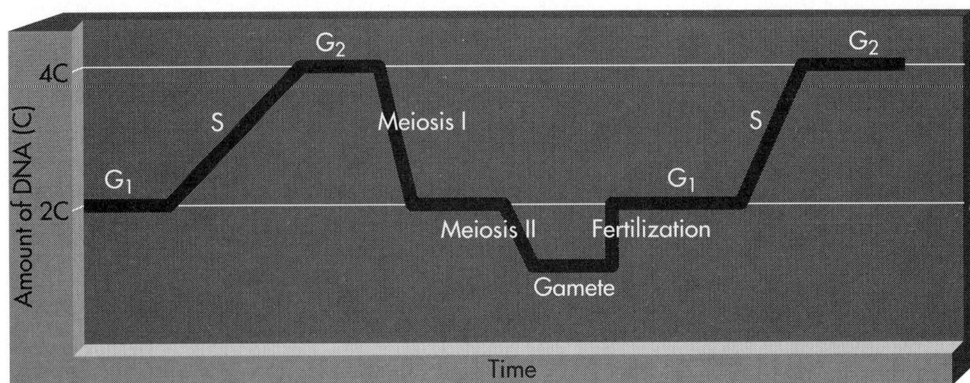

Fig. 3.7 Relationship of the cell cycle and meiosis to the amount of DNA in the nucleus. Before entering meiosis (or mitosis) the cell must replicate its DNA (pass through S). As a result of meiosis I (the reductional division) there is produced a cell (secondary spermatocyte or oocyte) that is haploid ($1n$) and contains 2C. As a result of meiosis II (the equational division) there is produced a haploid ($1n$) cell that contains 1C (spermatid or ootid). Fertilization restores the diploid ($2n$) chromosome number.

■ **Important Characteristics of Mitosis** During mitosis the homologous chromosomes do not pair. The chromosomes simply line up on the equatorial plate. During anaphase the chromatids of each chromosome separate. Before anaphase separation, one chromosome = two chromatids. After anaphase separation, one chromosome = one chromatid. Therefore each cell receives one chromatid from each metaphase chromosome. (Each cell receives 46 chromatids.) (These are now called *chromosomes*.) During the following S phase, the chromosomes duplicate so that there are 92 chromatids (46 chromosomes = 92 chromatids) at the beginning of the next mitosis.

■ **Important Characteristics of Meiosis** The paternally and maternally derived homologous chromosomes pair at the first meiotic division. The first meiotic division is a separation of these pairs of chromosomes. The chromatids of these chromosomes do not separate. The number of chromosomes is halved by this **reductional division.**

Without an intervening interphase (with no DNA synthesis occurring), the cells undergo a second division. During the second meiotic division, the chromatids of each chromosome separate. This is the **equational** division of meiosis. Each daughter cell receives 1 chromatid from each pair of chromosomes. This results in a cell with 23 chromosomes. This is the **haploid** chromosome number of man and is described as **n.**

At fertilization (fusion of sperm and egg) 23 egg chromosomes + 23 sperm chromosomes restore the number of chromosomes in the zygote to 46 chromosomes. This is the **diploid** chromosome number of man = **2n.** Since the segregation of maternal and paternal chromosomes is random at meiosis I, there is a possible 10,000,000 different chromosome combinations as the outcome of a single meiotic division. The number of possible genetic combinations is further augmented by the recombination (crossing over) that occurred during meiosis I.

— *The relation of meiosis to the amount of DNA in the cell (Fig. 3.7)*

- Before entering meiosis I, the cell passes through S phase attaining the G_2 amount of DNA (= 4C).
- As a result of meiosis I, the amount of DNA is halved (= 2C).
- There is no DNA replication between meiosis I and meiosis II.

- As a result of meiosis II, the amount of DNA is halved again (= C).
- Each gamete contributes C amount of DNA to the zygote.
- This would give rise to a cell with 2C amount of DNA.
- At fertilization DNA synthesis occurs to restore the G_2 amount of DNA (4C).
- Subsequent mitosis reduces this to the G_1 amount of DNA (2C).

Sex Determination and Sex Chromatin Cells of human females have 44 autosomes and 2 X chromosomes (46,XX). As a result of meiosis, a gamete (ovum) that has 22 autosomes and an X chromosome (23,X) is formed. Cells of human males have 44 autosomes and an X and a Y chromosome (46,XY). As a result of meiosis, two types of gametes (sperm) are formed. One has 22 autosomes and an X chromosome (23,X). One has 22 autosomes and a Y chromosome (23,Y).

Fertilization of an ovum by a Y-bearing sperm forms a male offspring (46,XY). The Y chromosome is a male determinant. Individuals lacking a Y chromosome develop female phenotype. Fertilization of an ovum by an X-bearing sperm forms a female offspring (46,XX). During early development, about 2 weeks in the human embryo, one of the X chromosomes in female cells becomes heterochromatinized (an example of facultative heterochromatinization). The heterochromatinized X chromosome is visible during interphase as the **sex chromatin body,** or **Barr body.** The presence or absence of sex chromatin bodies can allow one to tell the chromosomal sex of an individual. The number of Barr bodies = number of X chromosomes minus 1(XY = 0 Barr bodies, XX = 1 Barr body, XXX = 2 Barr bodies, etc).

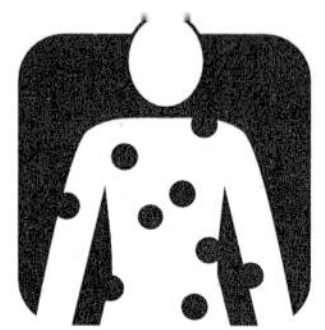

Abnormalities of Cell Division The following abnormalities can occur during either mitosis or meiosis. When they occur during meiosis, virtually all the cells in the resulting offspring will be affected and carry the aberration. When they occur during mitosis, **mixoploidy** (chromosome mosaicism) occurs, and some cells will show the aberration, and others will not.

Nondisjunction is the failure of a single pair of chromosomes (meiosis I) or a single pair of chromatids (meiosis II, or mitosis) to separate at cell division. This results in one daughter cell receiving two and the other daughter cell receiving none of the chromosomes or chromatids in question. When nondisjunction occurs during meiosis and the gamete is fertilized by a normal gamete, it results in an individual all of whose cells either lack one chromosome or have an additional chromosome (e.g., in Turner's syndrome, that individual lacks one sex chromosome: 45,XO); in Down's syndrome there is an extra chromosome number 21: 47,XX or XY,21$^+$).

Anaphase lagging is lagging of a chromosome (meiosis I) or a chromatid (meiosis II, or mitosis) behind the remainder of the chromosomes so that it is not included in the daughter cells. It results in one daughter cell that is normal and another that lacks a chromosome. When anaphase lagging occurs during meiosis and the resulting gamete is fertilized by a normal gamete, the result is an individual all of whose cells lack a single chromosome (e.g., Turner's syndrome: 45,XO).

Deletion occurs when a fragment of a chromosome breaks off. If it has no centromere, it is lost to the cell at cell division. When a deletion occurs during meiosis and the resulting gamete is fertilized by a normal gamete, the result is an individual all of whose cells have the normal chromosome number but one chromosome is lacking a piece (e.g., cri-du-chat syndrome: deletion of the short arm of chromosome number 5). When a deletion occurs during mitosis, the result is mixoploidy. Some cells have the normal chromosome complements; others are lacking a small piece of a single chromosome. (e.g., chronic myelocytic leukemia: deletion of chromosome number 22 in blood and bone marrow).

Translocation occurs when a piece is broken off of one chromosome and is attached to another chromosome that is not its homologe. There is a large number of possible translocations. Basically what happens is that a cell effectively has an extra piece of a single chromosome or is lacking a piece of that chromosome. (e.g., translocation Down's syndrome is the translocation of a large piece of chromosome number 21 to another chromosome. The cell effectively has an extra copy of chromosome 21). When translocation occurs during mitosis, there will be mixoploidy.

MULTIPLE CHOICE REVIEW QUESTIONS

1. A rapidly growing diploid human tumor (46 chromosomes), the cells of which are all continuous replicators is treated with colchicine, a drug that inhibits spindle formation. Assuming the gamete amount of DNA to be 1.5 picograms, how many picograms of DNA would there be in the tumor cell nuclei after a 10-hour treatment with colchicine.

   a. 1.5
   b. 3.0
   c. 4.5
   d. 6.0
   e. 12.0

2. Match the sex chromosome constitution with the number of sex chromatin bodies:

   _____ XO
   _____ XY
   _____ XYYY
   _____ XXX
   _____ XX

   a. No sex chromatin bodies
   b. 1 sex chromatin body
   c. 2 sex chromatin bodies
   d. 3 sex chromatin bodies
   e. 4 sex chromatin bodies

3. Chromosome analysis shows that the sex chromosome constitution in various tissues of a female patient is XO, XX, XXX. All cells have 44 autosomes. Assume that a single abnormal division accounts for these aberrations. What division process would account for these chromosome numbers?

   a. Meiotic nondisjunction
   b. Mitotic nondisjunction
   c. Meiotic anaphase lagging
   d. Mitotic anaphase lagging
   e. Mitoic translocation

4. A single male cell that has already undergone the first meiotic division would under normal conditions give rise to

   a. either two X-bearing or two Y-bearing spermatids.
   b. either four X-bearing or four Y-bearing spermatids.
   c. one X-bearing and one Y-bearing spermatid.
   d. two X-bearing and two Y-bearing spermatids.
   e. none of the above is correct.

5. Treatment of cells for 24 hours with toyocamycin, an antibiotic that blocks the conversion of the nucleolar 45S precursor of ribosomal RNA to 18S and 28S RNA but not the synthesis of the 45S ribosomal precursor would be expected to have what effects?

   a. An increase in the fibrillar components of the nucleolus.
   b. A decrease in the amount of nucleolar granules.
   c. A decrease in the number of cytoplasmic ribosomes.
   d. The number of ribosomal genes remains the same.
   e. All of the above are correct.

6. Certain polyanions interact with chromatin in the nucleus and remove histone from DNA and thereby convert heterochromatin to euchromatin. Which of the following effects would occur in cells treated with such polyanions?

   a. Decrease in the amount of heterochromatin in the nucleus.
   b. Increase in the total RNA synthesis.
   c. Expression of genes that were previously repressed.
   d. All of the above are correct.
   e. None of the above is correct.

7. Which of the following describe facultative heterochromatin?

   a. Relatively inert genetically.
   b. Inactive in RNA synthesis.
   c. Contains DNA and histone protein.
   d. All of the above are correct.
   e. None of the above is correct.

8. Match the structures of the nucleolus with their molecular counterparts:

   _____ Nucleolus organizer
   _____ Chromosomal secondary constriction
   _____ Fibrillar area of nucleolus
   _____ Granular area of nucleolus
   _____ Nucleolar membrane

   a. Nonexistent
   b. Site genes for rRNA
   c. Kinetochore
   d. Site of synthesis 45S precursor
   e. Contains 40S and 60S ribosome subunits

Chapter 4

Epithelial Tissue

GENERAL

Epithelia are tissues that are composed primarily of cells that cover or line the surfaces, cavities, and organs of the body (sheetlike epithelia) or perform secretory functions (glandular epithelia). Epithelia may be specialized to perform the functions of protection, absorption, transport, or secretion.

CLASSIFICATION OF EPITHELIA

There are two basic types of epithelia:

- Sheetlike, or membranous (Table 4.1)
- Secretory, or glandular

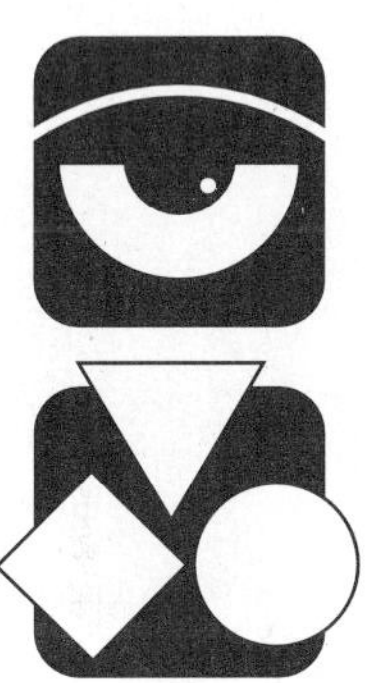

Membranous, or sheetlike, epithelia cover or line surfaces. Membranous epithelia may be simple or stratified (Fig. 4.1, Table 4.1).

Simple epithelia are composed of a single layer of cells and are classified on the basis of the shape of those cells.

- **Simple squamous epithelium** a single layer of flattened epithelial cells (e.g., endothelium, mesothelium)
- **Simple cuboidal epithelium** a single layer of cuboidal epithelial cells (e.g., lining of terminal bronchiole)
- **Simple columnar epithelium** a single layer of columnar epithelial cells (lining of gallbladder)
- **Pseudostratified columnar epithelium** a single layer of cells, some of which are tall columnar and others are short basal cells, all of which contact the basement membrane, giving to the epithelium a stratified appearance (e.g., lining of trachea)

Stratified epithelial are composed of more than one layer of cells and are named according to the shape of the surface cells.

- **Stratified squamous epithelium** Demonstrates squamous surface cells which may be
    - Dry (cornified, keratinized)—Cells are filled with keratin, and most cellular organelles are gone. Cell nuclei are not present in plaque-like remains of surface cell (e.g., epidermis).
    - Wet (noncornified, nonkeratinized)—Cells are filled with keratin. Cell nuclei are present in surface cells (e.g., lining of esophagus).
- **Stratified cuboidal epithelium** Surface cells are cuboidal.
- **Stratified columnar epithelium** Surface cells are columnar.
- **Transitional epithelium** Surface cells are large and accommodate stretch-

Classification of Sheetlike Epithelia

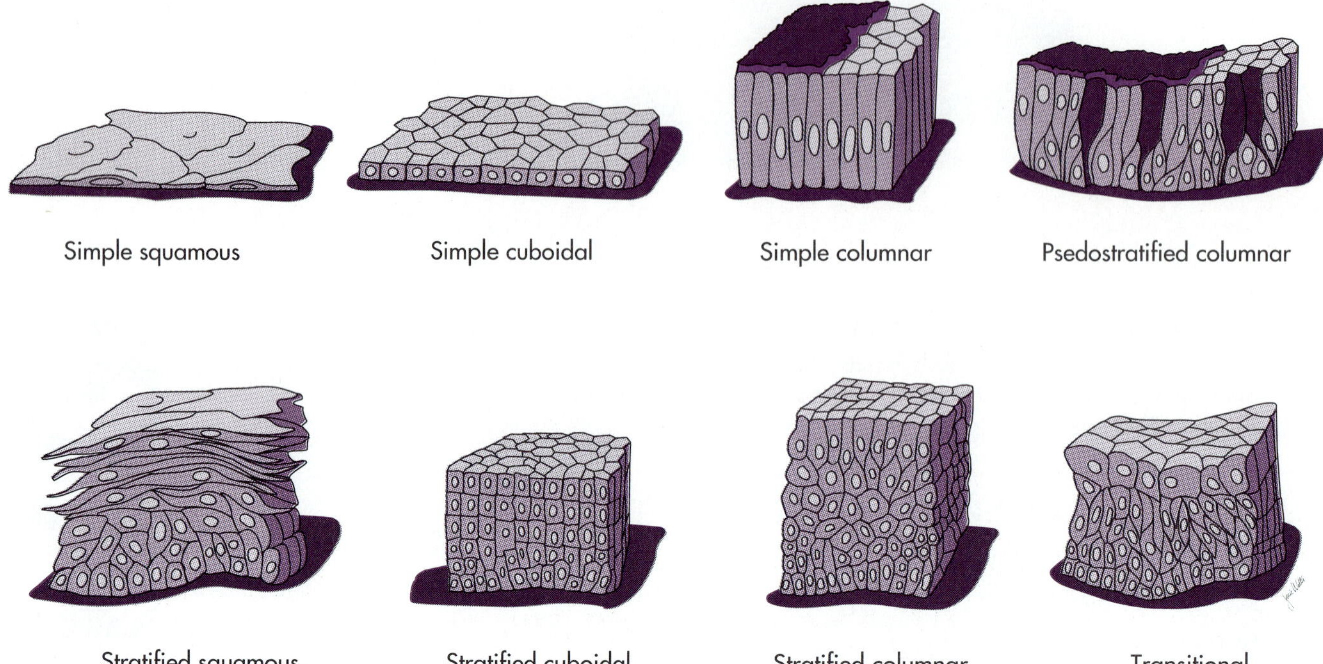

Fig. 4.1 Classification of sheetlike epithelia. Sheetlike epithelia are classified on the basis of the number of cell layers composing the epithelium and the morphology of the surface cells. *(Modified from Fawcett DW:* A textbook of histology, *Philadelphia, 1986, Saunders.)*

Table 4.1   *Classification of Sheetlike Epithelia*

| | NUMBER OF CELL LAYERS | | |
CELL SHAPE	SIMPLE	STRATIFIED	PSEUDOSTRATIFIED
Squamous	Simple squamous	Stratified squamous	
Cuboidal	Simple cuboidal	Stratified cuboidal	
Columnar	Simple columnar	Stratified columnar	Pseudostratified
		Transitional	columnar

ing or contracting of the organ by going from a flattened to a thickened state.

Glandular epithelia produce a secretory product. There are two types of glandular epithelia.

- Exocrine glands deliver their secretion externally (to a surface).
- Endocrine glands do not have ducts and deliver their secretion internally (into the bloodstream) and from there to other organs.

Exocrine glands with ducts are classified on the basis of branching of their ducts and the shape of the secretory unit (Fig. 4.2).

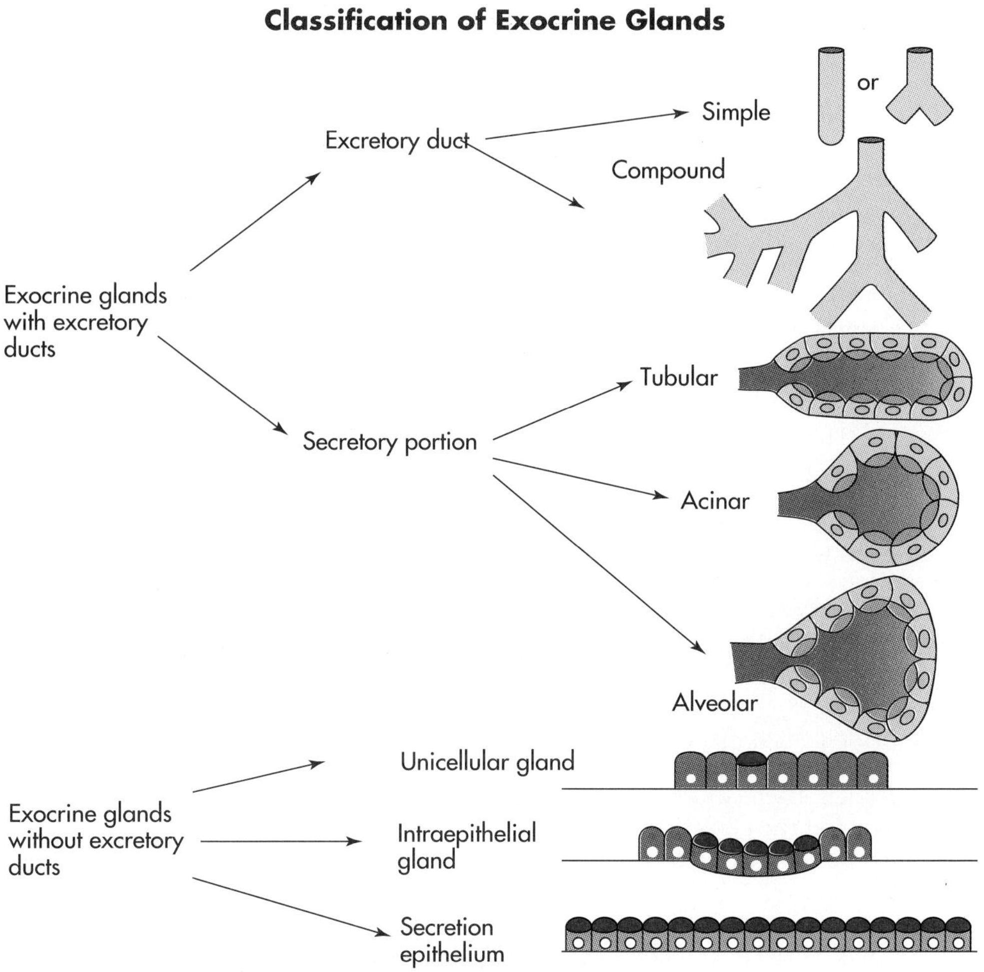

Classification of Exocrine Glands

Fig. 4.2 Classification of exocrine glands. Exocrine glands are classified on the basis of the duct system and the morphology of the secretory unit.

- Simple exocrine glands have unbranched ducts. Their secretory units can be tubular, acinar, or alveolar.
- Compound exocrine glands have a branched duct system. Their secretory units may be tubular, acinar, alveolar, or mixed.

There are other secretory cells of an exocrine type that are part of a sheetlike epithelium and deliver their secretion onto the surface without an intervening duct.

- Unicellular glands (e.g., goblet cells)
- Intraepithelial gland (e.g., urethral glands)
- Secretory epithelium (e.g., sheetlike epithelium lining the colon)

The cells in exocrine glands produce secretion in various ways.

- Holocrine secretion—The entire cell is the secretion (e.g., sebaceous gland).
- Apocrine secretion—The apical portion of the cell is the secretion (e.g., mammary gland epithelium).
- Merocrine secretion—The secretion (in secretory granules) is released from the cell by exocytosis (e.g., pancreatic exocrine cell).

SPECIALIZATION OF THE EPITHELIAL CELL SURFACE

■ **Special Configurations of Cell Membrane** Microvilli are fingerlike projections of the plasma membrane that cover the apical portion of the cell and project into the lumen.

- They measure 1.5 μm long and 0.1 μm thick.
- They form a "brush" or "striated" border with light microscopy.
- They are anchored in a microfilamentous terminal web, composed of keratin-like intermediate filaments.
- They function to increase the surface area for absorption.
- Each microvillus has a microfilamentous core.

Cilia are motile projections on the apical surface of the cell that contain microtubules.

- They measure 5 to 15 μm long and 0.2 μm thick.
- The body of cilium contains 9 doublet microtubules and 2 central single microtubules.
- The basal body of the cilium contains 9 triplet microtubules (no central).

Cilia of a cell or of a whole epithelium lash with an orderly beat in a constant direction. Each cilium moves the fluid surrounding it by lashing through it like an oar and then bending on the recovery stroke so as to offer less resistance. ATP provides the energy for ciliary beat. Isolated cilia show rhythmic beat. With the removal of ATP they become nonmotile. With replacement of ATP, they begin to beat.

Specialized attachment areas are frequently encountered in epithelial cells. They bind the individual cells into a mechanically and functionally coherent tissue.

- Occludens junctions (zonula, macula, and fascia)
- Adherens junctions (zonula, macula, and fascia)
- Nexus junctions

The **junctional complex** is generally found in columnar epithelia. It consists of several types of junctions arranged in a specific sequence acting together. Proceeding from the apical luminal side toward the basal end of the cell, we find the following:

- Zonula occludens
- Zonula adherens
- Macula adherens

EPITHELIAL CELL POPULATION KINETICS

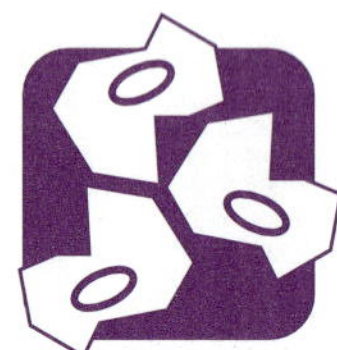

Like other differentiated cells, highly specialized epithelial cells are constantly undergoing loss because of cell death and replacement. A source of cells to replace the lost cells is provided in several different ways (Fig. 4.3). In simple epithelia consisting of relatively nonspecialized cells:

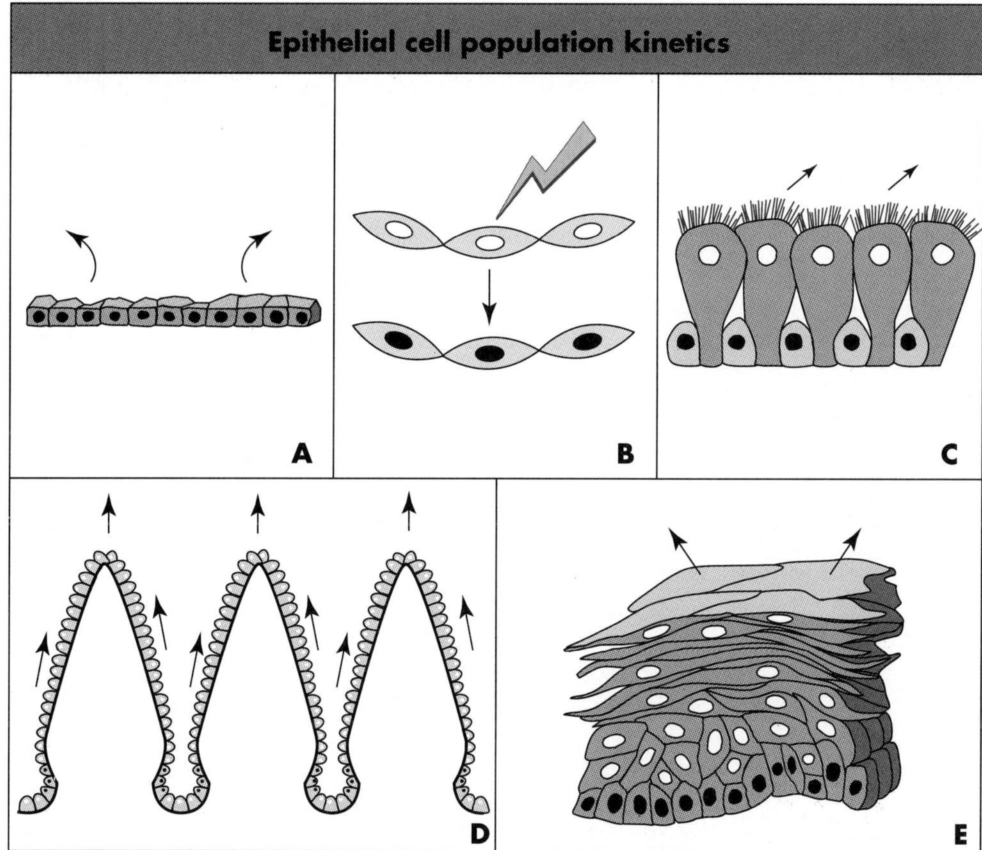

Fig. 4.3 Population kinetics of epithelial cells. Examples of the population kinetics of cells in simple (A-D) and stratified epithelia (E). Cells capable of synthesizing DNA are indicated by shading of the nucleus.

- Virtually all the cells may be of the continuous replicator type and are constantly replaced (e.g., cuboidal epithelium—bronchiole) (Fig. 4.3, *A*).
- Virtually all the cells may be of the occasional replicator type and are capable of replacing damaged cells (e.g., capillary endothelium) (Fig. 4.3, *B*). Under normal circumstances few cells are replicated, but in response to trauma or response to a specific signal the cells undergo replication and division.

In simple epithelia consisting of specialized cells the differentiated cells have lost the ability to divide and require a separate stem-cell population for replication and division. In pseudostratified epithelium the basal cells are of the continuous replicator type, and progeny are differentiated into glandular or ciliated cells (e.g., respiratory epithelium) (Fig. 4.3, *C*). Differentiated cells on the surface of an epithelium are continually sloughed. Cells in the necks of glands are of the continuous replicator type. They divide, and their progeny migrate to the surface where they replace the surface cells (e.g., intestinal epithelium) (Fig. 4.3, *D*).

In stratified epithelium, cells on the surface are continuously sloughed off (Fig. 4.3, *E*), cells in the basal layers are continuous replicators whose progeny may undergo the following:

- Both daughter cells differentiate and migrate to surface.
- Both daughter cells may remain in basal layers as continuous replicators.
- One daughter cell may remain in basal layer; the other migrates to surface.

In many such stratified epithelia the cells in layers immediately adjacent to the basal layers (intermediate layers) are good examples of DIM cells. In traumatic situations where the surface becomes denuded of epithelium occasional replicator cells in glands associated with epithelium may divide and differentiate to form epithelial cells.

EPITHELIAL CELL SPECIALIZATIONS

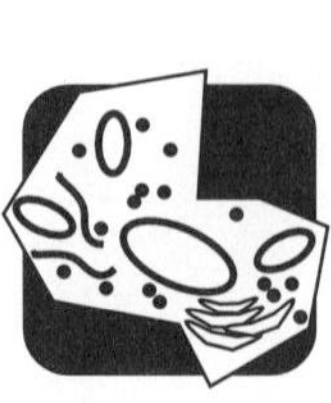

Epithelial cells demonstrate many modifications of their cellular organelles to enable them to carry out their cell-specific functions. Below are detailed some of the modifications that epithelial cells have that enable them to carry out some of these functions (Fig. 4.4).

- **Protection (e.g., Stratified Squamous Epithelium—Dry)** (Fig. 4.4, *A*)
  - Cell shape—flattened to provide maximal strength
  - Covered with macula adherens—adhesion
  - Cornified—loses cell organelles; packed with keratin; resists water loss

- **Absorption (e.g., Intestinal Epithelial Cell)** (Fig. 4.4, *B*)
  - Junctional complex maintains integrity of tissue.
  - Microvilli increase surface area for absorption.
  - Filamentous glycocalyx has a well-developed basal lamina and acts as a diffusion barrier.
  - Terminal web consists of supporting elements in apex of cell.
  - Polarization of cell.

- **Transport**
  - **Transport over cell surface (e.g., respiratory epithelium)** (Fig. 4.4, *C*)
    - Cilia beat to move material on surface
  - **Transport through cell (e.g., capillary endothelium)** (Fig. 4.4, *D*)
    - Cell shape thin and flattened for maximal surface area
    - Well-developed basal lamina acting as a diffusion barrier
    - Many pinocytotic vesicles that transport from one side of cell to other side. In some cases the cell may be fenestrated (i.e., contain holes that perforate the cell) (Fig. 4.4, *E*).

- **Secretion**
  - **Synthesis of protein (e.g., pancreatic exocrine cell)** (Fig. 4.4, *F*)
    - Well developed rough endoplasmic reticulum
    - Well developed Golgi apparatus
    - Many secretory granules in apical region of cell
  - **Synthesis of steroid hormones (e.g., granulosa lutein cell)** (Fig. 4.4, *G*)
    - Well developed smooth ER
    - Filled with lipid droplets

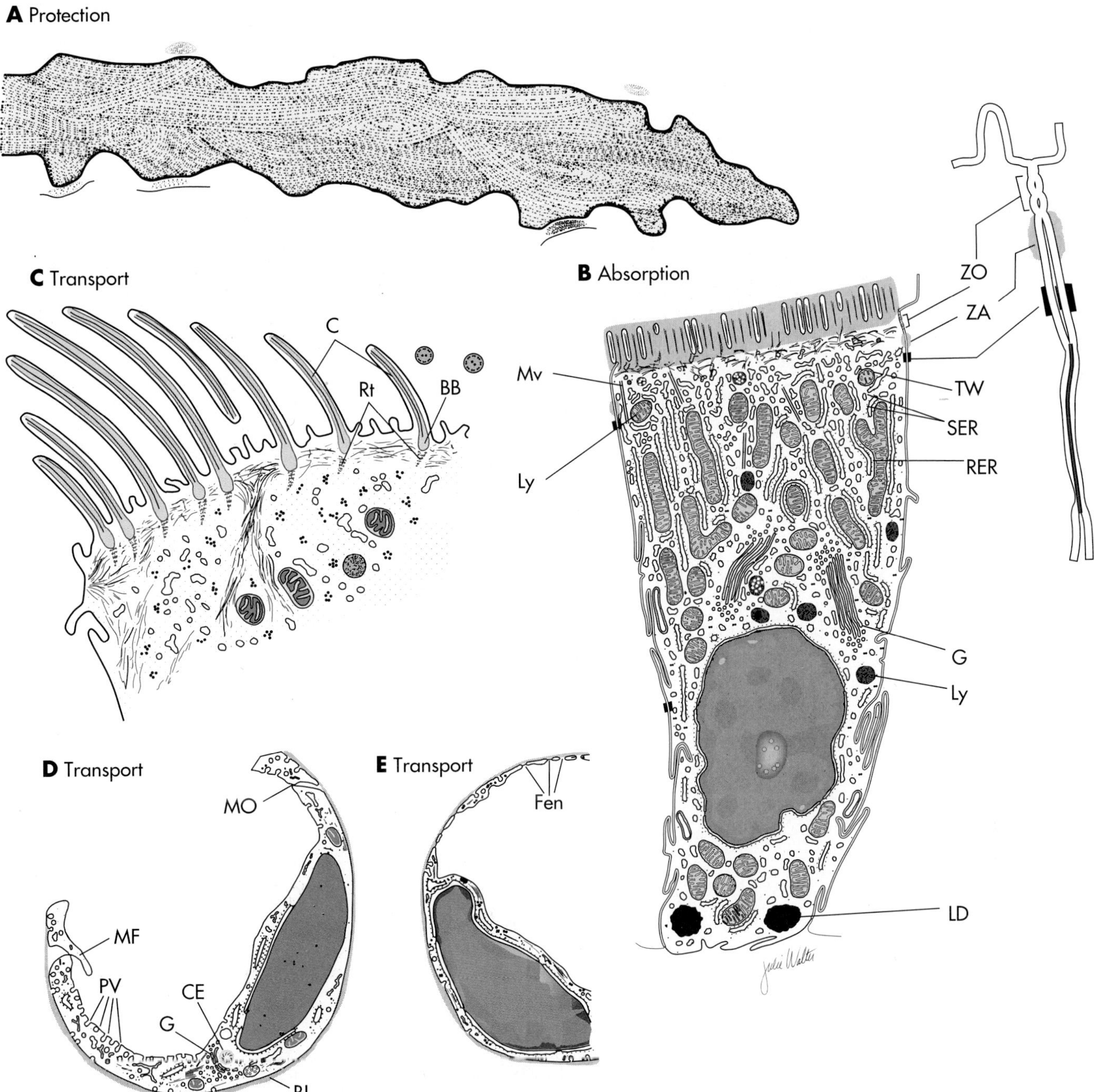

Examples of cellular specializations of epithelial cells. Cells illustrated demonstrate modifications of their cellular organelles, which enable them to carry out various cell functions. Protective function is illustrated by a cell from the stratum corneum of the epidermis; absorptive function by a simple columnar epithelial cell from the small intestine; transport over a surface by a ciliated simple columnar epithelial cell from the respiratory system; transport through a cell by a continuous capillary endothelial cell and a fenestrated capillary endothelial cell; secretion of a proteinaceous secretion by a pancreatic acinar cell and secretion of a steroid hormone by a lutein cell from the ovary. *BB,* Basal body; *BL,* basal lamina; *CE,* centriole; *C,* cilia; *CV,* condensing vacuole; *fen,* fenestra; *G,* Golgi body (or apparatus); *LD,* lipid droplet; *Ly,* lysosome; *M,* mitochondria; *MA,* macula adherens; *MO,* macula occludens; *Mv,* microvilli; *Pv,* pinocytotic vesicles; *RER,* rough endoplasmic reticulum; *Rt,* rootlet; *SER,* smooth endoplasmic reticulum; *Tw,* terminal web; *ZA,* Zonula adherens; *ZG,* zymogen granule; *ZO,* zonula occludens. *(Modified from Lentz T: Cell fine structure, Philadelphia, 1971, Saunders.)*   *Continued.*

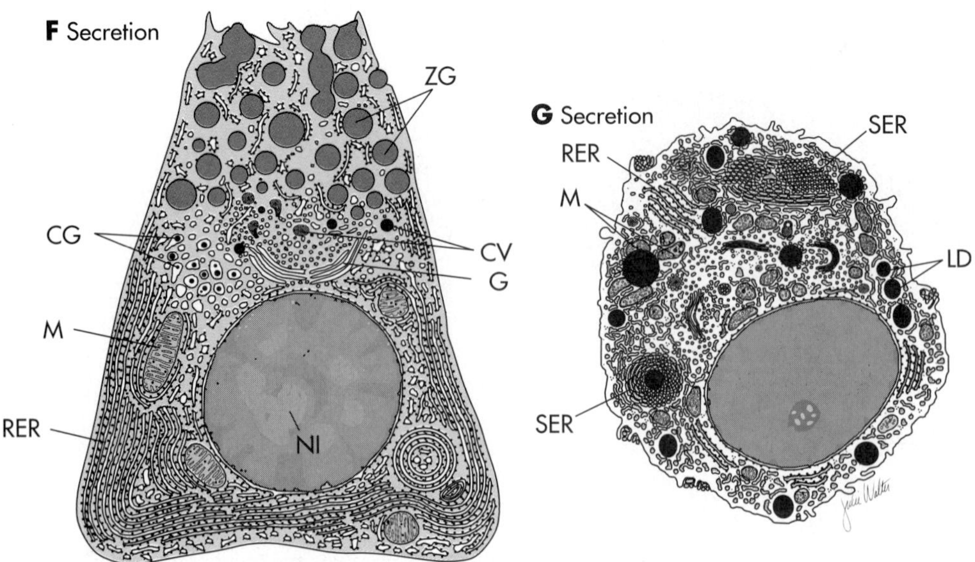

Fig. 4.4, cont'd. For legend see p. 51.

MULTIPLE CHOICE REVIEW QUESTIONS

1. Which of the following statements best describes the ultrastructural organization of the basal bodies of cilia and flagella?

    a. Composed of 7 doublet and 2 centrally located microtubules
    b. Composed of 9 doublet and 2 centrally located microtubules
    c. Composed of 9 triplet microtubules
    d. Composed of 9 doublet microtubules
    e. Composed of 9 doublet and 2 centrally located microtubules

2. Which cellular organelles would you expect to find in excessive amounts in a cell that is specialized to synthesize steroid hormone?

    a. RER
    b. SER
    c. Nucleus
    d. All of the above are correct.
    e. None of the above is correct.

3. In a typical stratified epithelium, where are most of the cells located that provide for renewal and replacement of the cells lost because of attrition or cell death?

    a. On the surface
    b. In the basal layer
    c. In the intermediate layers
    d. In all of the above
    e. In none of the above

4. Match the epithelial specialization with function:

    _____ Keratin
    _____ Well developed SER
    _____ Well developed Golgi apparatus
    _____ Nexus
    _____ Microvilli

    a. Absorption
    b. Direct intercellular communication
    c. Protection
    d. Detoxification of toxins
    e. Secretion protein

5. Match the epithelial cell with its type of cell life:

    _____ Basal cell in stratified squamous epithelium
    _____ Surface cell in stratified squamous epithelium
    _____ Capillary endothelial cell
    _____ Basal cell pseudostratified columnar epithelium
    _____ Epithelial cells at apex of intestinal villus

    a. Vegetative intermitotic cell
    b. Differentiating intermitotic cell
    c. Reverting postmitotic cell
    d. Fixed postmitotic cell

Chapter 5

Connective Tissue

GENERAL

Connective tissues are populations of cells and their products that hold other tissues together. They may be specialized to function in support, transport, storage, or protection.

Organs are composed of **parenchyma** and **stroma**. The parenchyma is the cellular population of an organ that performs the major function of that organ. (e.g., the epithelial cells in the salivary gland are the parenchyma; they secrete saliva. In skeletal muscles, the muscle cells represent the parenchyma; they contract.) The stroma is the connective tissue that supports and nourishes the parenchyma (e.g., the epimysium, perimysium, and endomysium are composed of connective tissue that surrounds the muscle cells in a muscle).

Since every organ is composed of parenchyma and stroma, connective tissue is distributed throughout all organs and systems of the body, playing important roles in the support, nutrition, and protection of these organs. It conveys materials to the various parenchyma blood vessels and nerves.

Connective tissue contains two basic elements:

- **Cells**
- **Intercellular matrix,** which is composed of ground substance (also called the amorphous ground substance) and fibers

THE CELLS OF CONNECTIVE TISSUE

■ Permanent Residents (Fig. 5.1)

- **Fibroblasts** Fibroblasts are responsible for the synthesis of connective tissue fibers as well as the proteoglycans and glycoproteins of the ground substance. Some workers distinguish fibroblasts from fibrocytes.

  - Fibroblasts are more immature cells that actively synthesize fibers.
  - Fibrocytes are more mature cells that have ceased fiber synthesis as in tendons.

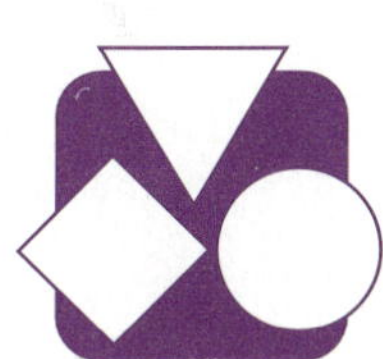

- **Adipose cells** Adipose cells store lipid triglycerides in the cytoplasm.

  - Unilocular adipose cells have only one large fat vacuole and are the most common form in adults.
  - Multilocular adipose cells have a large number of lipid droplets and are found in embryos and newborn humans.

- **Mast cells** Mast cells are filled with membrane-bound granules containing

  - heparin, an anticlotting factor
  - histamine, which increases vascular permeability
  - eosinophil chemotactic factor of anaphylaxis (ECFA)

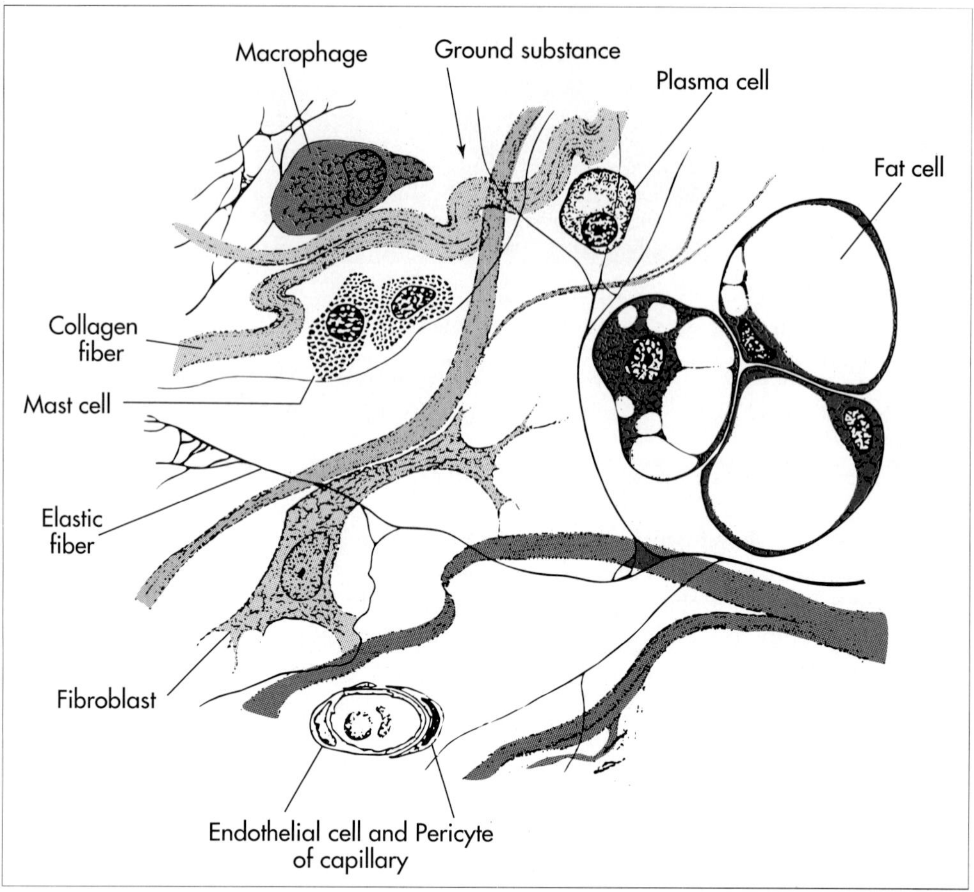

Fig. 5.1 The cells and fibers of loose connective tissue as seen in the light microscope. The microscopically identifiable components lie in the ground substance where they are continuously bathed by tissue fluid. *(Modified from Cormack DH:* Ham's histology, *Philadelphia, 1987, Lippincott.)*

Mast cells produce but do not store leukotrienes (slow-reacting substance of anaphylaxis, SRS-A). Mast cells contain receptors for IgE (The second exposure to an antigen causes degranulation and release of heparin, histamine, leukotrienes, and ECFA, leading to immediate hypersensitivity—anaphylaxis). Some workers believe that mast cells are precursor to the tissue basophil or *vice versa* (both contain ECFA and leukotrienes).

● **Macrophages** Macrophages are resident phagocytes of connective tissue. These cells were originally derived from blood monocytes.

● **Plasma cells** Plasma cells are an important part of the immunological defense system. They produce humoral antibodies. They arise from the B lymphocytes in circulating blood to become residents of the connective tissue.

● **Uncommitted mesenchymal cells** Uncommitted mesenchymal cells give rise to other cells of connective tissue. It is commonly believed that the pericyte performs this function. The pericyte is a flattened cell that lies adjacent to the capillary endothelial cell and is enclosed within its basal lamina.

■ **Migratory Residents** Other cells are **migratory residents,** which may increase under various conditions.

- Inflammation results in an increase in the number of leukocytes from peripheral blood.
- Neutrophils increase in acute infection.
- Monocytes and lymphocytes accumulate during chronic infections.
- Eosinophils are found at the site of allergic reactions.
- Both T and B lynphocytes accumulate during infection.

THE GROUND SUBSTANCE

The **ground substance** is the optically homogeneous material filling the space between cells and fibers. It is composed of proteoglycans and tissue fluid.

Proteoglycans are complex molecules consisting of a core protein to which hundreds of glycosaminoglycans side groups are attached. Glycosaminoglycans (GAGs) are unbranched polysaccharides made up of repeating disaccharide units. There are several main groups of GAGs.

- Hyaluronic acid (HA)
- Chondroitin sulfates
- Dermatan sulfate
- Heparan sulfate
- Keratan sulfates

Proteoglycans are an extremely diverse group of proteins whose functions are mediated by their core proteins and GAG chains. The common proteoglycans of the ground substance would include decorin in connective tissue, aggrecan in cartilage, and perlecan in the basal lamina.

Hyaluronic acid is a polysaccharide composed of a repeating disaccharide unit. (Glucuronic acid linked to *N*-acetylglucosamine). Hyaluronic acid is a GAG, but it is not attached to a core protein. Therefore it is not a proteoglycan. It is synthesized enzymatically by enzyme complexes embedded in the plasma membrane of the fibroblast. Its MW is 10^6 daltons; it measures up to 2.5 μm long and is coiled in the living state. Hyaluronate molecules interact with one another and with proteoglycans to provide a barrier to the movement of large molecules and bacteria in the connective tissue. This was demonstrated in a classic experiment.

- Bacteria injected into the hypodermal connective tissue remain localized at the injection site.
- If the enzyme hyaluronidase is injected with the bacteria, the bacteria spread throughout the connective tissue.
- Some bacteria produce their own hyaluronidase (spreading factor).
- Many tumor cells produce hyaluronidase enabling them to invade tissues.

Except for hyaluronic acid, the other GAGs are covalently attached to protein forming proteoglycans. The core protein is produced on the RER and the polysaccharide chains are added in the endoplasmic reticulum and Golgi by adding one sugar at a time using specific glycosyltransferases. The GAGs are further modified in the Golgi. In this way, up to hundreds of subunits are attached like the bristles on a test-tube brush to a backbone of core protein.

Proteoglycans associate to form aggregates in the extracellular space (Fig. 5.2). In the ground substance individual proteoglycan complexes of GAGs-core protein are bound to long hyaluronic acid molecules by linker proteins. Such an aggregate, which contains approximately 100 proteoglycan side groups attached to a single hyaluronic acid molecule, may attain a molecular weight of 10^8 daltons, occupying a volume equivalent to that

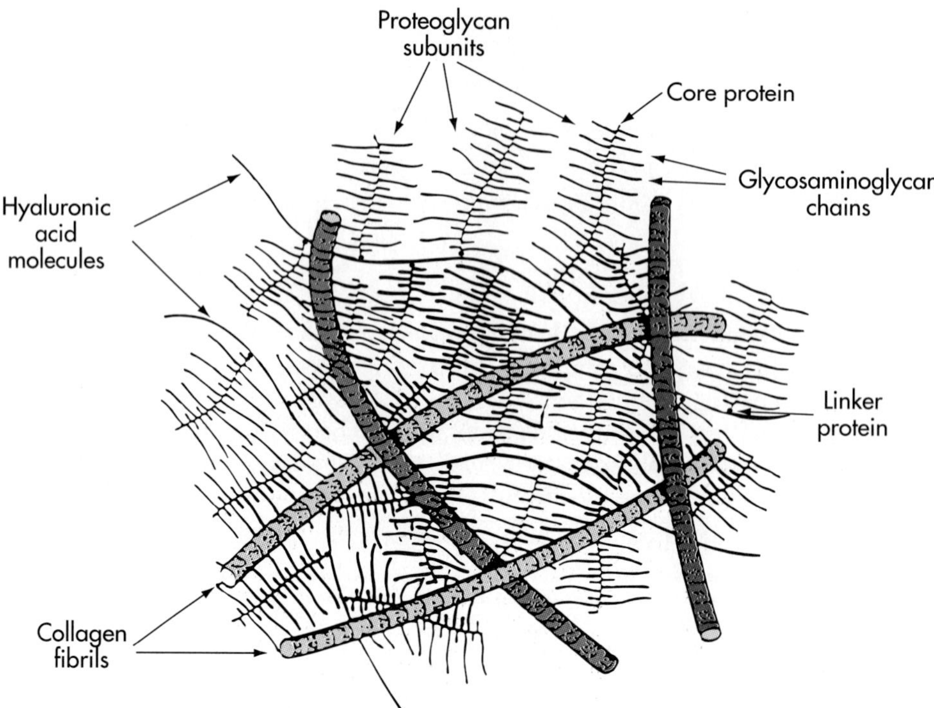

Fig. 5.2 Scheme of the organization of the extracellular matrix of cartilage. It is composed of collagen fibrils with intertwining proteoglycan conjugates. The extracellular matrix of connective tissues in general is believed to have a similar organization. *(Modified from Fawcett DW:* A textbook of histology, *Philadelphia, 1986, Saunders.)*

of a bacterium. The proteoglycan aggregate is made up of proteoglycan monomers.

- Proteoglycan monomer = GAG + Core protein
- Proteoglycan aggregate = Proteoglycan monomers + HA

Proteoglycans impart to the ground substance the staining property, metachromasia. The intercellular ground substance when stained with the basic dye toluidine blue exhibits metachromasia. When the dye is bound to randomly distributed negative groups, as it is in staining protein, the structure stains blue (orthochromasia). When bound to regularly repeating closely spaced negative groups, as it is in staining a nucleic acid or a GAG, the dye molecules stack, and there is a color shift to long wavelengths (red) (metachromasia). Removal of GAGs from connective tissue causes loss of metachromasia.

The functions of proteoglycans in connective tissue are

- to act as a supporting matrix for cells and fibers
- to attract and hold tissue fluid
- to permit diffusion of small molecules in solution
- to obstruct the movement of large molecules

The proteoglycans of connective tissue are turned over (i.e., they are constantly synthesized and degraded). Their breakdown is dependent on specific lysosomal enzymes in macrophages. The core protein is synthesized by the fibroblast on RER where the GAG side units are added. They are further processed and secreted by the Golgi apparatus. Some proteoglycans are not secreted into the matrix but remain associated with the plasma membrane with the core protein acting as an intrinsic membrane protein. Among these proteoglycans are the syndecans. Syndecans, found on the surface of fibroblasts and other cells, serve as receptors for collagen to which the cell binds.

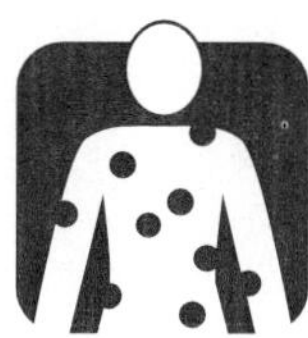

The breakdown of the proteoglycans is dependent on lysosomal enzymes. There are diseases in which there is a deficiency of a given lysosomal enzyme and concomitant accumulation of proteoglycans in connective tissue and brain (e.g., Gaucher's disease and lack of glucosidase). Breakdown of some of the proteins of the ground substance is accomplished by extracellular proteases secreted by cells.

Fibronectins are structural glycoproteins of connective tissue. They are protein dimers, with each subunit having a molecular weight 250kDa. Fibronectins are produced by fibroblasts as well as by other cell types in the body. The protein has specific domains that bind to

- cells
- collagen
- fibrin (involved in blood clotting)
- heparin

By attaching cell to collagen, fibronectin acts as an anchor for the cell. There are intrinsic membrane proteins that bind actin on their cytoplasmic side through talin and vinculin, and fibronectin on their external surface thereby increasing the cell's rigidity. Intrinsic membrane proteins of this type are called *integrins.* Similar attachments occur with fibrin and the intrinsic proteins in the membrane of platelets.

Fibronectin is also important in the processes of cell movement or migration lining the routes that cells travel during development.

Laminin is another structural glycoprotein of the connective tissue. It is found in the basal lamina and is partially responsible for adhesion of epithelial cells to the basal lamina.

FORMATION OF TISSUE FLUID

In addition to proteoglycans the ground substance contains soluble proteins. Some of these are synthesized by fibroblasts and others by connective tissue cells. Some of these proteins are derived from blood plasma. The fluid part of the ground substance is tissue fluid. Tissue fluid is derived from blood. (The formation and resorption of tissue fluid is discussed later in more detail with blood). Blood contains cells and a liquid part called plasma. The blood plasma consists of fluid, macromolecules, dissolved small molecules, and gases.

As blood passes through the terminal portions of the vascular system, the thin-walled capillaries, hydrostatic pressure forces the fluid part of plasma, dissolved gases, and small ions out at the arterial end of the capillaries. Cells and large molecules are retained in the capillary lumen. The fluid thus formed is called *tissue fluid.*

■ Functions of Tissue Fluid

- It provides for circulation of metabolites and breakdown products of metabolism.
- It provides a diffusion medium in intercellular space.

The fluid and some of its contents are resorbed at the venous end of the capillary and by lymphatics, providing for a constant turnover of tissue fluid. Resorption at the venous end of the capillary is accounted for by the osmotic draw of fluid and dissolved solutes back into the capillary, and such a process results in

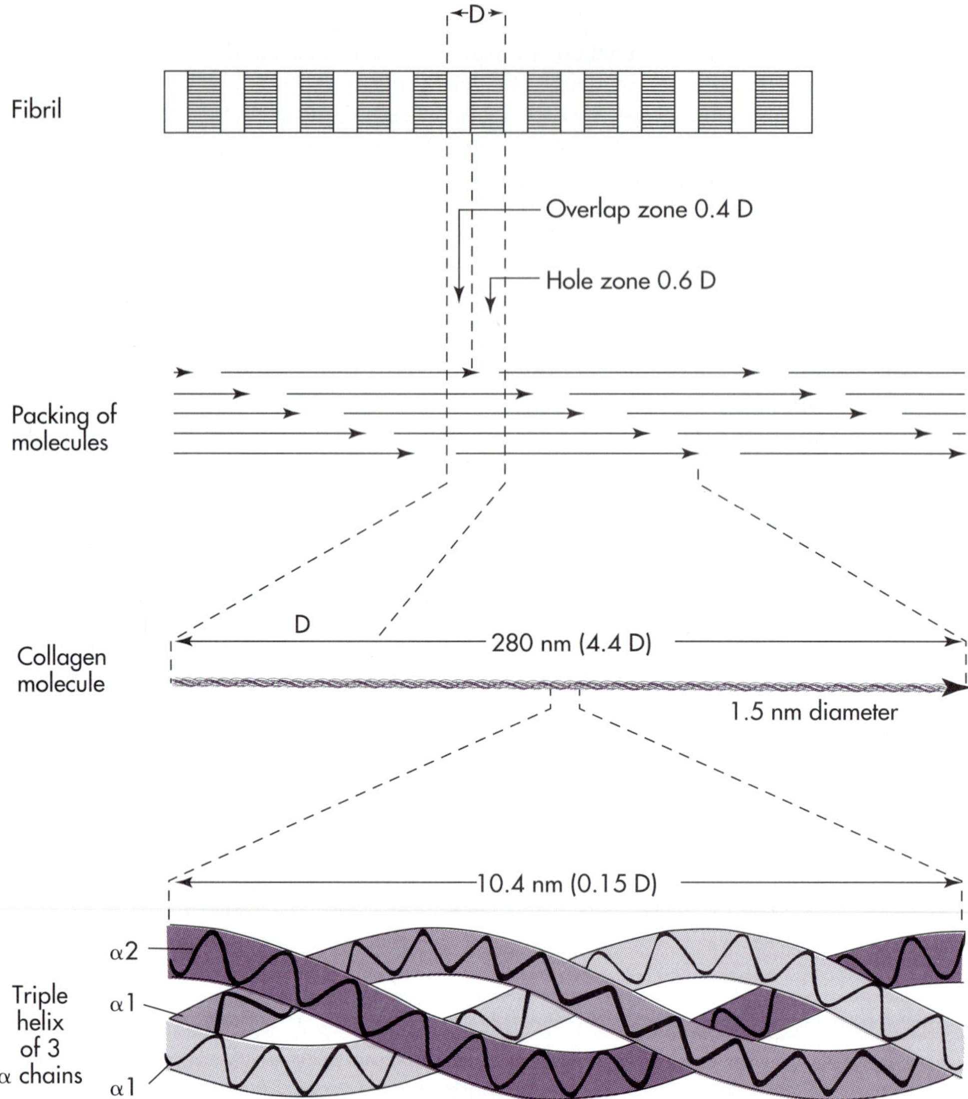

Fig. 5.3 Organization of tropocollagen in the collagen microfibril. A collagen fibril displays a characteristic periodicity (*D*) of 64 nm. It is made of tropocollagen molecules organized in a quarter 1-staggered array. The tropocollagen molecule is three polypeptide chains (alpha chains) organized in a triple helix. *(Modified from Ross RB, Reith EJ:* Histology: a text and atlas, *New York, 1985, Harper & Row.)*

the increased concentration of protein in the plasma because of the loss of fluid at the arterial end of the capillary.

THE FIBERS OF CONNECTIVE TISSUE

The connective tissue contains three morphologically distinguishable types of fibers.

- **Collagen Fibers** Collagen fibers measure 1 to 12 µm in thickness. They are inelastic and flexible and have high tensile strength (Fig. 5.3). They are composed of microfibrils visible in the electron microscope (20 to 100 nm thick). A constant feature of the collagen microfibril is a repeating dark and light unit. This dark and light unit repeats itself each 64 nm (64 nm periodicity). This periodicity is an expression of subunit structure of collagen. If collagen is treated with alkali, the collagen microfibril is disrupted to yield tropocollagen. (The following description is generalized for fibrous collagen.)

Tropocollagen (300 kDa) (280 nm long) is a long, rigid molecule. Each tropocollagen molecule is composed of three polypeptide chains (alpha chains) helically coiled about one another (MW, = 100 KDa). The amino acid composition of tropocollagen is unusual: 30% glycine, 25% **proline** and **hydroxyproline.** Each tropocollagen molecule has a head region and a tail region. If tropocollagen is allowed to aggregate into fibers under manipulated conditions, it can form

- "segment long-spacing (SLS) collagen," which are tactoids having about a 240 nm periodicity (approximately the same length as a collagen molecule)
- "fibrous long-spacing (FLS) collagen," with a 240 nm periodicity
- reaggregated fibers with a 64 nm periodicity (native collagen)

The data indicate that native collagen consists of tropocollagen molecules organized so that the ends are polarized and the molecules overlap in a quarter-staggered array.

The periodicity of the fiber is accounted for by the fact that the tropocollagen molecules are staggered in such a way that the gaps between ends of the tropocollagen molecules in the fiber always fall in a dark segment whereas the light segments have no gaps.

- ● **Collagen formation in vivo** Polypeptide chains (pro–alpha chains) are synthesized on fibroblast RER (proline and lysine are hydroxylated in RER and the hydroxyl groups of these molecules form intramolecular hydrogen bonds) → (addition of carbohydrate in RER) → (3 stranded procollagen formed by formation disulfide bonds in RER) → (SER → Golgi → secretion vesicle → on the surface of the cell procollagen peptidases remove peptides from the amino and carboxyl end of procollagen) to form tropocollagen.

  Tropocollagen aggregates to form collagen fibers extracellularly. The formation of the collagen fibers appears to be a self-directed self-assembly. Subsequently the fibers are stabilized by lysyl oxidase, which cross-links lysine in adjacent tropocollagen molecules. Lysyl oxidases deaminate hydroxylysine and lysine moieties to form highly reactive aldehyde groups, which spontaneously form covalent bonds within and between tropocollagen molecules.

  There is little turnover of collagen in adult tissue. In adult bone, for example, collagen molecules persist for years. As collagen ages, it increases cross-linking and as a result becomes more insoluble in an aqueous solution. About 25 distinct collagen alpha chains have been identified, each encoded by a separate gene and demonstrating variations in amino acid sequence. Different gene combinations are expressed in different tissues. Although in principle more than 10,000 types of triple-stranded molecules could be assembled from the 25 alpha chains, only about 20 have been identified so far. Different combinations of alpha chains in the triple helix are responsible for the different types of collagen (I, II, III, etc.). The description above is general for fibrous collagen.

  More than 20 biochemically different types of collagen have been described up to now. Each differs in the combination of alpha chains in the triple helix. The important ones are

  - Type I collagen (found in dermis, bone, tendon, fascias, fibrocartilage) has low-level interaction with dermatan sulfate.
  - Type II collagen (found in hyaline and elastic cartilage) interacts with chondroitin sulfates.

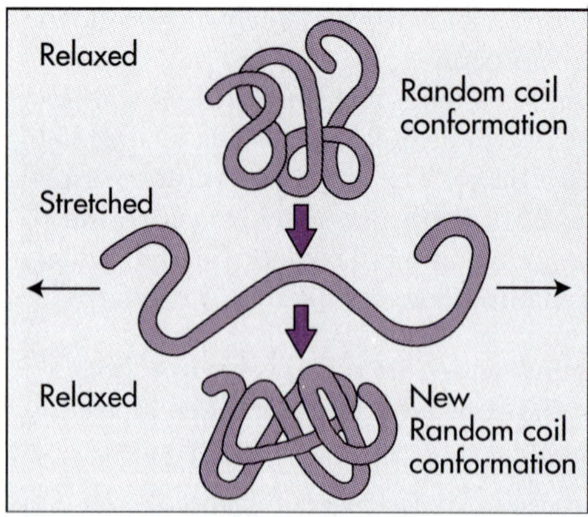

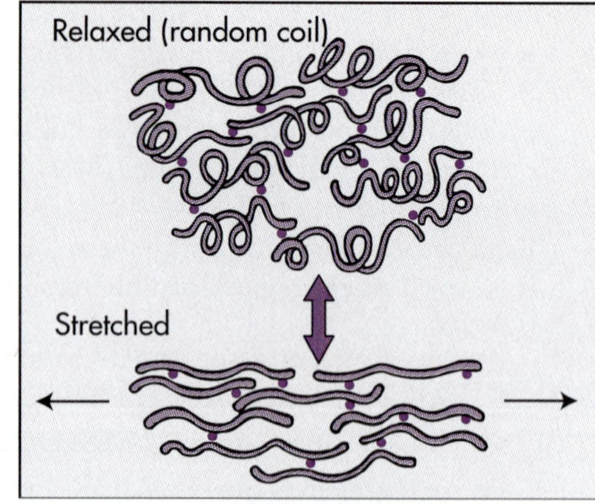

Fig. 5.4 Stretching and recoiling of elastin. Tropoelastin has a random coiled structure in the relaxed state that can stretch but reforms as a different random coil on relaxation. Tropoelastin molecules are covalently linked into elastin in elastic fibers, which can reversibly stretch and recoil. (*Modified from Stevens A, Lowe. JS:* Histology, *Brookfield, Vt., 1992, Gower Medical {London}.*)

- Type III collagen (found in reticular fibers associated with the endoneurium, liver, spleen, kidney, lung) interacts with heparan sulfate.
- Type IV collagen (found in basal lamina) interacts with heparan sulfate.

■ **Reticular Fibers** Reticular fibers are very fine collagenous fibers that have the following characteristics:

- They are high in proline and hydroxyproline (like collagen).
- They have a 64 nm periodicity (like collagen).
- They stain with periodic acid–Schiff and silver stains (unlike most collagen fibers).
- Reticular fibers are believed to be a variant of collagen (type III), which has more carbohydrate residues.

■ **Elastic Fibers** Elastic fibers can be readily deformed or stretched by a small force and reversibly recover their original dimensions after considerable deformation or stretching. There are two components of elastic fibers.

- A microfibrilar component that measures 11 nm in diameter. The microfibrils demonstrate no periodicity. They contain little hydroxyproline (unlike collagen).
- An amorphous component (elastin)

Unlike collagen, elastin contains little proline and no hydroxyproline. Elastin contains about 60% nonpolar hydrophobic amino acids, and so it is relatively insoluble (Fig. 5.4). Elastin is made up of tropoelastin subunits. Tropoelastin is composed of 5.5% lysine (a basic amino acid). Unlike other proteins, which adopt a unique stable structure, tropoelastin exhibits random coiling. Cross-linking of lysine in adjacent tropoelastin molecules through lysyl oxidase activity forms elastin. In addition to such cross-linking, very elaborate cross-links involving 4 lysine molecules occur. (The complex amino acid is called *desmosine.*) It is this aggregate's ability to expand and contract as a highly cross-linked random coil that accounts for the fiber's elasticity.

● **Formation of elastic fibers** The first elements to appear during embryogenesis are microfibrils (which do not contain elastin). (The fibers are called

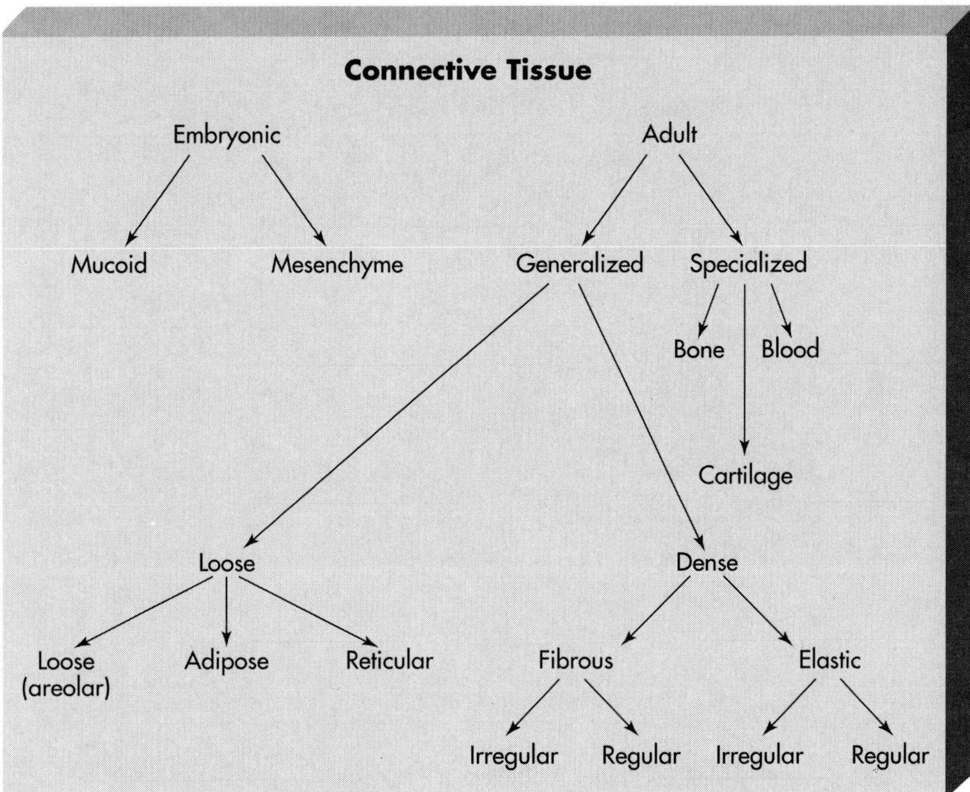

Fig. 5.5 Classification of connective tissue. All connective tissues are composed of cells, fibers, and ground substance and are classified on the basis of the organization of these components.

oxytalan.) Microfibrils first appear on the cell's surface. Microfibrils are not a precursor of elastin. They act as a mold for shaping amorphous elastin into a fibrous configuration.

As development proceeds, the elastin begins to appear (forming elaunin). Adult elastic fibers are predominantly elastin. Tropoelastin is synthesized on RER $\rightarrow$ Golgi $\rightarrow$ intercellular matrix. In the intercellular matrix the tropoelastin is converted to elastic fibers by the cross-linking of lysine to form desmosine. Microfibrils shape amorphous elastin into a fibrous configuration.

Although composed of cells, fibers, and ground substance, connective tissue is further specialized to form several functionally and morphologically different types. They accomplish this by altering the types and relative amounts of cells, fibers, and ground substance components (Fig. 5.5).

■ **Basement Membrane** The basement membrane lies at the interface between epithelium and connective tissue. The basement membrane is rich in carbohydrate (PAS positive). Proteins include a type of collagen (type IV) and a peculiar glycoprotein *laminin* (which is important in adhesion) as well as a large heparan sulfate–containing proteoglycan called perlecan. Type IV collagen does not form fibers but associates by their tropocollagen molecules forming head-to-head dimers at their carboxyl end and an extended latticework with side-by-side and amino-terminal associations. Three major structural elements are associated with basement membranes:

- The cell coat (lamina lucida)

Table 5.1	*Special Terms Describing Epithelia and Connective Tissues*

			SITE	EPITHELIUM	SUBJACENT CONNECTIVE TISSUE	EPITHELIUM AND CONNECTIVE TISSUE
B O D Y			Covering exterior surface of body	Epidermis	+ Dermis	= Skin
	Open to exterior		Alimentary Urinary Respiratory	Epithelium (may or may not have glands)	+ Lamina propria	= Mucosa
C A V I T I E S	Closed cavity		Coelomic cavity (peritoneal, pericardial, and pleural)	Mesothelium (no glands)	+ Submesothelium	= Serosa
			Cardiovascular cavity	Endothelium	+ Subendothelium	= Intima (vessels) Endocardium (heart)

    • Basal lamina (0.1 µm thick, adjacent to epithelium) (basement membrane proper) (lamina densa). Some fibers (3 to 4 nm thick) of type IV collagen. This layer is believed to be produced by the epithelium.

    • Lamina reticularis, rich in collagen and reticular fibers embedded in the ground substance. This layer is believed to be a product of underlying connective tissue.

The basement membrane plays an important role in determining what enters and leaves connective tissue. It is a barrier to the transport of large molecules. The basement membrane separates connective tissue from the epithelial cell environment. It provides elastic support and determines cell polarity and may induce differentiation. The basal lamina is found in cells other than epithelial cells. It is synthesized, for example, by muscle cells, adipose cells, and Schwann cells.

● **Composition of the basal lamina**
    • Type IV collagen
    • Perlecan-containing heparan sulfate GAGs
    • Laminin—a cross-shaped glycoprotein that binds to type IV collagen

Table 5.1 describes special terms for describing epithelium and its subjacent connective tissue.

FUNCTIONS OF CONNECTIVE TISSUE

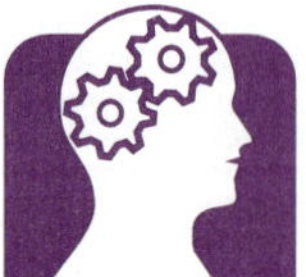

Connective tissue supports and binds together the structures of the body (largely a function of fibers). It transports metabolites to cells and waste products to the vascular system. (This is largely a function of the ground substance and tissue fluid.) Connective tissue is responsible for the storage of lipid in fat cells, water, and electrolytes in ground substance.

Connective tissue also provides protection. The ground substance is a barrier to the spread of microorganisms. The mast cells release histamine (inflammation) and increase vascular permeability. The leukocytes emigrate from blood to engulf bacteria. The macrophages ingest dead cells, bacteria, and debris. Connective tissue provides for repair. Fibroblasts multiply and begin to synthesize matrix.

MALFUNCTIONS
OF CONNECTIVE TISSUE

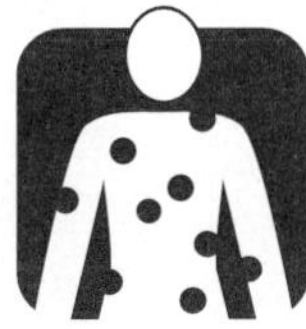

Lathyrism is a disease resulting from inhibition of the enzyme that cross-links lysine (lysyl oxidase). This may result from severe Cu^{++} deficiency required for enzyme activity or be caused by treatment with the drug β-aminopropionitrile. The disease causes a deficiency particularly in collagen in bone and elastin in blood vessels. Lathyrism may result in rupture of the aorta. There may be a buildup of tropoelastin and a decrease in elastin. The tropoelastin is not converted to elastin (because of decreased activity in the cross-linking enzyme lysyl oxidase).

Scurvy is a disease of connective tissue (particularly bone) that is caused by a deficiency in Vitamin C. Collagen metabolism is severely impaired. Fibroblasts revert to an immature state and collagen synthesis decreases. The conversion of proline to hydroxyproline ceases. Collagen is not formed.

Ehlers-Danlos syndrome demonstrates the absence of N-terminal peptidase. (Procollagen is not converted to tropocollagen, resulting in increased articular mobility.)

Marfan's syndrome is caused by a mutation in the gene coding for the microfibrillar component of elastic fibers. In severely affected individuals, the aortic wall is prone to rupture.

MULTIPLE CHOICE
REVIEW QUESTIONS

1. Match the connective tissue cell with its characteristic:

   _____ Plasma cell
   _____ Mast cell
   _____ Fibroblast
   _____ Adipose cell
   _____ Macrophage

   a. Phagocytosis
   b. Store lipid
   c. Synthesize heparin
   d. Synthesize tropocollagen
   e. Synthesize antibody

2. Arrange in proper sequence for collagen formation:

   _____ Proline hydroxylated
   _____ Procollagen
   __a__ Pro–alpha chain synthesized
   _____ Collagen fiber
   _____ Tropocollagen

3. A specific agent is known to interfere with the cross-linking of tropoelastin to form elastin but not with the synthesis of tropoelastin. What would you expect to be the effect of long-term treatment (2 months) with the drug?

   a. Increase elasticity of the tissue
   b. Increase in the amount of elastin in connective tissue
   c. Increase in the amount of tropoelastin in connective tissue
   d. Decrease in the amount of tropoelastin in connective tissue
   e. None of the above

4. Place A beside those things that increase,
   B beside those things that decrease,
   C beside those things that remain the same:

   _____ The relative number of monocytes in chronic infection
   _____ Collagen synthesis during vitamin C deficiency
   _____ Amount of cross-linking of collagen fibers during aging
   _____ Effect of hyaluronidase on movement of large molecules in connective tissue.
   _____ The relative number of neutrophils in acute infections

5. Which of the following statements is correct?

   a. Tropocollagen measures 280 nm in length.
   b. Tropocollagen is 64 nm long.
   c. Tropocollagen shows a 64 nm periodicity.
   d. Tropocollagen lacks proline and hydroxyproline.
   e. None of the above is correct.

Chapter 6

Nervous Tissue

GENERAL

Nervous tissue comprises a population of neurons and associated supporting cells, which is specialized to receive stimuli (irritability) and transmit impulses (conductibility). The nervous system is organized into three major components.

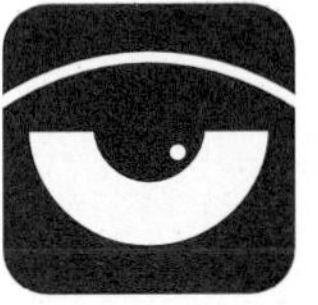

1. The **central nervous system (CNS),** which is composed of

    - the brain
    - the spinal cord

The major components of the CNS are segregated into gray and white matter. The gray matter consists of the cell bodies of neurons, neuron processes, and supporting (glial) cells. The white matter does not contain any cell bodies of neurons. It contains glial cells and a large number of neuron processes, most of which are covered with myelin.

2. The **autonomic nervous system (ANS),** which is composed of

    - autonomic ganglia (which contains the cell bodies of neurons)
    - autonomic nerves
    - autonomic endings

3. The **peripheral nervous system (PNS),** which is made up of

    - peripheral ganglia (which contain the cell bodies of neurons)
    - peripheral nerves
    - nerve endings

THE NEURON

The **neuron** is the fundamental unit and the **basic genetic unit** of the nervous system. Neurons arise embryologically from specialized neuroepithelial cells (in neuroectoderm). Neuroepithelial cells are continuously replicating cells (VIMs). They give rise to neuroblasts (FPMs). A specialized region of the neuroectoderm, the neural crest, gives rise to the neurons of the PNS. Neuroblasts differentiate into neurons, which are nonreplicating cells (FPMs). The neuroepithelial cells that give rise to neurons are present only during prenatal development. They are not present after birth. Consequently, if the cell bodies of neurons are destroyed, these cells are not replaced.

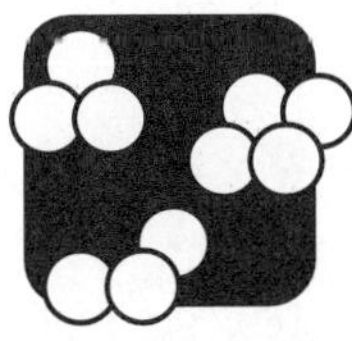

The neuron is also the **basic structural and functional unit** of the nervous system. It is composed of the cell body and processes, which extend from the cell body (axons and dendrites). The cell body, or perikaryon, contains the cell nucleus and surrounding cytoplasm. The neuronal processes include

1. **Axons**

Anatomically this is a single, usually long and branched process. Axons are some-

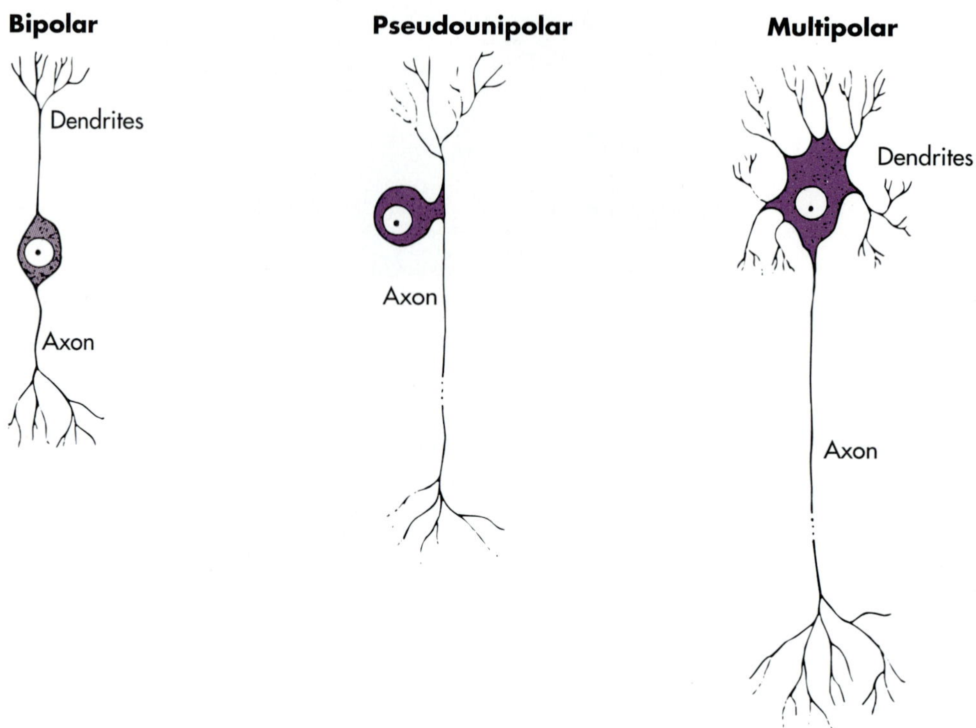

Fig. 6.1 The three main classes of neurons classified on the basis of their cell shape.

times referred to as nerve fibers. Physiologically they conduct impulses away from the cell body.

2. **Dendrites**

Anatomically these are multiple processes, usually short and branched. Physiologically they conduct impulses toward the cell body.

Neurons vary in the number of processes (See Fig. 6.1).

- **Unipolar** neurons have a single process that usually divides into two branches. One branch functions like an axon and the other like a dendrite.
- **Bipolar** neurons have two processes, an axon and a dendrite.
- **Multipolar** neurons have multiple processes, one axon and many dendrites.

Specialized organelles of the neuron include

- **Nissl substance,** which is composed of RER and free ribosomes, and is localized in the cell body.
- the **Golgi apparatus,** which is distributed around the nucleus in the cell body.
- **neurofilaments and neurotubules,** which are intermediate filaments and microtubules that extend from the cell body into the axon.
- **lipofuscin granules,** which are the result of lysosomal activity. They increase during aging and are related to the cell's being a nonreplicative cell.

Synapses are specialized junctions between neurons and other cells. There are two types of synapses.

1. The **chemical synapse** has three components.

   - The **presynaptic terminal** of the axon has numerous mitochondria and synaptic vesicles containing neurotransmitters.
   - A **synaptic cleft** measuring 20 to 40 nm separates the presynaptic from the postsynaptic components.
   - The **postsynaptic component** may be an axon, a dendrite, or the cell soma of another neuron.

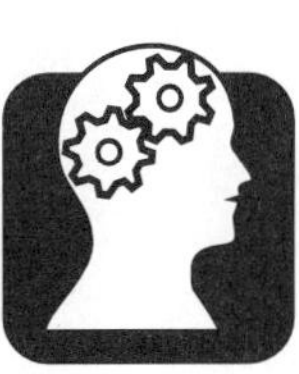

Nerve impulses are transmitted from one neuron to the next by neurotransmitters, which are released at synapses. When an action potential reaches the end of an axon, Ca^{++} enters the axonal ending. Ca^{++} ions facilitate fusion of synaptic vesicles containing neurotransmitters (e.g., acetylcholine) with the presynaptic membrane. The transmitter is released into the synaptic cleft by exocytosis.

The transmitter diffuses across the synaptic cleft to receptors on the postsynaptic membrane. Binding of the neurotransmitter to the receptors increases the permeability of the postsynaptic membrane, causing its depolarization and generation of an action potential in the postsynaptic cell.

2. An **electrical synapse** (or **ephatic synapse**) is a gap junction that enables ions to flow from the cytoplasm of one cell to the cytoplasm of the other. The two cells are electrically linked. No neurotransmitters are involved because the action potential sweeps over the two cells linked by a gap junction.

Axoplasmic transport provides a constant transport of materials between the cell body and the axon termination.

Anterograde transport transports material from the cell body to the axon terminal. A fast component (50 to 400 mm per day) transports cytoplasmic proteins and macromolecules required for metabolic and synaptic activity. A slow component (1 to 4 mm per day) transports cytoskeletal components down the axon.

Retrograde transport moves membranous components of the synaptic vesicles from the axon terminal back to the cell body. It is the mechanism by which viruses (e.g., rabies) or toxins (e.g., tetanus toxin) are transported from the periphery to the CNS.

■ Functional Classes of Neurons

   - **Sensory neurons** transmit impulses from sensory receptors to the CNS (surface to CNS).
   - **Motor neurons** transmit impulses from the CNS to a motor effector organ (a muscle or gland).
   - **Interneurons** transmit within the CNS and connect the two other cell types.

The neuron is the trophic unit of the nervous system. Neurons, or other cells, may be dependent on synaptic contact with a neuron. Some muscle cells are dependent on synaptic contact with a neuron. (Denervation causes muscle atrophy.) Some neurons are dependent on synaptic contact with other neurons. (Denervation causes transneuronal degeneration.)

The cell processes of a neuron are dependent on the integrity of the cell body. Damaging the cell body destroys the neuron. Damaging neuronal cell processes demonstrates the following changes:

   - Wallerian, or anterograde, degeneration refers to changes in the distal portion of the axon (the portion separated from the cell body). The axon begins to swell and degenerate, the myelin sheath fragments, and phagocytes remove cellular debris. After 1 week Schwann cells proliferate and form tubes for the axonal sprouts.

- Chromatolysis refers to changes in the neuron cell body. The cell body swells. The Nissl body disperses. The nucleus is displaced peripherally.

Recovery and regeneration of peripheral neurons occurs if the lesion is at a distance from the cell body. The end of the axon produces fiber sprouts that seek the tubes formed by Schwann cells and will likely regenerate.

NEUROGLIA

The term neuroglia means "supporting tissue of the nervous system (neuro = nerve, glia = glue).

■ **Neuroglial Elements of the CNS** Oligodendrocytes are the predominate cell type of white matter. In the gray matter oligodendrocytes are closely associated with the cell body (satellite cells) and provide a sheath (unmyelinated) around several axons. In the white matter, they produce the myelin sheath of the myelinated fiber. Each oligodendrocyte myelinates several axons.

Astrocytes are "star-shaped" neuroglial cells. In the white matter, they are **fibrous** and unbranched. In the gray matter, they are **protoplasmic** and branched. Astrocytes are closely apposed to neurons and have end feet, or pedicels, that terminate on capillaries. Capillaries of the CNS are completely enveloped and ensheathed by foot processes of astrocytes. Similar pedicels are present at the periphery of brain and spinal cord, forming a layer under the pia mater. Several functions have been proposed for astrocytes.

- Astrocytes regulate the composition of the intercellular environment or entry of substances into it.
- They provide structural support.
- They store neurotransmitters.
- They mediate the exchange of nutrients and metabolites between the blood and neurons.

Ependymal cells form a ciliated cuboidal layer of cells that lines the ventricles of the brain and the central canal of the spinal cord. The choroid plexus cell is a special type of ependymal cell and is the principal secretory agent of cerebrospinal fluid (CSF).

Microglia are phagocytic cells derived from embryonic mesoderm.

Developmentally, the **neuroepithelial cells** (VIMs) of the neuroectoderm give rise to the glioblasts (DIMs); the glioblasts give rise to the astrocytes and oligodendrocytes (RPMs).

Meninges are protective layers around the CNS. There are three distinguishable layers.

- The **dura mater** is the outer layer of meninges that blends with the periosteum of the skull but is separated from the vertebra of the spinal column by the epidural space. It is composed of dense fibrous connective tissue that is lined by a discontinuous mesothelium. It is separated from the underlying arachnoid by the subdural space.
- The **arachnoid** is a fibrous layer with weblike strands that extend into the underlying subarachnoid space. The inner and outer surfaces of the arachnoid are

lined with mesothelium. The subarachnoid space contains arteries and veins surrounded by CSF.

    • The **pia mater** is attached to the brain and spinal cord. It consists of a delicate layer of fibroblasts and collagen fibers. Blood vessels penetrate the CNS through tunnels covered by pia mater and called perivascular spaces. The pia disappears as blood vessels are transformed into capillaries. In the CNS the capillaries are completely covered by the foot processes of astrocytes.

    • The **blood-brain barrier** is a functional barrier that prevents passage of certain substances from blood to nervous tissue. The barrier is a reflection of reduced permeability of endothelial cells. The capillaries of CNS are not fenestrated. The endothelial cells are surrounded by the zonula occludens, forming a permeability seal. The foot processes of astrocytes completely envelope these capillaries.

■ Neuroglial Elements of the PNS

    • Neuroglial elements of the PNS are derived from the neural crest. Satellite cells (amphicytes) form a capsule of cells around neuron cell bodies in the peripheral ganglia. Schwann cells elaborate the myelin sheath of fibers in the PNS. The **myelin sheath** differentiates from the cell membrane of the oligodendrocyte (CNS) or a Schwann cell (PNS) (Fig. 6.2). Myelin consists of many layers of modified plasma membrane. It has a higher proportion of lipids than other membranes. CNS myelin contains two major proteins:

    • Myelin basic protein
    • Proteolipid myelin

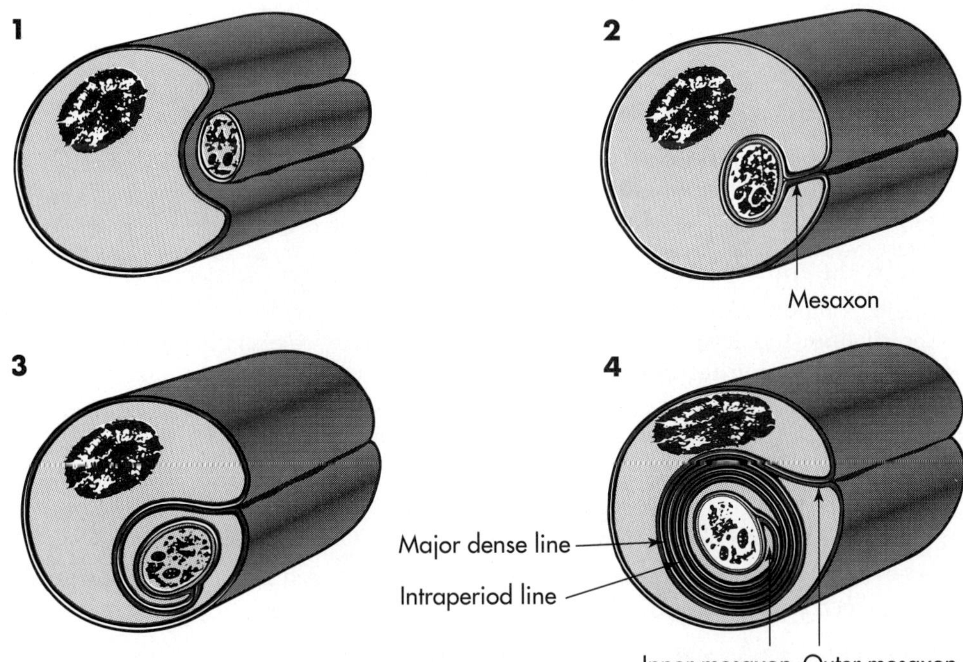

Fig. 6.2 The formation of myelin in the peripheral nervous system. The Schwann cell wraps around the axon, and the Schwann cell cytoplasm is extruded from the wrapping portion. *(Modified from Junqueira LC, Carneiro J:* Basic histology, *ed 7, East Norwalk, Conn., 1992, Appleton & Lange.)*

The formation of the myelin sheath starts with the invagination of the axon into the cytoplasm of the neuroglial cell, eventually surrounding it and completely forming the mesaxon. The mesaxon lengthens and forms a spiral around the axon. The cytoplasm sandwiched between consecutive spirals is squeezed out.

Fusion of the inner (protoplasmic) surfaces of the Schwann cell plasma membrane forms the **principal dense line,** which is visible in the electron microscope.

Fusion of the adjacent external surfaces of the membrane results in the **intraperiod line,** which is visible in the electron microscope.

Axons in gray matter may be surrounded by oligodendrocytic cytoplasm but are not myelinated. A single oligodendrocyte surrounds or myelinates several axons. The Schwann cell myelinates but a single axon. Because each Schwann cell or oligodendrocyte myelinates only a segment of an axon, there are small interruptions in the myelin sheath called **nodes of Ranvier.** At these points the axon is exposed. Dendrites are not myelinated.

■ Elements of the Peripheral Nervous System

Ganglia are collections of neuron cell bodies outside the CNS. There are three types of ganglia:

- Cranial
- Spinal (dorsal root ganglia)
- Autonomic

Sympathetic ganglia are located paravertebrally. Parasympathetic ganglia are located within or near the target tissue. Ganglia are composed of

- cell bodies of neurons located outside of the CNS
- nerve fibers
- satellite cells (amphicytes), which surround the cell bodies of neurons
- the usual elements of connective tissue

Peripheral nerves are composed of connective tissue and neuroglial elements. They contain bundles (or fascicles) of nerve axons, myelin sheaths, and connective tissue. The connective tissue elements are organized into

- the **epineurium,** which is the external fibrous coat of a nerve
- the **perineurium,** which surrounds bundles of nerve fibers, contains an epithelium-like layer, the cells of which are joined by **macula occludens** providing a permeability barrier to the perineurium
- the **endoneurium,** which surrounds individual nerve processes (outside of the myelin sheath)

The neuroglial elements are

- **Schwann cells,** which in an unmyelinated fiber envelop the axon.
- Schwann cells form **myelin sheaths** in myelinated nerves. Most peripheral nerves consist of myelinated and unmyelinated fibers.

Nerve fibers can be classified according to function.

Sensory fibers are processes of neurons transmitting impulses from peripheral receptors to the CNS. Cell bodies are located in the peripheral ganglia. **Motor fibers** are processes of neurons transmitting impulses from the CNS to effector organs (muscle and glands). Cell bodies are located in the CNS or autonomic ganglia. Most peripheral nerves contain motor and sensory fibers.

There are two types of **peripheral nerve endings. Motor endings** are the terminations of nerves on muscles or glands. The motor end plate is such a termination. The release of a chemical neurotransmitter changes the permeability of the effector cell (muscle-gland) causing a wave of depolarization to sweep over the effector cell bringing about contraction or secretion. **Sensory endings** are modality specific. Mechanoreceptors are stimulated by stretch, touch, or pressure. Chemoreceptors are stimulated by taste or smell. Radiant receptors are stimulated by light. Free nerve endings are stimulated by temperature and pain.

Multiple Choice Review Questions

1. Place A beside those elements found principally
   in gray matter,
   B beside those found principally in white
   matter,
   C beside those found in gray and white
   matter,
   D beside those found in neither white nor
   gray matter:

   _____ Oligodendrocyte
   _____ Collagen fibers
   _____ Neuron cell body
   _____ Myelin sheath
   _____ Endoneurium

2. Match the cell with its function:

   _____ Neuron
   _____ Astrocyte
   _____ Oligodendrocyte
   _____ Microglia
   _____ Schwann cell

   a. Phagocytosis
   b. Synthesize neurotransmitter
   c. Formation myelin sheath
   d. Nutrition and transport
   e. Synthesis of tropocollagen

3. Place A beside these things that increase,
   B beside those that decrease,
   C beside those that remain the same:

   _____ Amount of Nissl material in cell body after
   severing axon
   _____ Total number of neurons in CNS between 3
   and 5 years of age
   _____ Amount of connective tissue elements in
   gray versus white matter

4. Two weeks after a sublethal dose of x irradiation
   to a portion of the brain, one would expect to find
   in that portion of the brain:

   a. a decreased number of microglia.
   b. a decreased number of oligodendrocytes.
   c. a decreased number of neurons.
   d. all of the above.
   e. none of the above.

5. Arrange in sequence from neuron outward:

   _____ Epineurium
   _____ Plasma membrane of axon
   __a__ Perineurium
   _____ Endoneurium
   _____ Myelin sheath

Chapter 7

Muscular Tissue

GENERAL

Muscular tissues are populations of cells that are specialized to perform the function of movement or locomotion through the processes of contraction and relaxation. There are three basic types of muscular tissue.

- **Skeletal muscle,** which is striated and constitutes the muscles of the skeleton
- **Cardiac muscle,** which is also striated and is the muscle of the heart
- **Smooth muscle,** which is not striated and provides the muscle of the blood vessels, internal organs, and viscera

The term **fiber** applied to muscle refers to the muscle cell itself and not to extracellular material (as in connective tissue) or cell processes (as in nervous tissue).

The term *muscle* is also used to refer to the organ as in *biceps brachii muscle.* Such an organ, in which the parenchyma is skeletal muscle, is composed of muscle, nerve, and connective tissue. The connective tissue enveloping the entire muscle is the epimysium. Perimysium separates individual fascicles of the muscle, and endomysium is the connective tissue enveloping each muscle fiber.

■ Properties of the Muscle Fiber Enabling Its Basic Functions (i.e., Movement or Locomotion)

- *Excitability* is the ability of the fiber to respond to a stimulus.
- *Conductivity* is the ability of the fiber to propagate a limited stimulus.
- *Contractility* is the ability of the fiber to shorten and thicken.
- *Elasticity* and *viscosity* enable the fiber to return to its original shape after contraction.

SKELETAL MUSCLE

Skeletal muscle consists of large multinucleated fibers (up to 30 cm long and 100 μm thick). The cytoplasm (sarcoplasm) of the cell is filled with myofibrils. The skeletal muscle fiber is a multinucleate cell that arises in the embryonic connective tissue mesenchyme. The earliest muscle cell is called the **myoblast.** The fusion of many myoblasts gives rise to a tubelike cell with many nuclei, the **myotube.** As the cell differentiates, it lays down myofilaments, which organize into striated myofibrils. As the number of myofibrils increase, the nuclei are displaced to the periphery of the cell under the plasma membrane.

Growth of muscle after puberty occurs by an increase in the size of muscle fibers (hypertrophy) rather than an increase in the number of fibers (hyperplasia).

Myofibrils run parallel to the long axis of the fiber and give to the fiber a cross-banded (striated) appearance. Each myofibril itself, like the fiber, is cross-striated. There are dark **A bands** (anisotropic), and adjacent to each A band is a light **I band** (isotropic). A **Z line** bisects each I band. The **sarcomere** is the functional unit of

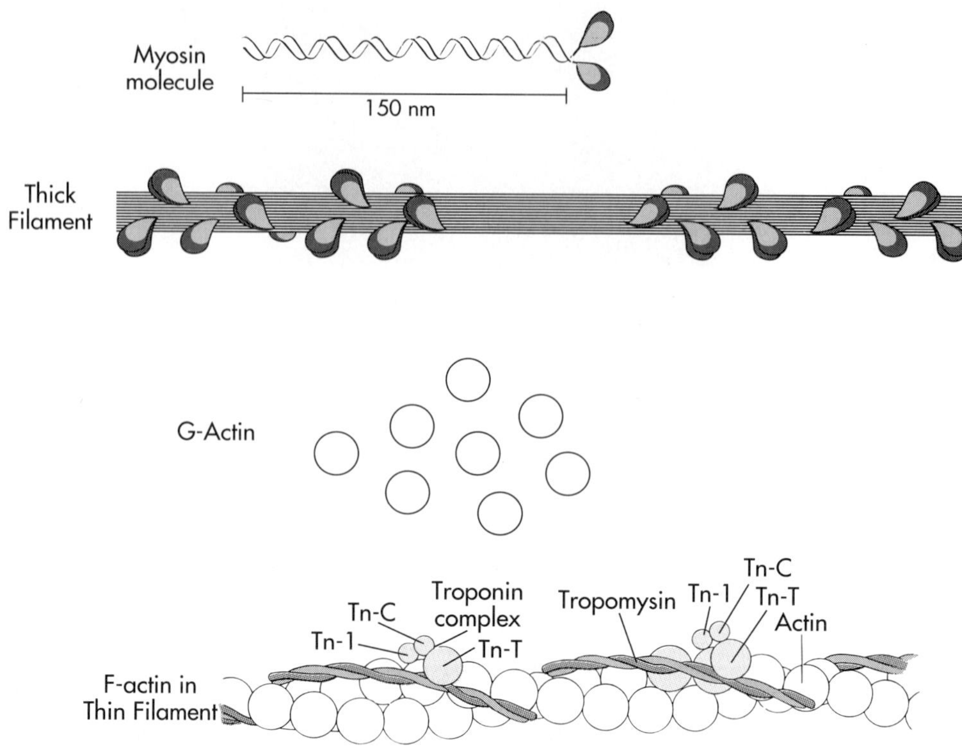

Fig. 7.1 Organization of actin and myosin in thick and thin filaments. The myosin molecules are laid down in the thick filaments so that their tails are parallel and their heads project from the surface of the thick filament. The molecules at one end of the thick filament are oriented at 180 degrees relative to the molecules at the other end. Therefore the middle region of the thick filament (shown) is devoid of heads. The thin filaments are composed of *F*-actin. The locations of tropomyosin and the three troponin peptides (TN-T, TN-I, and TN-C) are shown. *(Modified from Darnell JE: Molecular cell biology, New York, 1986, Scientific American Books.)*

the fiber and is the distance between two Z lines. It is the smallest unit capable of contraction.

Myofilaments are the basic components of myofibril. There are two types of myofilaments, as shown in Fig. 7.1.

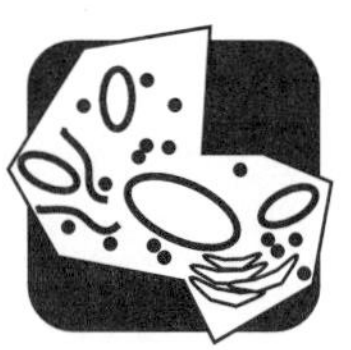

■ **Thick Filaments (Myosin-containing Myofilaments)** Each thick myofilament is about 1.5 μm long, 14 nm thick, and contains hundreds of myosin molecules. Myosin is a thin, rodlike protein with a globular head region and a long tail. Its molecular weight is 500 kDa, and it measures 150 nm in length.

   In the thick filament, the tails of the myosin molecules associate to form cigar-shaped structures such that the molecules at one end of the thick filament are oriented 180 degrees opposite to the molecules at the other end. The heads of the myosin molecules project from the thick filament, and they attach to actin in the thin filament. The heads bind and hydrolyze ATP.

■ **Thin Filaments (Actin-containing Myofilaments)** Each thin filament measures 1 μm long, 8 nm thick. Thin filaments are composed of 300 to 400 units of the globular protein actin (G-actin) (MW 42 kDa). These spherical particles of G-actin are arrayed like a twisted double-helical strand of beads in fibrous actin (F-actin).

   Tropomyosin is a long filamentous protein that runs over several actin subunits along the groove in the helix. Each tropomyosin molecule spans seven

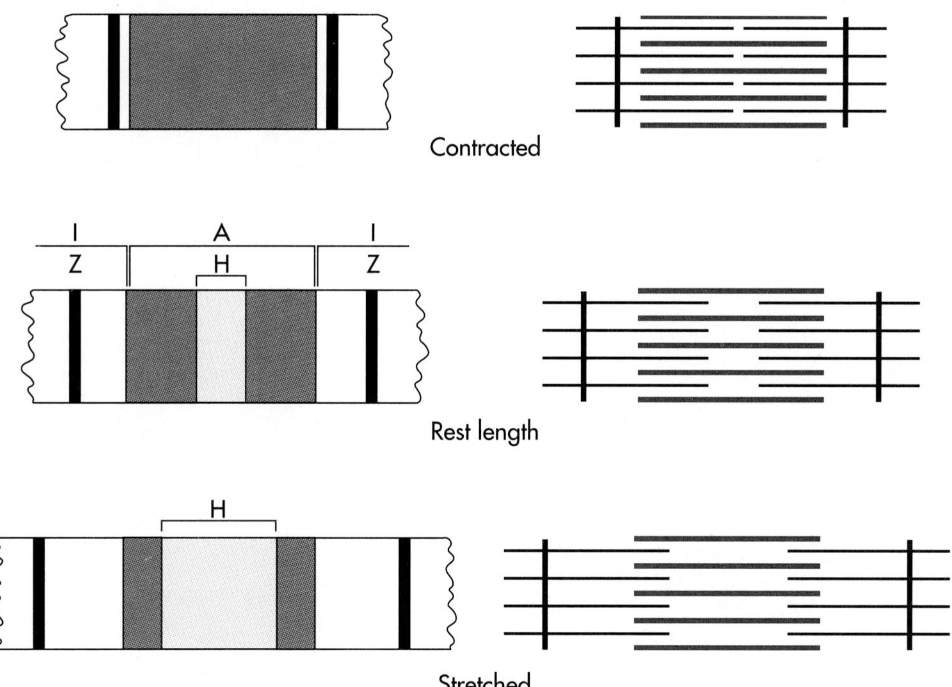

Fig. 7.2 Changes in the cross striations of a myofibril reflecting contraction, relaxation, and stretching. Changes in the interdigitation of thick and thin filaments are responsible for these changes. *(From Fawcett DW: A textbook of histology, ed 11, Philadelphia, 1986, Saunders.)*

actin molecules. Troponin is a globular protein complex that attaches to a specific site on each tropomyosin molecule. There is one troponin complex/tropomyosin molecule. The troponin complex has 3 subunits.

- TnT, which attaches to tropomyosin
- TnC, which binds Ca^{++}
- TnI, which inhibits the actin-myosin interaction

Each G-actin monomer contains a myosin-binding site. If thin filaments are isolated, intact and then incubated with the heads of myosin molecules, the thin filaments bind the myosin heads. The myosin heads bound on one side of the Z line are oriented at 180 degrees to those on the other side of the Z line, indicating a polarity in the thin filaments.

■ The Organization of Myofilaments in the Myofibril (at Rest) (Fig. 7.2)

Thick filaments are limited to the A band. Thin filaments extend from the Z line through the I band and into the A band. The thin filaments are firmly attached to the Z line. Alpha actinin anchors the actin-containing filaments to the Z line. They interdigitate with the thick filaments. The thin filaments overlap the thick filaments extending into the A band where they form a hexagonal array about each thick filament. The thin filaments are absent from the H zone. In the center of the H zone is the M line.

The "A" and "I" bands of adjacent myofibrils are in register, giving to the entire fiber a cross-striated appearance. Intermediate filaments (desmin) form a delicate framework linking myofibrils together laterally and keeping the A and I bands in register. At Z bands, desmin filaments form a planar network that interacts with alpha actinin at the Z line and extends laterally to the plasma membrane (sarcolemma). The protein dystrophin links the desmin-actinin complex

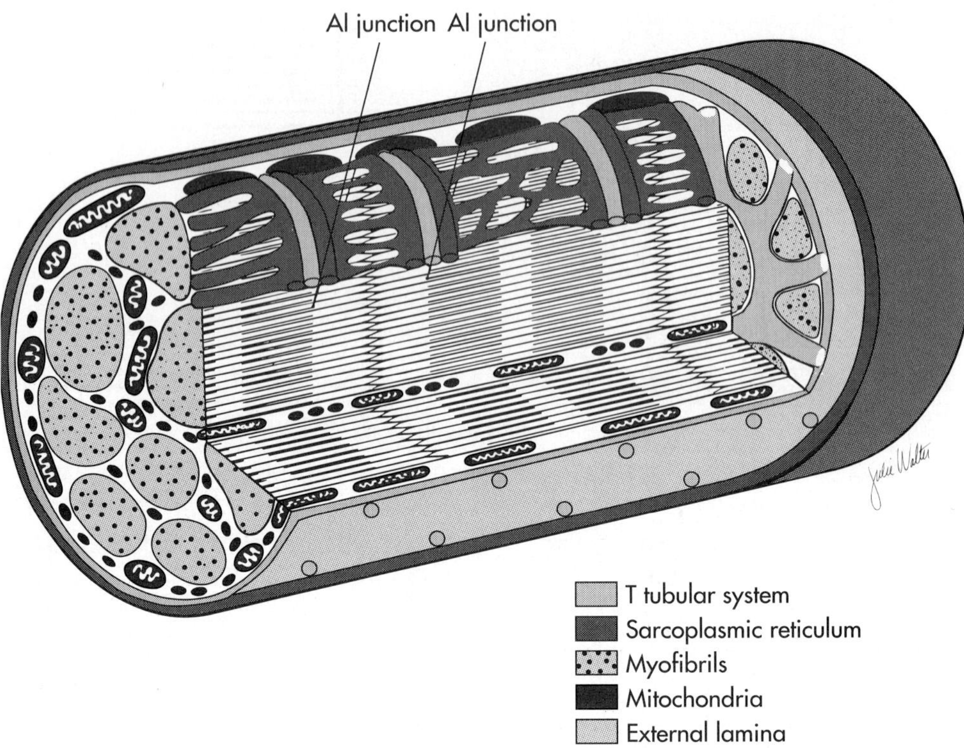

Fig. 7.3 The organization of the transverse tubules and sarcoplasmic reticulum in the skeletal muscle fiber. *(From Stevens A, Lowe JS:* Histology, *Brookfield, Vt., 1992, Gower Medical {London}.)*

to the plasma membrane (sarcolemma). Dystrophin is absent or defective in individuals with muscular dystrophy.

■ **The Sarcoplasmic Membrane System (Fig. 7.3)** The plasma membrane of skeletal muscle is referred to as the *sarcolemma.* The sarcolemma is continuous with a series of transverse tubules (T tubules) that extend into the cytoplasm (sarcoplasm) at the A-I intercept and surround each of the individual myofibrils. Closely associated with the T tubules but not in direct continuity with them is a modified smooth endoplasmic reticulum (sarcoplasmic reticulum). A parallel array of membrane-lined cisternae extends over each myofibril. The cisternae fuse at the region of the A-I intercept to form the greatly expanded terminal cisterna (i.e., there is a terminal cisterna on two sides of each transverse tubule). The association of the two terminal cisternae and the T tubules is called a *triad.* A network of tubules extends over the myofibril connecting the terminal cisternae of two separate triads.

The space between the myofibrils is occupied by sarcoplasm (cytoplasm). Mitochondria are arranged at regular intervals along myofibrils. They are more prominent in I bands. Mitochondria encircle the myofibrils at the I band.

■ **Muscle Contraction** ATP provides the immediate source of energy for muscular contraction. During contraction ATP causes cyclic changes in the binding of the myosin to actin. At the start of a contraction cycle, a myosin head (lacking a nucleotide) is attached to actin in a thin filament. ATP binds to the myosin head and causes a conformational change in it, reducing the affinity of the head for actin. ATP is hydrolyzed (but ADP and P_i, inorganic phosphate, remain bound to the head). A change in the shape of the head causes the head to be

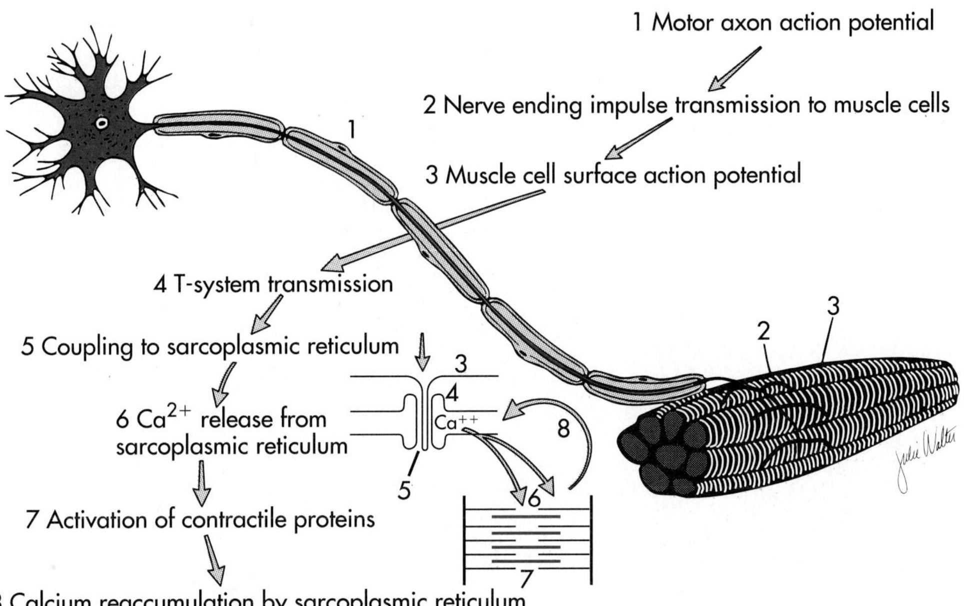

Fig. 7.4 Diagram summarizing the events leading to contraction of skeletal muscle. *(From Ross RB, Reith EJ, Histology: a text and atlas, New York, 1985, Harper & Row.)*

displaced along the thin filament. The release of P_i causes the tight binding of the head to another actin, and a change in the shape of the head when the head loses ADP causes it to swivel. This results in the myosin head walking along the thin filament in one direction. The myosin head pulls the actin-containing thin filament, causing the thin filament to slide over the thick filament.

Contraction of skeletal muscle is regulated by Ca^{++} and its interaction with troponin. In resting muscle, the binding of TnI to actin moves tropomyosin, through its interaction with TnT, to a position on the actin-containing filament that is occupied by myosin heads, inhibiting the interaction of myosin with actin. When the level of Ca^{++} increases, the binding of Ca^{++} to TnC causes TnT to release its hold on actin, allowing a shift in position on the thin filament so that myosin can bind to actin.

The sequence of events in the contraction of the muscle fiber is shown in Fig. 7.4. The neurotransmitter substance acetylcholine is released at the neuromuscular junction (motor end plate). Each muscle fiber is innervated by a motor end plate. A wave of depolarization sweeps over the sarcolemma and T tubules and is relayed across a gap between the T tubule and the terminal cisternae. The terminal cisternae contain large Ca^{++}-release channels that are voltage sensitive. The action potential causes these channels to open and release Ca^{++} from the sarcoplasmic reticulum. The release of Ca^{++} causes the myofibrils to contract. Ca^{++} is rapidly pumped back into the sarcoplasmic reticulum by the Ca^{++}-ATPase in the sarcoplasmic reticulum membrane.

When the myofibril contracts, the thin filaments slide over the thick filaments in such a manner that the distance between the Z lines decreases (i.e., the sarcomere decreases in length) (Fig. 7.2). Some consequences of this shortening are that

- the A bands remain a constant length.
- the I bands decrease in length.
- the overlapping of thick and thin filaments in the A bands increases.

Unlike the actin and myosin in other cell types, which are labile, myofilaments in muscle are very stable, giving rise to the differentiated state of muscle tissue. Other proteins important in the contractile machinery of striated muscle are

- titin, which extends from the Z line to the thick filament, centering the thick filament in the sarcomere
- myomesin, which holds thick filaments in a lattice in the region of the M line

Fibers making up individual muscles are not uniform in size or appearance. There is a range of fibers described as red, white, and intermediate. Red fibers are capable of sustained activity over long periods of time (slow twitch). They are rich in myoglobin and in mitochondria. White fibers are capable of quick contractions or bursts of activity (fast twitch). They have little if any myoglobin but are rich in glycogen.

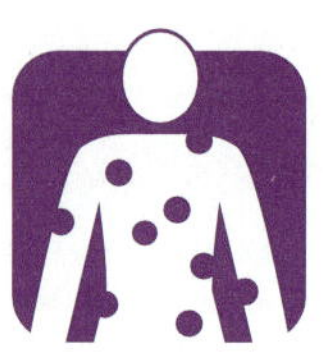

■ **Disorders of Skeletal Muscle** There are two major classes of muscle disorders.

• Myopathies are degenerative diseases of muscle not involving loss of innervation. In the case of myopathies, the weakness is generally proximal and symmetrical.

• Neuropathies are degenerative diseases of muscle caused by a loss of innervation. In the case of neuropathies the weakness is generally distal and asymmetrical.

In both types of malfunction, the muscle fibers atrophy. There is a decrease in the cross-sectional area of muscle fibers and a decrease in the number of myofibrils. Other causes of atrophy are aging, malnutrition, and immobilization.

CARDIAC MUSCLE

There is a single nucleus per cardiac muscle cell or fiber. Like skeletal muscle, cardiac muscle is striated. Its cytoplasm is filled with myofibrils composed of thick (myosin-containing) and thin (actin-containing) filaments that are held in register giving the cardiac muscle fiber a cross-striated appearance.

Cardiac muscle cells are joined tightly to one another by intercalated disks = junctional complexes. The transverse parts of intercalated disks, which are at right angles to the long axis of fiber, demonstrate fascia adherens, macula adherens, and macula occludens. The lateral parts of intercalated disks are parallel with the long axis of the fiber and demonstrate nexi (gap junctions). There are 3 important functions of intercalated disks.

- To attach one cell to the adjacent cell
- To connect actin filaments in the myofibrils of one cell to the next
- To provide a means for transmitting the action potential from one cell to the next, since each cell is not individually innervated (as in the motor end plate of skeletal muscle)

Like skeletal muscle, cardiac muscle fiber has a transverse tubular system. The T tubules are located at the Z line instead of A-I intercept. Small, discontinuous terminal cisternae of sarcoplasmic reticulum are associated with the T tubules. Only one terminal cisternae is associated with each T tubule forming a diad. There is not an elaborate sarcoplasmic reticular network.

The contraction mechanism for the cardiac muscle is the same as that of skeletal muscle. The cardiac muscle fiber is a fixed postmitotic (FPM) cell for which there is no stem cell compartment; therefore these cells are not replaced if killed or destroyed. Associated with aging there is an increase in lipofuscin granules (see lysosomes). A large number of such granules gives rise to brown atrophy of the heart.

SMOOTH MUSCLE

Each smooth muscle cell or fiber contains a single, centrally located nucleus. Smooth muscle fibers contain thin (actin-containing) and thick (myosin-containing) filaments, but the fibers are not striated. The filaments are more loosely arranged along the long axis of the cell, attaching obliquely to the plasmalemma. The cytoplasm of the smooth muscle fiber is distinguished by dark bodies or patches (located on the surface and within the fiber). Bundles of 10 nm filaments extend from one dark body to another. These intermediate filaments are composed of desmin. When the muscle fiber contracts, the plasma membrane becomes covered with bubbles as cytoplasm under pressure pushes the plasma membrane between patches. This results in a shortening and thickening of the cell in an accordion manner. There is no T-tubular system in smooth muscle. Caveolae on the cell surface are perhaps analogous to the T-tubules. Smooth muscle fibers have an abundance of gap junctions (nexi) on their surface. This enables the cell to transmit an action potential, since each fiber is not individually innervated as in the motor end plates of skeletal muscle (Table 7.1).

Table 7.1   *Characteristics of Muscle Fibers*

	SKELETAL	CARDIAC	SMOOTH
Structure			
Location	Muscles of skeleton	Heart	Vessels, organs, and viscera
Connective tissue component	Epimysium, perimysium, endomysium	Endomysium	Sheaths and bundles
Fibers	Single large cells	Branched single cells	Single cells
Striations	+	+	−
Nucleus	Many peripheral	Single central	Single central
T tubules	A-I junction	Z lines	Replaced by caveolae
Cell junctions	−	Zonula adherens, zonula occludens, nexus	Nexus
Special features	Sarcoplasmic reticulum well developed	Intercalated disk	
Function			
Regulation of contraction	Voluntary	Involuntary	Involuntary
Type of contraction	All or none (red and white fibers)	All or none, rhythmic	Slow, partial
Efferent Innervation	Somatic efferent, motor end plate	Autonomic efferent (nexi)	Autonomic efferent (nexi)
Growth and Regeneration			
Mitosis	−	−	+
Response to demand	Hypertrophy	Hypertrophy	Hypertrophy
Regeneration	Limited, satellite cells (pericytes)	−	+

+, Presence; −, absence.

MULTIPLE CHOICE REVIEW QUESTIONS

1. Arrange in order of increasing size:

    __a__ Carbon atom
    _____ Myofibril
    _____ Myofilament
    _____ Myosin
    _____ G-actin

2. Which of the following statements describe the thick filaments of skeletal muscle?

    a. Localized in A band.
    b. The thick filament is the same as a single myosin molecule.
    c. Attached to Z line.
    d. All of the above are correct.
    e. None of the above is correct.

3. Place an A beside those things that increase,
    B beside those things that decrease,
    C beside those things that remain the same:

    _____ Length of A band during contraction of skeletal muscle
    _____ Length of H zone during relaxation of skeletal muscle
    _____ Length of I band during contraction of skeletal muscle
    _____ Amount of Ca^{++} bound to sarcoplasmic reticulum during contraction
    _____ Thickness of muscle fiber during contraction

4. Match the following:

    a. A band
    b. I band
    c. Z lines
    d. A-I intercept
    e. Thick filaments

    _____ Location of T tubules in skeletal muscle
    _____ Composed principally of contractile protein myosin
    _____ Remains same length during relaxation of muscle
    _____ Location of T tubules in cardiac muscle
    _____ Area composed principally of contractile protein actin

5. Which of the following structures are not found in smooth muscle?

    a. Actin and myosin
    b. Transverse tubules
    c. Gap junctions (nexus)
    d. Mitochondria
    e. All of the above

Chapter 8

Integumentary System

GENERAL

The integumentary system includes the skin and its appendages. The skin covers
the body and comprises the **epidermis** and the **dermis**. The epidermis is a stratified
squamous keratinized epithelium (dry), in which up to five cellular layers (strata) are
distinguished.

- The **stratum basale** is a single layer adjacent to the basement membrane. Desmosomes and hemidesmosomes attach one cell to another and to the basement membrane.

- The **stratum spinosum** is composed of flattened polyhedral cells. Tonofibrils
terminate in desmosomes. The term **stratum germinativum** is used to describe the
combination of stratum basale and stratum spinosum, which are both composed of
proliferative cells.

- The **stratum granulosum** is distinguished by keratohyalin granules. Lamellar
granules of lipids are numerous. The cells secrete glycolipids and sterols into the intercellular space to form the lipid barrier of skin.

- The **stratum lucidum** is evident in thick skin. It is a thin, translucent region
underlying the stratum corneum.

- The **stratum corneum** is composed of flattened cornified cells. The desmosomes have a thick electron-dense intermediate layer. The cell contents are replaced
by cross-linked keratin filaments embedded in a globular amorphous matrix. The inner cell membrane is thickened because of the deposition of the cross-linked
involucrin.

The **dermis** is separated from the epidermis by a basement membrane composed
of a basal lamina and a lamina reticularis. It is composed of two layers.

- The **papillary layer** is composed of loose connective tissue arranged in fine interlacing bands of thin collagenous bundles. Cells are more abundant in the papillary
dermis than in the reticular dermis.

- The deeper **reticular layer** is composed of dense fibrous irregular connective
tissue arranged in thick interlacing bands.

- The **hypodermis** lies beneath the skin but is not really a part of it. Its other
names are the **subcutaneous tissue or superficial fascia.** It is composed of loose
areolar connective tissue, which is continuous with the dermis. When it is composed
of primarily adipose tissue, it is termed **panniculus adiposus.**

In addition to the usual elements of connective tissue, the dermis and hypodermis
contain smooth muscle, nerves, nerve endings, and blood vessels, as well as derivatives extending from the epidermis.

- Hair follicles
- Sweat glands
- Sebaceous glands

The thickness of skin is variable. It can be accounted for by variation in the thickness of the dermis. The dermis is very thick on the back and very thin on the abdomen. The thickness can also be accounted for by variations in thickness of the epidermis. Thin skin (most of body) is 0.07 to 0.15 mm thick, and thick skin (palms and soles) is 0.4 to 1.4 mm thick.

CELL TYPES OF THE EPIDERMIS

■ **Keratinocytes** Keratinocytes synthesize large amounts of the intermediate filament keratin. Different keratins are synthesized at different stages:

- Cells in the **stratum basale** synthesize low-molecular-weight keratins.
- Cells in the **stratum spinosum** synthesize high-molecular-weight keratins.
- Keratins become cross linked with disulfide bonds as cells migrate toward the surface.

The proteinaceous involucrin envelope is formed on the inner layer of the plasma membrane.

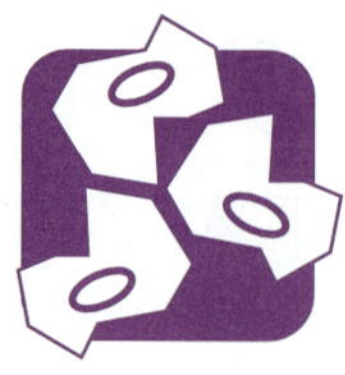

● **Cell population kinetics and differentiation in the epidermis** Cytomorphosis of the keratinocyte takes 20 to 30 days. There are both continuously replicating (vegetative intermitotic) and occasionally replicating (reverting postmitotic) cells in the basal layer. The continuously replicating cells give rise to differentiating cells, which move into the stratum spinosum, and nondifferentiating cells, which maintain the supply of continuously replicating and occasionally replicating cells in the stratum basale. Some of the newly formed continuously replicating cells move into the stratum spinosum.

  On entering the stratum spinosum the cells continue differentiation. The cells in the stratum spinosum are continuous replicators (differentiating intermitotics). Further differentiation occurs as the cells enter the stratum granulosum. Cells in the stratum granulosum are no longer capable of replication or division. They are nonreplicating Fixed postmitotic (FPM) cells. Release of lysosomal contents results in the destruction of cellular organelles (autophagy), but the keratin filaments and remaining keratohyalin are not digested as the cells move into the stratum corneum. Cells in stratum corneum remain nonreplicating, fixed, postmitotic cells. It is principally a dead layer that is continually exfoliated. Cellular organelles including the nucleus have disappeared.

■ **The Melanocyte** synthesizes melanin, the pigment of the skin. Melanocytes are located in the stratum basale, papillary dermis, and hair follicles. They are derived from embryonic neural crest cells. The melanocyte is derived from the melanoblast.

● **Synthesis of melanin** Protyrosinase enzyme (in the promelanosome) is converted to tyrosinase enzyme (in the melanosome).

$$\text{Tyrosine} \rightarrow \text{Dopa} \rightarrow \text{Dopaquinone} \rightarrow \text{Melanin}$$

● **The distribution of melanin granules** Melanin granules are distributed to the cytoplasm of basal and spinous cells (melanophores) by cytocrine secretion by means of the melanocyte cell process. Chromatophores in the dermis obtain melanin by phagocytosis.

  The color of skin is determined by

- carotene in the stratum corneum and in the adipose cells of the dermis (yellow)

- oxyhemoglobin (red) in the blood
- melanin (black to brown)

■ **Langerhans' Cells** are dendritic cells located particularly in the stratum spinosum. Dendritic processes form a network throughout the epidermis. Desmosomes, melanosomes, and tonofibrils are absent. These cells are involved in the immune response.

■ **Merkel Cells** are located in the stratum basale near the well-vascularized, highly innervated dermis. They contain dense-cored granules in cytoplasm. They are involved in sensory reception and may be paraneurons.

APPENDAGES OF SKIN

Hair follicles are located in the dermis and hypodermis. There are 10 morphologically distinguishable layers in a hair follicle. Growth of hair occurs at the base, not the tip of the hair. Growth is cyclic.

- Resting (club) hair (catagen and telogen)
- Growth phase (anagen)

The arrector pili muscle is the smooth muscle connecting the papillary dermis with the connective tissue sheath of the hair follicle. Contraction of the arrector pili muscles erects the hair follicle and depresses the skin causing "gooseflesh."

Nails are located in the epidermis. The nail plate covers the nail bed. Its root is proximal and positioned in the nail fold. The proximal whitish crescent is termed the *lunula.* Nail synthesis occurs in the nail matrix. The proliferative cells are found in the epithelium of the nail root and underlying lunula. The growing nail slides over the nail bed. The thickened epithelium under the free distal edge of the nail is termed the hyponychium. The epithelium of the nail fold is termed the *eponychium.* The blood vessels in the dermis are visible through the translucent nail plate as a pink color. This permits clinical diagnosis (e.g., cyanotic heart disease).

GLANDS

■ **Sebaceous Glands** Sebaceous glands are located in the dermis. They are simple branched glands with short ducts and alveolar acini. Their holocrine lipid secretion is termed *sebum.* Their ducts are lined by stratified squamous epithelium continuous with the hair external root sheath and epidermis. Epithelial cell mitosis occurs primarily near the duct walls. Sebaceous glands usually open into a hair follicle. There are no sebaceous glands at mucocutaneous junctions.

Sweat glands are located in the dermis and hypodermis. *Eccrine* (merocrine) sweat glands are located in the dermis and hypodermis. They are simple coiled, tubular glands opening to the epidermis. There are dark cells and clear cells in the secretory portion of the gland. Their ducts are lined with stratified cuboidal epithelium. When the cholinergic nerve that innervates a sweat gland is stimulated, the glands produce hypotonic sweat for thermoregulation. *Apocrine* sweat glands are located in the hypodermis. They open into hair follicles. When the adrenergic nerve innervating the gland is stimulated, the gland produces an apocrine type of viscous secretion. Apocrine glands begin to function at puberty; their activity is linked to the menstrual cycle in females. Apocrine sweat glands are present in the axilla, mons pubis, mammary gland areola, and circumanal region.

VASCULATURE

Blood vessels are absent from the epidermis. There are two arterial plexuses in the dermis. The one at the dermis/hypodermis border is termed the **rete cutaneum.** The one at the papillary/reticular layer border is termed the **rete subpapillare.** Each papilla has a single capillary loop with an ascending arterial and a descending venous limb. Hair follicles, arrector pili muscles, sebaceous glands, and sweat glands are well supplied by capillaries or small arteries. Arteriovenous anastomoses occur in the skin for thermoregulation. Lymphatic vessels and capillaries parallel blood vessels.

Nerves

Motor nerve fibers of the integumentary system are postganglionic fibers of sympathetic ganglia. Sensory nerve fibers include vertical projections of free nerve endings into papillae, as well as corpuscular receptors, such as

- Meissner's corpuscles
- Merkel's corpuscles
- Pacinian corpuscles
- genital corpuscles

Hair follicles also serve as mechanoreceptors with nerve fibers at the epidermal openings and on the root sheath below the sebaceous gland.

Functions of Skin

As a **barrier,** skin keeps in fluids and keeps out foreign substances. (It is impermeable to most substances, with the notable exceptions of methanol and nickel.) Skin **filters** ultraviolet radiation. It disperses light through its keratinized layers. Melanin absorbs light in the UV region of the spectrum. One reaction to sunlight is that melanocytes increase in tyrosinase activity, increasing the skin's pigmentation (melanin content).

- Skin functions in **wound healing.** Reepithelialization occurs from the margin of a wound from the hair follicle keratinocytes and from cells in the ducts of glands. The connective tissue matrix is repaired by fibroblasts in the underlying dermis. Neovascularization is provided by capillary endothelial cells.
- Skin helps to **regulate body temperature.** This is a function of the capillary network in the dermis and surface evaporation of fluid from the eccrine sweat glands.
- Skin functions in the **regulation of blood pressure.** The opening of the capillary network in the dermis increases the total cross-sectional area of the circulatory system and lowers blood pressure. The closing of the capillary network decreases the total cross-sectional area and raises blood pressure.
- It functions in the **excretion of metabolic waste products.**
- It embodies the **senses** of touch, pressure, temperature, and pain.
- It defines the **surface features** of the body.

Histologic Disorders of Skin

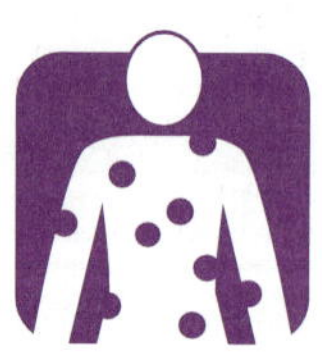

Psoriasis is the increased proliferation of keratinocytes in the basal layer of the epidermis. The normal differentiation of keratinocyte does not occur. The epidermis becomes thickened. The normal time for a keratinocyte to move from the basal layer through the stratum corneum is 20 to 30 days; in psoriasis, it is 3 to 7 days. Psoriasis is related to normal wound healing events; it usually appears at sites of abrasion.

Solar or senile elastosis is the loss of skin elasticity with aging. It is caused by exposure to UV rays. There is an increase in stainable elastic fibers in the dermis. Also there is a loss of elastic fiber elasticity.

MULTIPLE CHOICE
REVIEW QUESTIONS

1. Match the cell with its type of cell life:

    _____ Cell in stratum granulosum
    _____ Cell in stratum spinosum
    _____ Cell in duct of sweat gland
    _____ Cell in stratum basale
    _____ Chromatophore

    a. Vegetative intermitotic
    b. Differentiating intermitotic
    c. Reverting postmitotic
    d. Fixed postmitotic

2. Long-term treatment with cytosine arabinoside (20 days) would have what effect on skin?

    a. Skin would become thinned.
    b. Number of mitotic figures in basal layer would decrease.
    c. Hair would stop growing.
    d. All of the above are correct.
    e. None of the above is correct.

3. Cells capable of synthesizing melanin pigment are called

    a. melanophores.
    b. melanocytes.
    c. chromatophores.
    d. none of the above.

4. Arrange in sequence from outside of body in

    __a__ Stratum corneum
    _____ Papillary layer
    _____ Stratum spinosum
    _____ Reticular layer
    _____ Stratum basale

5. Cells containing melanin granules are to be found in

    a. dermis.
    b. stratum spinosum.
    c. stratum basale.
    d. all of the above.
    e. none of the above.

Chapter 9

Cartilage, Bone, and Joints

GENERAL

Cartilage and bone are examples of specialized connective tissue. Bone is vascularized, but cartilage is avascular. Cartilage contains an antiangiogenesis factor, which prevents invasion of this tissue by blood vessels. Both bone and cartilage differentiate from mesoderm and mesenchyme. If a piece of cartilage is covered with an investment of fibrous connective tissue, this layer is called a *perichondrium.* If a piece of bone is covered by connective tissue, it is called a *periosteum.* The only exception to this rule is that of articular cartilage, which faces a joint cavity filled with synovial fluid. In this case there is no perichondrium.

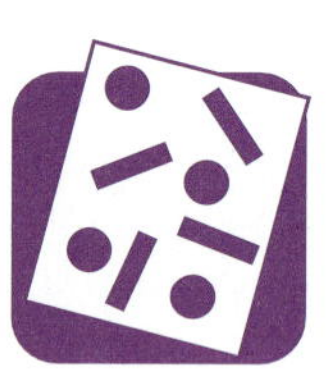

■ **Cartilage**

● **Cells** The cells of all types of cartilage are **chondrocytes.** They differentiate from stellate mesenchymal cells. During this differentiation the developing **chondroblasts** pull in their cytoplasmic processes and become round. Chondroblasts are the cells actually synthesizing and releasing the **intercellular matrix.** They contain significant amounts of RER and a prominent Golgi apparatus. Chondrocytes represent chondroblasts that have assumed a less active role. When chrondroblasts surround themselves with the intercellular matrix that they produce, they are forced to live in little lakes or **lacunae,** in the matrix.

● **Matrix** Extracellular fibers and an amorphous ground substance.

— *Fibers: Collagen (type II), elastic and reticular*

— *Ground substance*

  • Glycosaminoglycans (GAGs) of the proteoglycans
  • Hyaluronic acid
  • Chondroitin sulfate
  • Keratan sulfate

The sulfate groups are basophilic on H & E. The highest concentration of newly synthesized GAGs is in the matrix immediately surrounding the chondroblast or chrondrocyte. This rim of intense basophilia is the **capsular,** or **territorial, matrix.** The less basophilic matrix between adjacent areas of capsular or territorial matrix is **interterritorial matrix.**

— *Bound water* Chondroblasts and chondrocytes receive their nutrients, raw materials, oxygen, and so on, by diffusion through the water component of the ground substance. If this life line is compromised the cells will die. This cell death plays an important role in the process of endochondral ossification.

Because cartilage can survive quite well in avascular environments, pieces of articular cartilage that break off into the joint cavity have no trouble surviving and can live for years. In this situation they are called *joint mice.*

TYPES OF CARTILAGE

- **Hyaline** The matrix appears glassy and smooth in the light microscope, even though we know the matrix has collagen fibers in it. In fact, the matrix appears so smooth and glassy that if you were small enough you could ice skate on the interterritorial matrix without fear of tripping. Hyaline is found in most laryngeal cartilages, costal cartilages, tracheal rings, articular cartilages, and in the fetus as models of all of the long bones.

- **Elastic** The predominate fiber type is the elastic fiber, not the collagen fiber. The elastic fibers are discernible on H & E and are refractile if the slide is moved out of focus. Because of this, one would risk breaking a leg trying to ice skate on the interterritorial matrix of elastic cartilage. Elastic cartilage is found where a semirigid structure normally needs to be quite flexible, such as the core of the epiglottis, pinna of the external ear, and the cuneiform and corniculate cartilages of the larynx.

- **Fibrocartilage** In this type of cartilage the excessive amount of collagen fibers relative to the number of parenchymal cells (chondrocytes) imparts to it its name. Fibrocartilage is found in pubic symphysis and the intervertebral disks.

GROWTH OF CARTILAGE

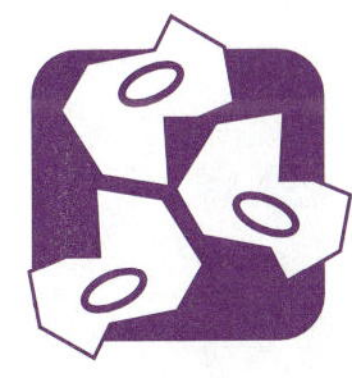

- **Interstitial Growth** Chondrocytes and chondroblasts undergo mitotic events while in their lacunae surrounded by matrix. Since they can't get out of the lacuna they were born in, they form **isogenic or isogenous groups** of cells. Growth in the length of the piece of cartilage by interstitial growth, e.g., hyaline cartilage model of a long bone in the fetus.

- **Appositional Growth** New cartilage cells and matrices are added onto the surface of the piece of cartilage by chondrogenic activity in the **perichondrium.** The outermost half of a perichondrium is the **fibrous perichondrium** and is fibrous connective tissue. The inner half of the perichondrium, or that part of the perichondrium closest to the cartilage itself, is the **chondrogenic layer** of the perichondrium. In this layer or region, undifferentiated mesenchymal cells continue to differentiate into chondroblasts and slowly add themselves and the matrix they produce to the outside of the piece of cartilage. The vessels contained within the perichondrium represent the source of nutrients, and they work by diffusion through the bound water of the ground substance for the chondrocytes and chondroblasts composing the piece of cartilage, which is avascular.

CALCIFICATION OF CARTILAGE

A normal process important for endochondral ossification in hyaline cartilage models of the long bones in a fetus and in the epiphyseal plate is *calcification.*

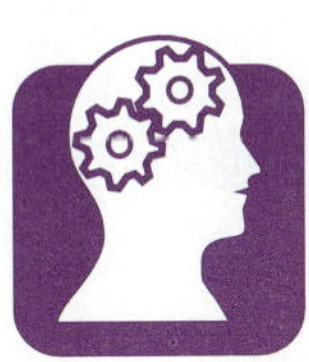

- **Mechanism** Chondrocyte **hypertrophies** and releases **alkaline phosphatase,** which increases the isoelectric point in the surrounding matrix. This causes the precipitation of **calcium phosphate** in the matrix. The nutrient supply to the chondrocyte is increasingly compromised by this calcification of the matrix. The chondrocyte dies (has committed suicide) and eventually disappears from its lacuna. Small pieces of calcified matrix dissolve. Larger or thicker pieces of the calcified matrix remain and become the scaffolding used in the process of endochondral ossification.

BONE: ADULT STRUCTURE

■ Cells

● **Osteoblasts** Osteoblasts differentiate from stellate mesenchymal cells; as this occurs, the cell keeps its stellate morphology, i.e., has cytoplasmic processes. This is in direct contrast to the differentiation of chondroblasts from stellate mesenchymal cells in which the cell pulls in its processes and rounds up. Osteoblasts are matrix makers by the synthesis of collagen fibers (type I) and **ground substance,** which contains **GAGs, glycoproteins, osteonectin** (anchors mineral component to collagen fibers), and **osteocalcin,** a calcium-binding protein. Osteoblasts contain prominent RER and Golgi body—so much RER that the cytoplasm is basophilic. Ground substance contains water, protein, and **mucopolysaccharide.**

The **osteoid** consists of the collagen fibers and the ground substance. It is an acidophilic material before it becomes mineralized. **Mineralization** of the matrix is not just calcification of osteoid; it involves the deposition of many different minerals to form **hydroxyapatite** crystals, $Ca_{10}(PO_4)_6(OH)_3$.

Vitamin C is necessary for the osteoblast to synthesize osteoid. **Vitamin D** is necessary for proper intestinal absorption of calcium.

Osteoblasts are found on the surface of a developing spicule of endochondral or intramembranous ossification. In this position they can add matrix to the surface of the developing spicule, i.e., a form of **appositional growth.**

● **Osteocytes** As osteoblasts synthesize and secrete osteoid around themselves, many of them get trapped or surrounded by matrix (like falling into wet cement with your arms and legs stuck out). Since they maintain their stellate shape, the matrix hardens around the cytoplasmic processes forming tiny tunnels or **canaliculi,** which contain cell processes.

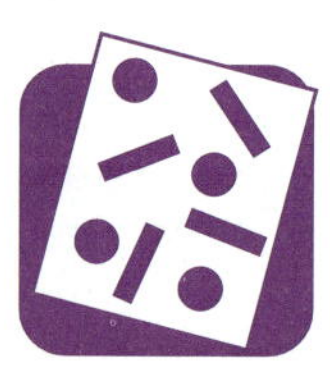

Osteocytes are the cells of bone trapped in little **lacunae** in the matrix, but with their "arms and legs" stuck out into the canaliculi. The cytoplasmic processes of adjacent osteocytes actually meet, contact, and form **gap junctions.** Between the plasmalemma of the osteocyte processes and the wall of the canaliculus is a small space that contains tissue fluid. The cytoplasm contains a small amount of RER because, relative to the osteoblast, the osteocyte is metabolically quite inactive.

Some metabolic activity accounts for their capability to remove some calcium from the matrix and thereby raise the blood calcium level. This process is **osteocytic osteolysis.** They are nondividing while in the osteocyte morphology; therefore there is no interstitial growth possible in bone.

● **Osteoclasts**

- Large, multinucleated, giant cells formed by the fusion of several **monocytes.**
- Major resorbers of bone matrix.
- Found on resorptive surfaces.
- Actually resorb out a depression in the surface they are "working on" or eroding (**Howship's lacuna**).
- Contain an extensive **ruffled border** on the resorptive surface of the cell.

- Many mitochondria, Golgi bodies, vesicles, and RER.
- Vesicles or lysosomes released between the ruffles.
- **Lysosomal hydrolyases** (collagenase) digest bone matrix and release minerals (calcium) in a locally acid environment.
- Nondividing but nuclear DNA synthesis without accompanying cytokinesis occurs.
- Resorptive activity is enhanced by the presence of **parathyroid hormone.**
- Resorptive activity is diminished by the presence of **calcitonin.**
- Easy to find on diaphyseal ends of spicules of endochondral bone and in **resorption tunnels** during the remodeling of adult compact bone.
- Neoplasm of these cells = osteoclastoma.

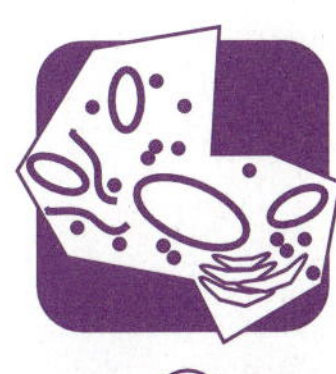

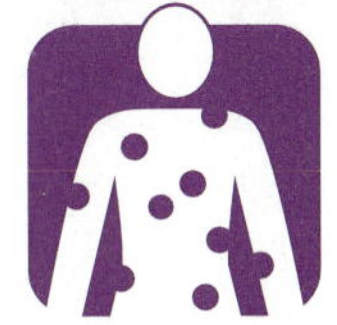

● **Osteoprogenitor or osteogenic cells** These are small spindle-shaped mesenchymal cells found on both the periosteal and endosteal surfaces of bone. On the inside of the fibrous layer of the vascular **periosteum,** the osteoprogenitor cells constitute the **osteogenic layer** of the periosteum. They constitute most of the **endosteum,** a single layer of osteogenic cells with osteoblasts and osteoclasts present in regions of bone resorption and can differentiate into osteoblasts. Malignancy of these cells leads to osteogenic sarcoma and may show some attempt at spicule formation.

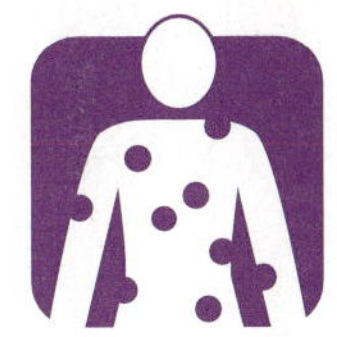

■ **Compact Bone (as in a Typical Long Bone)**

- Covered by a vascularized periosteum on the outside with its fibrous and osteogenic layers. Collagen fibers from the periosteum sweep into and get trapped in the matrix deep to the osteogenic layer of the periosteum. These **Sharpey's fibers** hold periosteum tightly to the bone matrix. Orthopedic surgeons use a periosteal elevator to cut Sharpey's fibers and elevate the periosteum from the surface of the bone.

- Lined by **endosteum** on all internal surfaces
- Matrix laid down in rows or **lamellae** with osteocytes trapped in lacunae throughout (Fig. 9.1). *Outer circumferential lamellae* are those produced by the osteogenic layer of the periosteum. These lamellae encircle the outer aspect of the bone. *Inner circumferential lamellae* are those produced by the endosteum and encircle the inner aspect of the bone, i.e., surround the marrow cavity. *Haversian lamellae* are found between the outer and inner circumferential lamellae. Haversian lamellae form concentric rings around a canal containing blood vessels and nerves. All of the concentric lamellae surrounding one Haversian canal, plus the canal itself, constitute a *Haversian system,* or *osteon. Interstitial lamellae* are chunks of older Haversian systems remaining after remodeling of compact bone by osteoclastic activity. Interstitial lamellae are the oldest lamellae of compact bone.

The **Haversian system,** or **osteon,** is a group of concentric lamellae surrounding a Haversian canal. The outer edge of an osteon is identifiable by the presence of a **cement line,** which is a thin zone of matrix that does not contain canaliculi. Haversian systems can be formed after osteoclasts resorb bone matrix in a **resorption tunnel.** The tunnel or hole in the bone is filled in from the outside toward the center. In this way the first and therefore the oldest lamella of bone in an osteon is that lamella just inside the cement line. The youngest lamella in an osteon would be the one surrounding the Haversian canal. Haversian systems run parallel to the long axis of the bone. **Volkmann's canals** are tunnels in compact bone that carry blood vessels and nerves at various angles

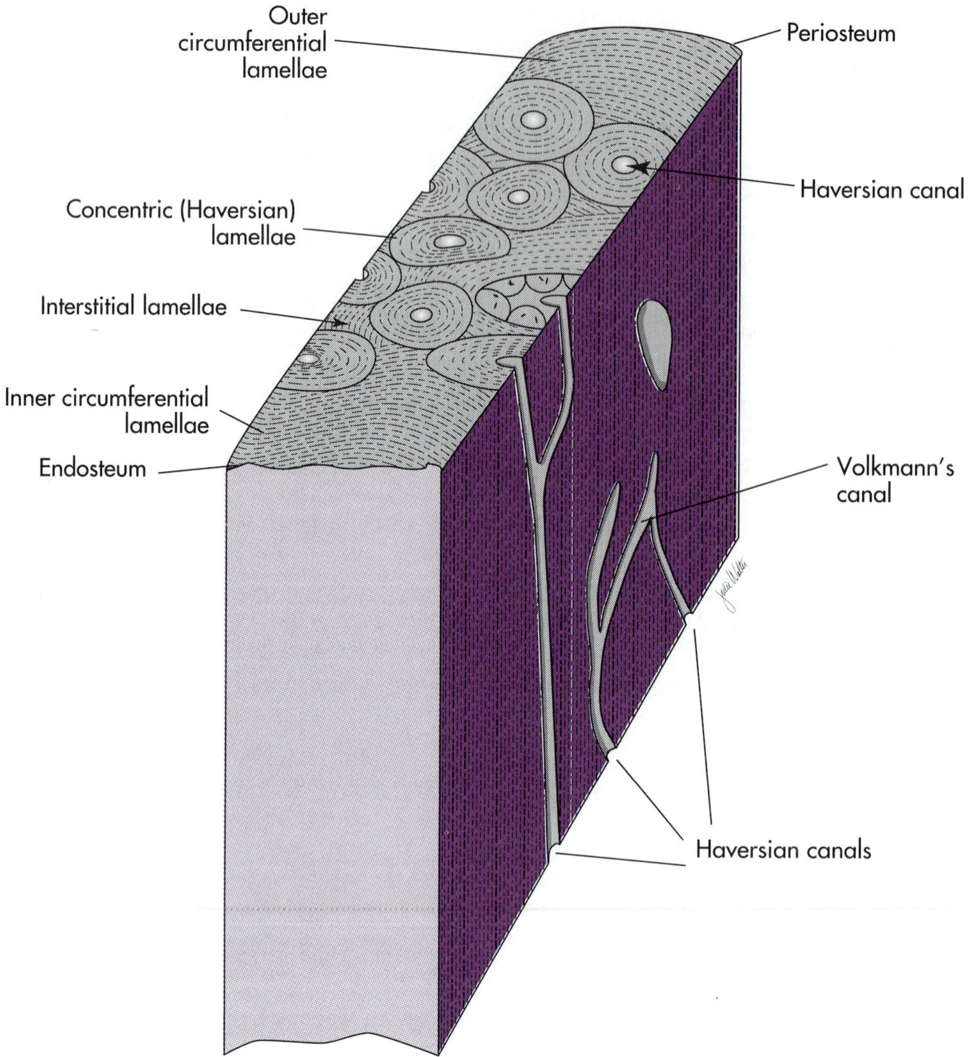

Fig. 9.1 Diagram of a section through the diaphysis of a long bone. The endosteal or bone marrow or internal surface faces toward us. The periosteal surface faces away from us.

from one osteon to the next. Volkmann's canals are not surrounded by concentric lamellae.

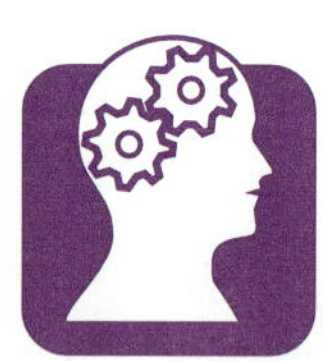

- **Remodeling of compact bone** Osteoclasts gather and resorb matrix, "cutting" a tunnel in compact bone in a fashion similar to drilling a hole in a rock with the drill bit being the area of concentration of the osteoclasts, i.e., the **cutting cone.** This proceeds generally parallel to the long axis of the bone. Behind the cutting cone is a **closing cone** in which osteoblasts begin to lay down matrix from the periphery of the newly formed tunnel toward the center, eventually forming a Haversian canal.

Cancellous or Spongy Bone

- Spicules of bone surfaced by endosteum
- Bone marrow is present between spicules
- A component of both endochondral and intramembranous ossification in the fetus
- Also found adjacent to the epiphyseal plate

INTRAMEMBRANOUS OSSIFICATION

Mesenchyme differentiates directly into cancellous bone, which can become compact bone without an intervening cartilage step. Stellate mesenchymal cells differentiate into osteoblasts, which make osteoid, and some cells get trapped to become osteocytes and some cells stay on the surface of the spicule as osteoblasts. The first or oldest osteoid produced slowly becomes mineralized; therefore the center of the developing spicule has a basophilic color relative to the acidophilic color of the fresh, unmineralized osteoid lying adjacent to and underneath the osteoblasts on the surface of the spicule. Spicules anastomose with each other and get remodeled by osteoclastic activity. Anastomosing spicules eventually enclose mesenchymal areas, which contain blood vessels and nerves. **Appositional deposition** can be greatest on the side of the spicule nearest the vessels and nerves and thereby form an immature osteon.

First bone, or **immature bone,** is not obviously lamellar; collagen fibers are randomly arranged and loosely packaged giving a woven appearance (**woven bone**), and there are many more osteocytes per unit of area of matrix than those in mature bone. Immature bone found mostly in the fetus gets "reworked" or "remodeled" into mature or lamellar bone in which the collagen fibers in each lamella all run in the same direction, which is different from collagen fibers in the adjacent lamellae. The cell density in mature bone is less than in immature bone. Flat bones of the cranial vault are produced by this type of ossification.

ENDOCHONDRAL OSSIFICATION

The hyaline cartilage model of a long bone is surrounded by a perichondrium, except at the ends where **articular cartilage** will form. The entire composition of the model is chondrocytes and matrix. The model increases in length by **interstitial growth** and in width by **appositional growth**. The perichondrium becomes vascularized, and this vascularization probably induces the differentiation of osteoblasts in this region, thereby changing the perichondrium to a periosteum. The osteogenic layer of this new periosteum produces a collar of bone of the intramembranous type around the diaphysis.

With bone deposition on the outside of the collar and bone resorption on the inside of the collar, the thickness of the collar can be maintained, and at the same time the diameter of the diaphyseal marrow cavity will increase. Variations in bone deposition and resorption of the **diaphyseal collar** can result in increasing or decreasing its thickness.

A vascular bud, the **periosteal bud,** develops in the diaphyseal periosteum and invades into the center of the hyaline cartilage model where chondrocytes are dying and cartilage matrix is calcifying (Fig. 9.2). In the center of the hyaline cartilage model, chondrocytes hypertrophy, calcify their neighboring matrix, and die, leaving empty lacunae and spicules of calcified cartilage. Osteoprogenitor cells accompany the periosteal bud as it invades the center of the model. Osteogenic cells leave the periosteal bud and and attach themselves to the surfaces of the spicules of calcified cartilage. Thus a **primary center of endochondral ossification** is formed. Pin piercing this from outside of the spicule to the core of the spicule = osteogenic cell→calcified cartilage.

Once on the surface of the spicule of calcified cartilage the osteogenic cells differentiate into osteoblasts, which begin to lay down fresh, or unmineralized, osteoid (acidophilic). Pin piercing this = osteoblast→fresh osteoid→calcified cartilage.

As time proceeds, the amount of osteoid deposited on the spicule of calcified cartilage increases and the first or oldest osteoid produced becomes mineralized (basophilic). Pin piercing this = osteoblast→unmineralized osteoid→mineralized osteoid→calcified cartilage (Fig. 9.3).

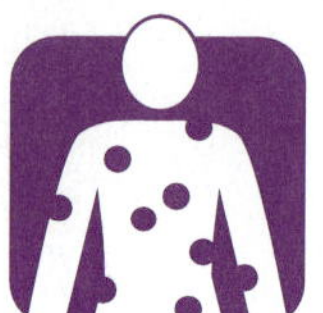

• If there is a vitamin C deficiency, very little matrix is present, but there is mineralization of what has been produced. **Vitamin C deficiency = scurvy** (the "c" in scurvy provides a hint which leads to vitamin "C" and "c"ollagen).

• If there is a **vitamin D deficiency,** lots of unmineralized matrix is present because of the presence of vitamin C, but this matrix cannot be mineralized, thus producing **rickets** ("D" provides a hint for *"d"* calcification).

The endochondral process proceeds toward both epiphyseal ends of the bone. Chondrocytes proliferate by interstitial growth, their progeny hypertrophy and

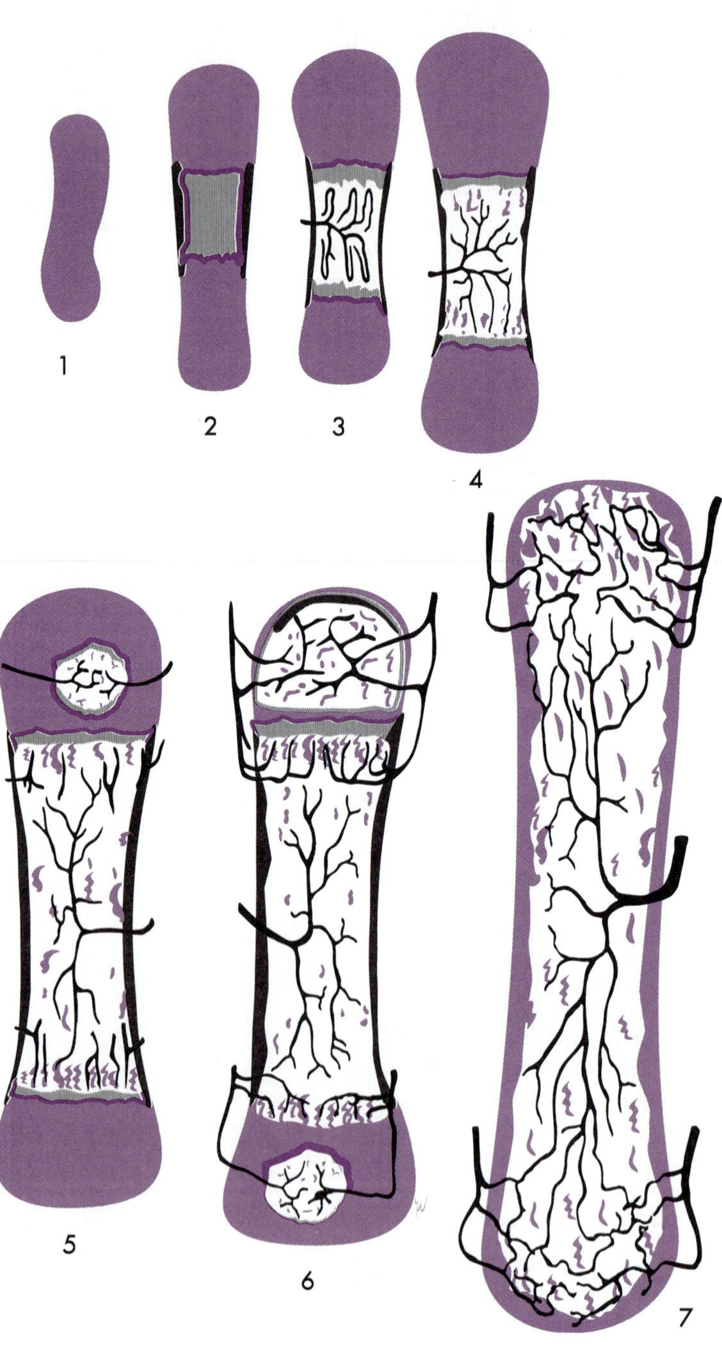

Fig. 9.2 Diagram of the different steps in the development of a long bone. *1,* Hyaline cartilage model of the future bone is differentiated from area mesenchyme. *2,* A periosteal collar of intramembranous bone has differentiated from the connective tissue surrounding the center of the model. The center of the cartilaginous model has undergone calcification because of hypertrophy of the chondrocytes in this region. *3,* Blood vessels and connective tissue cells have invaded the spaces (primitive marrow cavity) created by the death of the chondrocytes caused by the earlier calcification of the matrix. This establishes the primary center of ossification. *4,* Endochondral ossification proceeds outward toward both ends of the cartilage model, progressively enlarging the marrow cavity at the expense of the hyaline cartilage of the original model. The dark line and areas represent regions of hypertrophied-calcified cartilage undergoing endochondral ossification. *5,* A secondary center of ossification forms in the upper epiphyseal region. *6,* Further development of the secondary center of ossification fashions an epiphyseal plate of hyaline cartilage between the epiphyseal and the diaphyseal centers of ossification. A little later another epiphyseal center of ossification forms in the lower epiphyses. This will also form an epiphyseal plate. The bone will grow in length by endochondral ossification in these epiphyseal plates until the adult height of the individual is established. *7,* Then the epiphyseal plates disappear, i.e., closure of the epiphyses.

die, and the naked spicules of calcified cartilage are used as a lattice for the deposition of bone matrix. In this way the model of the long bone increases in length at the same time that endochondral ossification is increasing in the primary center of ossification. Ends of the spicules of endochondral bone are resorbed by osteoclasts leaving an ever-increasing diaphyseal marrow cavity.

After birth **secondary or epiphyseal centers of ossification** appear in both epiphyses. This isolates a strip of hyaline cartilage between the diaphyseal and epiphyseal centers of ossification; this is the **epiphyseal plate.** Epiphysis will increase in length by interstitial growth in the articular cartilage followed by endochondral ossification of this new cartilage in the secondary (epiphyseal) center of ossification.

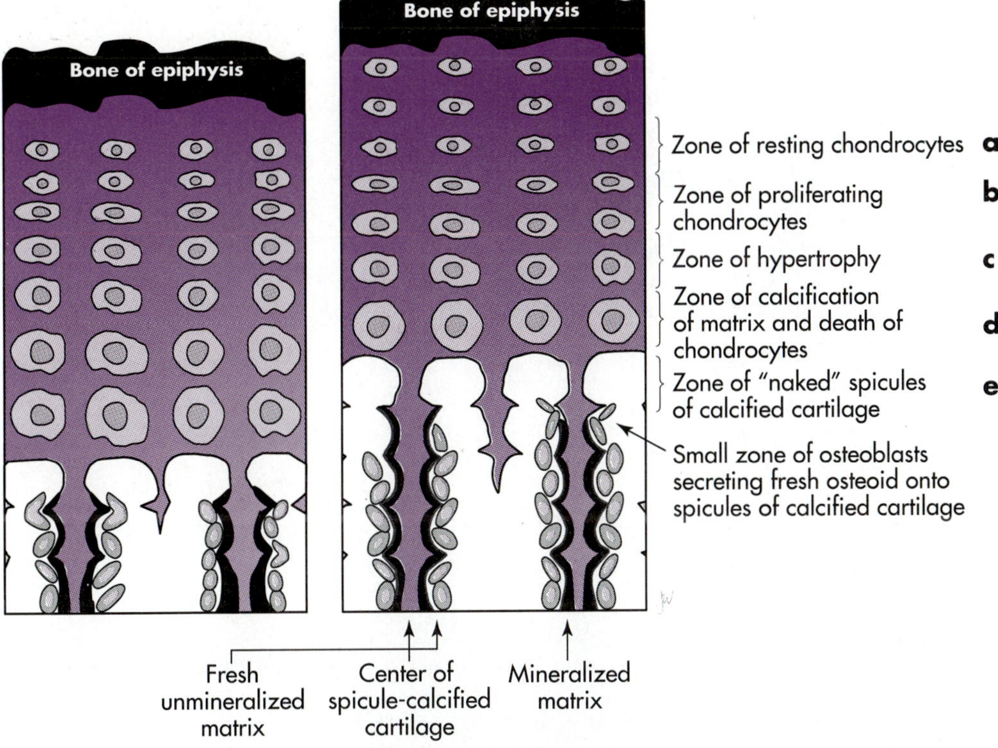

Fig. 9.3 Two views of the same region of endochondral ossification in an epiphyseal plate in a growing long bone. The diagram on the left is earlier in time than that on the right. From the bone of the epiphysis, extending through the epiphyseal plate of hyaline cartilage to the epiphyseal bone marrow cavity one can distinguish several zones: a, zone of resting chondrocytes; b, zone of proliferating chondrocytes; c, zone of hypertrophied chondrocytes; d, zone of calcified cartilage matrix and dying chondrocytes, and e, the zone of spicules of calcified cartilage temporarily not covered (naked) by any cell. Then osteoblasts attach themselves to the surface of the calcified spicules and begin to secrete unmineralized osteoid onto the surface of the calcified spicule of cartilage. In hematoxylin and eosin–stained sections fresh osteoid is eosinophilic. In time, the first osteoid produced (now the oldest), which is closest to the calcified cartilage, becomes mineralized and takes on a basophilic tint. At the bottom of each diagram, mature spicules of endochondral ossification can be seen. Each has a central core of calcified cartilage, covered by an increasingly larger region of mineralized osteoid in turn surfaced by a thin layer of fresh, unmineralized osteoid and then surfaced by osteoblasts. At the diaphyseal end of these spicules of endochondral bone formation one would find (not illustrated) osteoclasts "eating" the newly formed spicules, thereby forming the enlarging, diaphyseal marrow cavity.

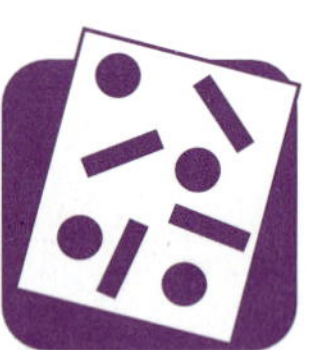

■ Epiphyseal Plate (Fig. 9.4)

- Responsible for most of the growth in length of a long bone
- Positioned between the epiphyseal and diaphyseal marrow cavities
- Composed of several zones from epiphyseal to diaphyseal side

1. **Zone of resting cartilage**
2. **Zone of proliferating cartilage** (interstitial growth)
3. **Zone of hypertrophying cartilage** (alkaline phosphatase)
4. **Zone of calcifying cartilage** matrix and dying or dead chondrocytes
5. **Zone of ossification** where osteoblasts attached themselves to naked spicules of calcified cartilage and begin to deposit osteoid

By continuous addition of new cartilage to the epiphyseal plate at one end, there is the eventual replacement of this cartilage by endochondral ossification at

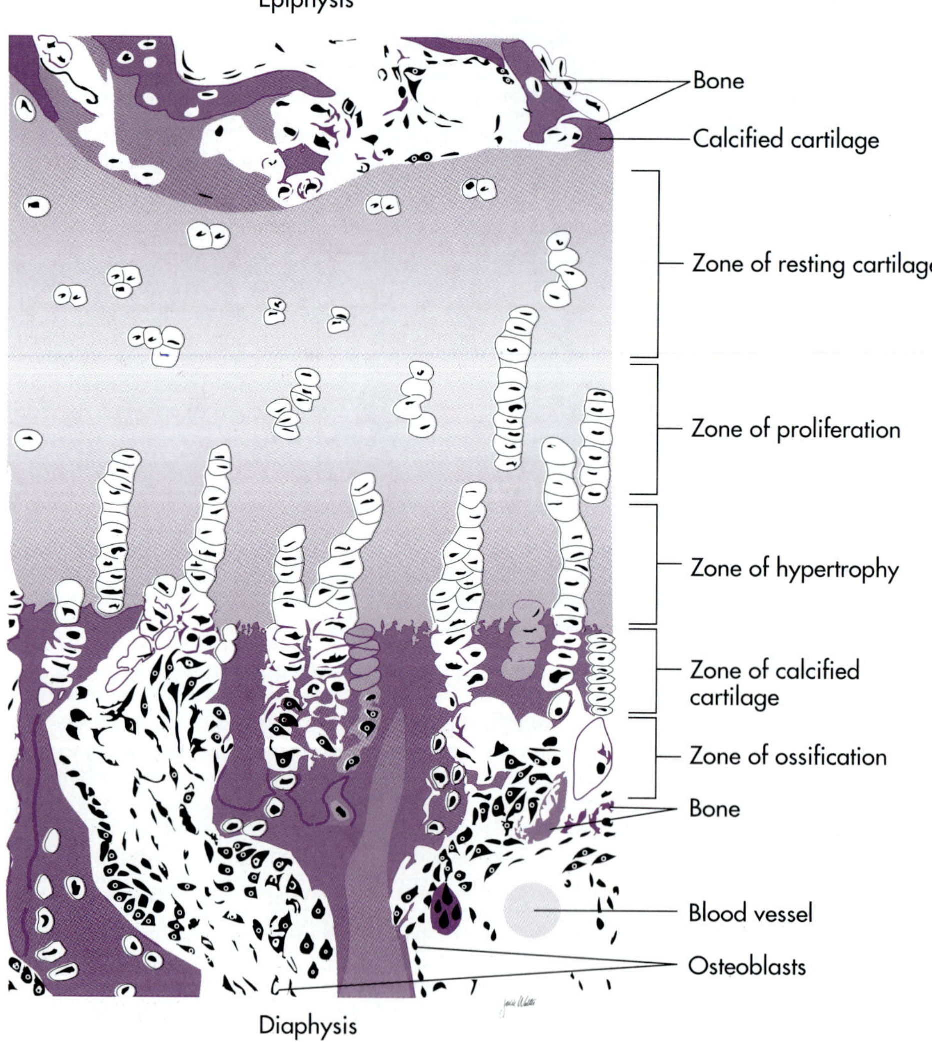

Fig. 9.4 Lower power view of endochondral ossification in an epiphyseal plate placed between an epiphysis and the diaphysis of a long bone. At the very top is the epiphyseal marrow cavity, and at the bottom is the diaphyseal marrow cavity.

the other end. Most of this new cancellous bone is removed forming an enlarging diaphyseal marrow cavity; thus the length of the bone increases, but the thickness of the epiphyseal plate remains the same. Epiphyseal plates become nonfunctional during the mid-20s and lead to **closure of the epiphyses.** In some small long bones there are no epiphyseal plates. In this case the articular cartilage serves as a kind of epiphyseal plate.

■ Functions of Bone

- Skeleton of body, **physical support**
- **Protection** of vital organs (brain, heart, lungs, liver, etc.)
- Home for red and yellow bone marrow
- **Calcium reservoir**

Because of constant remodeling, bone is replaced completely. Haversian systems can be resorbed and completely replaced in a matter of years.

Excessive amount of resorption leads to **osteoporosis.**

Excessive amount of deposition leads to **osteopetrosis.**

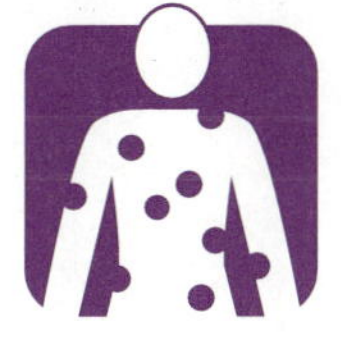

Broken Bones

- **Fracture** occurs, of which there are several types.
- **Thrombus** forms at the wound site.
- PMNs and macrophages arrive and remove debris.
- Broken blood vessels in the region of the break cause **anoxia** of the bone matrix distal to loss of blood supply.

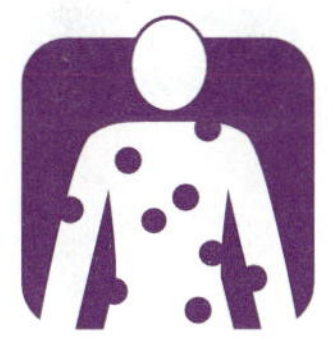

Osteocytes die in osteons. Vascularization of both endosteum and periosteum is better than in osteons, and so osteogenic capabilities of endosteum and periosteum remain. Osteoprogenitor cells in endosteum and periosteum differentiate into chondroblasts and chondrocytes.

A cartilagenous bridge, or **callus,** forms across the break. **External callus** bridges or covers the break on the outside; the cell source is from periosteum. **Internal callus** bridges the break internally, the cell source is mostly from endosteum. Hyaline cartilage of the callus turns into cancellous bone by means of endochondral ossification. Cancellous bone eventually is remodeled into compact bone. Stress forces (weight bearing) eventually cause remodeling of the ossified callus area to original architecture, and the callus slowly disappears. **Wolff's law** states that a bone develops the structure most suited to resist the forces acting on it.

Types of Joints

- ● **Classification of different types**
    - — *Synarthrosis*
        Syndesmoses. Bone joined to bone by dense fibrous connective tissue; e.g. sutures of the skull during childhood
        Synchrondroses. Bone joined to bone by cartilage; epiphyseal plate
        Synostoses. Bone joined to bone by bone; sutures of skull in adult
        Symphysis. Bone joined to bone by fibrocartilage; pubic symphysis
    - — *Diarthrosis* **Synovial** joints have **synovial fluid** in them
        - Articular cartilage surfaces oppose each other

- No perichondrium on articular surface
- Collagen fibers in cartilage matrix closest to synovial fluid; run parallel to each other
- Deep to the parallel layer; run in arches or arcades
- Fibrous joint capsule spans joint.
- **Synovial membrane** on inner aspect of joint capsule

  1. Innermost layer of synovial cells (not an epithelium)
     - Cells secrete hyaluronic acid
     - Can be phagocytic
     - Play a role in allowing dialysate of blood to enter joint cavity and help form synovial fluid

  2. Supporting layer to synovial cell layer
     - Fibrous type withstands pressure
     - Areolar type allows sliding
     - Adipose type is more of a cushion
     - Some synovial joints have varying shaped cushions of fibrocartilage in them called **menisci**

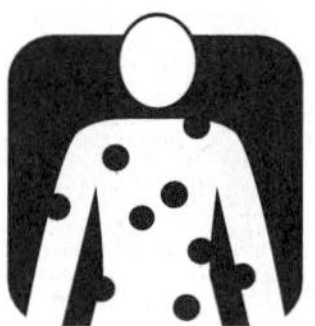

— *Osteoarthritis* Degeneration of articular cartilage with age is accompanied by inflammation, which causes pain and stiffness.

MULTIPLE CHOICE REVIEW QUESTIONS

1. Volkmann's canals

   a. contain the processes of osteocytes.
   b. interconnect lacunae.
   c. interconnect Haversian canals.
   d. are components of a Haversian canal.
   e. are components of interstitial lamellae.

2. The cells in a developing long bone that are most sensitive to growth hormone are

   a. in the zone of calcifying cartilage.
   b. in the zone of proliferating cartilage.
   c. in the periosteum.
   d. the osteoblasts of the metaphysis.
   e. the osteoclasts.

3. Arrange the following regions in proper sequence for a pin passing through the diaphysis of a long bone from skeletal muscle on the outside to bone marrow on the inside: 1 = skeletal muscle; 2 = endosteum, 3 = osteogenic layer of periosteum, 4 = Haversian canal, 5 = inner circumferential lamellae, 6 = megakaryocyte.

   a. 1-2-3-4-5-6
   b. 1-2-3-5-4-6
   c. 1-3-4-5-2-6
   d. 1-3-5-2-4-6
   e. 1-4-3-5-2-6

4. Arrange the following in correct sequence for a pin passing into the center of a developing spicule of endochondral bone from the bone marrow outside the spicule: 1 = promyelocyte, 2 = fresh, unmineralized osteoid, 3 = osteoblast, 4 = calcified cartilage, 5 = mineralized osteoid.

   a. 1-3-2-5-4
   b. 1-2-3-4-5
   c. 1-2-5-3-4
   d. 1-5-3-4-2
   e. 1-4-3-2-5

5. Exocytosis of lysosomal hydrolyases so that they can be effective in an acid environment is best associated with which of the following?

   a. Hypertrophied chondrocyte
   b. Osteocyte performing osteocytic osteolysis
   c. Osteoprogenitor cell
   d. Osteoclast
   e. Osteogenic cell in osteogenic layer of perichondrium

Chapter 10

Respiratory System

GENERAL

The respiratory system has two major divisions.

- A **conducting portion** in which no gas exchange occurs. This is a system of chambers and tubes designed to remain patent so air can be delivered to the respiratory portion in which actual gas exchange occurs. It is composed of the **nasal cavity, nasopharynx, oropharynx, larynx, trachea, bronchi,** and the **bronchioles** through the **terminal bronchioles.**
- A **respiratory division** that begins with the respiratory bronchioles, which have alveoli in their walls, and includes the **alveolar ducts, alveolar sacs,** and the individual **alveoli.** Gas exchange occurs between air in the alveolus and blood in the capillaries in the alveolar wall.

Respiratory epithelium lines most of the larger conducting structures. **Pseudo-stratified ciliated columnar epithelium** (PCCE) with mucus-producing **goblet cells** contains 4 cell types in addition to the mucus-producing goblet cell (Fig. 10.1):

- **Ciliated columnar cells**
- **Columnar cells with no cilia** but microvilli **(brush cell)**
- **Undifferentiated basal cells,** which are the source for the other cell types
- Small granule containing **neuroendocrine cells,** which release catecholamine

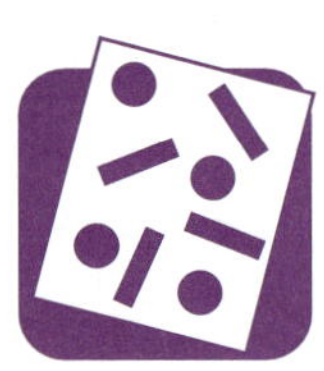

The goblet cells secret a mucus film, which traps inhaled particles such as dust particles, pollen granules, and bacteria. The mucus film is moved by the action of the cilia. The cilia beat toward the oropharynx whether the conducting structure is superior or inferior to the oropharynx. At the oropharynx the constantly arriving mucus film is swallowed.

The tall PCCE epithelium changes over to a progressively shorter and thinner epithelium as one proceeds down the narrower conducting structures into the respiratory structures, ending with a very thin simple squamous epithelium lining the inside of each alveolus.

Under the epithelial lining of the larger structures of the respiratory system is the **lamina propria,** a typical loose areolar connective tissue area containing many defense system cell types such as plasma cells, lymphocytes, macrophages, mast cells, eosinophils, and neutrophils. Inspired air contains many bacteria, viruses, and other foreign substances; it is no surprise to find lymphoid tissue here.

NASAL CAVITY AND NASOPHARYNX

Spaces are lined with PCCE under which the lamina propria contains mucous and serous glands. The lamina propria contains a large number of blood vessels, which help to warm the inspired air. The watery secretion of the serous glands helps to moisten the inspired air.

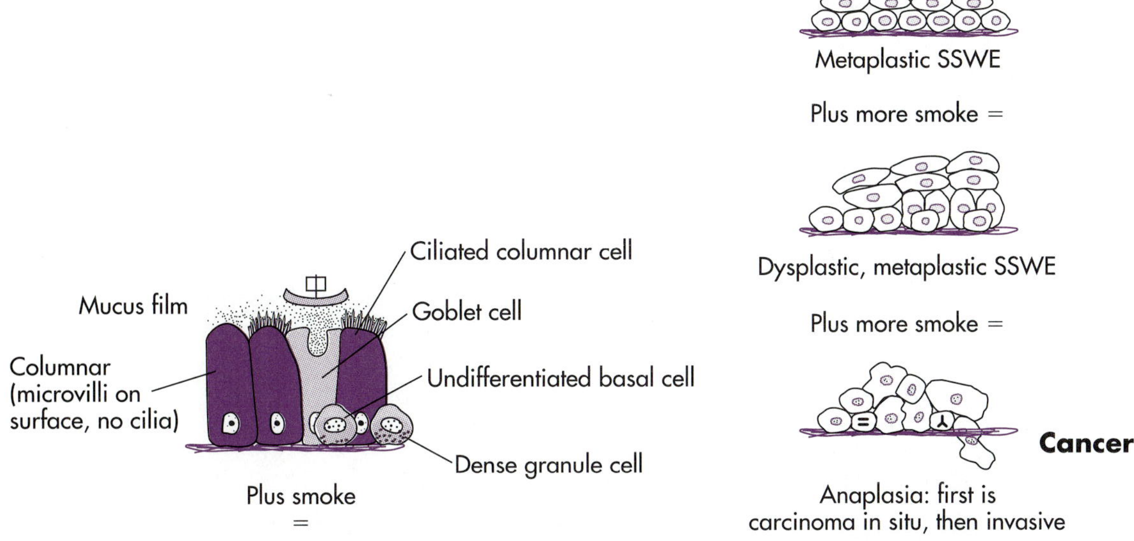

Fig. 10.1 Changes in the pseudostratified ciliated columnar epithelium with goblet cells that occur during smoking. In the normal "respiratory" epithelium, five cell types are found: mucus-producing goblet cell; undifferentiated basal stem cell; columnar brush cells, which have an apical surface devoid of cilia but full of microvilli; columnar ciliated cells, which have cilia and some microvilli on their apical surface; and dense granule cells, which are neuroendocrine cells. The mucus film traps inhaled particles such as dust and bacteria. The mucus film is constantly moved toward the oropharynx by the action of the cilia. In the presence of cigarette smoke the normal epithelium undergoes changes from metaplasia to dysplasia to anaplasia. *SSWE,* Stratified squamous wet epithelium.

In the superior aspect of each of the nasal cavities lies the **olfactory mucosa,** which is an organ of special sense. The olfactory mucosa is discussed in Chapter 20.

All regions of the nasopharynx are lined by PCCE except for those areas that experience wear and tear, such as the uvula. Here the PCCE is replaced by nature's toughest "wear-and-tear" wet epithelium, stratified squamous wet epithelium (SSWE).

Larynx

The **epiglottis** is the superior extension of the larynx. Since it folds on itself and closes the glottis during swallowing, it is both a component of the conducting portion of the respiratory system and a digestive system structure. It has a core of elastic cartilage surrounded by a lamina propria, which in turn is surfaced by either PCCE or SSWE depending on whether the surface is involved in a digestive function such as transport of food over its surface or is a respiratory structure. The anterior or lingual aspect of the epiglottis is covered by SSWE for it is this surface that is exposed to food during swallowing when the epiglottis folds posteriorly on itself to close the glottis. The SSWE continues inferiorly on the posterior or pharyngeal surface about halfway down the organ. The inferior half is covered with PCCE.

Two **vocal folds** on each side are separated by a space, the **laryngeal ventricle.**

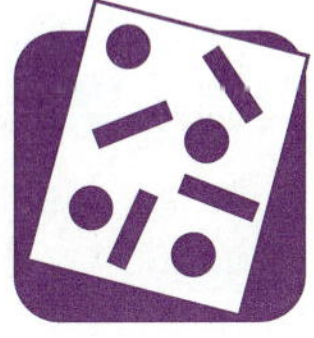

- **False vocal folds** are the superior pair of folds. They do not play a role in phonation, are covered by PCCE, and have a lamina propria of loose areolar connective tissue that contains seromucous glands.

- **True vocal folds** are involved in phonation and are surfaced by SSWE on their apices but PCCE elsewhere. The lamina propria is devoid of seromucous glands but does contain a mass of elastic tissue, the **vocal ligament.** Deep to the vocal ligament lies a mass of skeletal muscle, the **vocalis muscle.**

TRACHEA AND EXTRAPULMONARY BRONCHI

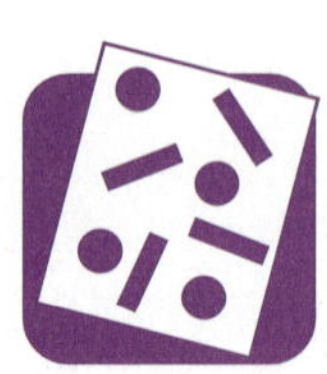

These organs are lined by a mucosa that contains a PCCE with a distinct histologic basement membrane overlying a typical lamina propria. At the interface between the lamina propria and the underlying submucosa there is a concentration of elastic fibers forming an **elastic membrane.** The submucosa contains seromucous glands. Deep to the submucosa is a C-shaped mass of hyaline cartilage covered by a perichondrium. The opening in the C faces posteriorly and is bridged by smooth muscle (**trachealis**). Outside of the perichondrium is a typical adventitia.

INTRAPULMONARY BRONCHI

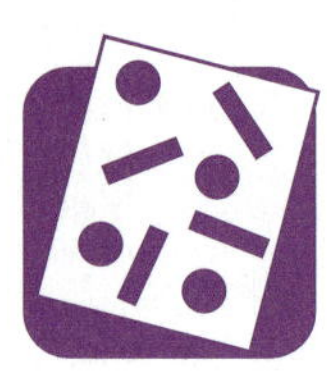

The robust structures and layers of the large conducting structures need to be removed as we move out the respiratory tree. The first indication of this "getting thinner" routine is that the C-shaped masses of hyaline cartilage break up into blocks of hyaline cartilage, which then get progressively smaller. All the other histologic layers of the main bronchi also begin to diminish in thickness, and even the PCCE begins to decrease in height. This lessening of everything continues until the conducting structure reached contains no cartilage in its wall, i.e., the bronchiole.

BRONCHIOLES

In these conducting structures, in addition to the loss of the cartilage, there are no seromucous glands, the epithelium is now a ciliated columnar to cuboidal epithelium, and there remains a significant amount of smooth muscle. The presence of smooth muscle and the absence of cartilage sets the scene for possible collapse of the bronchioles if the tonus of the smooth muscle is excessive as in the case of an asthma attack.

The last member or branch of the conducting tree is the **terminal bronchiole.** It terminates into the first component of the respiratory division or the respiratory bronchiole. Terminal bronchioles still contain ciliated cuboidal cells, but mucus-producing goblet cells and glands are absent. It is very important to have cilia farther out the tree than mucus production because this permits movement of the mucus film by the cilia from deep in the lung. If the opposite were true, i.e., mucus production deeper into the lung than cilia, pneumonia would result.

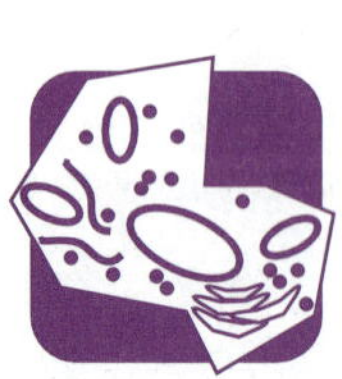

In the bronchiolar epithelium a special cell type is present, the **Clara cells.** They increase in number as the ciliated cells decrease in number as one proceeds out the bronchiolar tree. Clara cells have a dome-shaped apex and are ultrastructurally sophisticated, having well developed SER, RER, Golgi body, and secretory granules. They secrete a **lipoprotein,** which is a surface-active agent preventing collapse of the terminal bronchioles especially during exhalation.

Respiratory bronchioles have a general structural plan similar to the terminal bronchiole with one major difference and that is the presence of alveoli. This makes this structure the first member of the respiratory division. Between the alveoli in the wall of the respiratory bronchiole are tabs of smooth muscle. Clara cells are more frequent than ciliated low cuboidal cells. Each respiratory bronchiole and its subsequent divisions, i.e., the **alveolar ducts, alveolar sacs,** and individual **alveoli,** compose a pulmonary lobule.

At the center of a **pulmonary lobule** is a respiratory bronchiole that is accompanied by a branch of the **pulmonary artery** bringing **deoxygenated blood** into the capillary bed of the lobule. The veins that drain the respiratory lobule are located at its periphery, which is discernible by the presence of a small amount of delicate connective tissue. On a good chest film one can see delicate connective tissue extensions arise from the visceral pleura and enter the lung parenchyma. This is the connective tissue that is at the periphery of the respiratory lobule.

ALVEOLI

The alveolus is the structural and functional unit of the lung. The respiratory bronchioles give way to **alveolar ducts,** which are elongated airways that communicate with **alveolar sacs.** An alveolar sac has a bunch of alveoli opening into it. The entire system is designed to bring air and deoxygenated blood together for gaseous exchange in the alveolus.

There are about 300 million alveoli per lung. Alveoli are actually air spaces. They can open into an alveolar sac, an alveolar duct, or the lumen of a respiratory bronchiole.

The septum, or partition, between adjacent alveoli is the **interalveolar septum,** which contains capillaries supported by elastic and reticular fibers. The interalveolar septum has **pores (of Kohn)** through which adjacent alveoli normally share air but, in pneumonia, can share bacteria.

Facing the air in the alveolus is a very thin simple squamous epithelium, the cells of which are **type I pneumonocytes.** These cells have a basal lamina, which may or may not be fused with the basal lamina of the endothelial cell of the alveolar capillary in the thinnest portion of the interalveolar septum. Collagen, elastic, or reticular fibers can be interposed between the pneumonocytes and the endothelium making this region of the interalveolar septum thicker and less efficient in gaseous exchange.

Another type of pneumonocyte, the **type II pneumonocyte,** or **great alveolar cell,** can be found mixed in with the type I pneumonocytes lining the alveolus. Although there are equal numbers of type I and type II pneumonocytes in an alveolus, the type II cells constitute only about 5% of the surface area of the alveolus, with the other 95% being accounted for by the type I pneumonocytes because they are so thin and cover so much more surface area. Type II pneumonocytes are secretory cells that bulge into the alveolus in a manner reminiscent of how Clara cells bulge into the lumen of the bronchioles. Type II pneumonocytes have granules in their apical cytoplasm that have a lamellar arrangement within them and therefore are called **lamellar bodies.** They contain **phospholipids,** which after secretion coat the surface of the type I pneumonocytes and serve to decrease the surface tension. This surface active agent is **surfactant.** With less than normal amounts of surfactant the surface tension in the alveoli would be great enough that the alveoli would collapse on expiration.

RESPIRATORY DISTRESS SYNDROME (RDS)

RDS is a condition found in premature infants in which the surfactant-producing cells have not fully differentiated and the amount of surfactant is minimal. RDS is a common cause of death in premature infants. It can be treated by giving surfactant to the infant. For this treatment surfactant has been isolated from minced animal lungs and from human amniotic fluid.

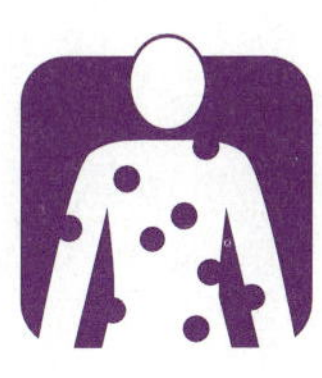

AIR-BLOOD BARRIER

We now review the histophysiology of gaseous exchange by tracing the path a molecule of oxygen has to take from air in the alveolus to hemoglobin in the RBC across the air-blood barrier (Fig. 10.2).

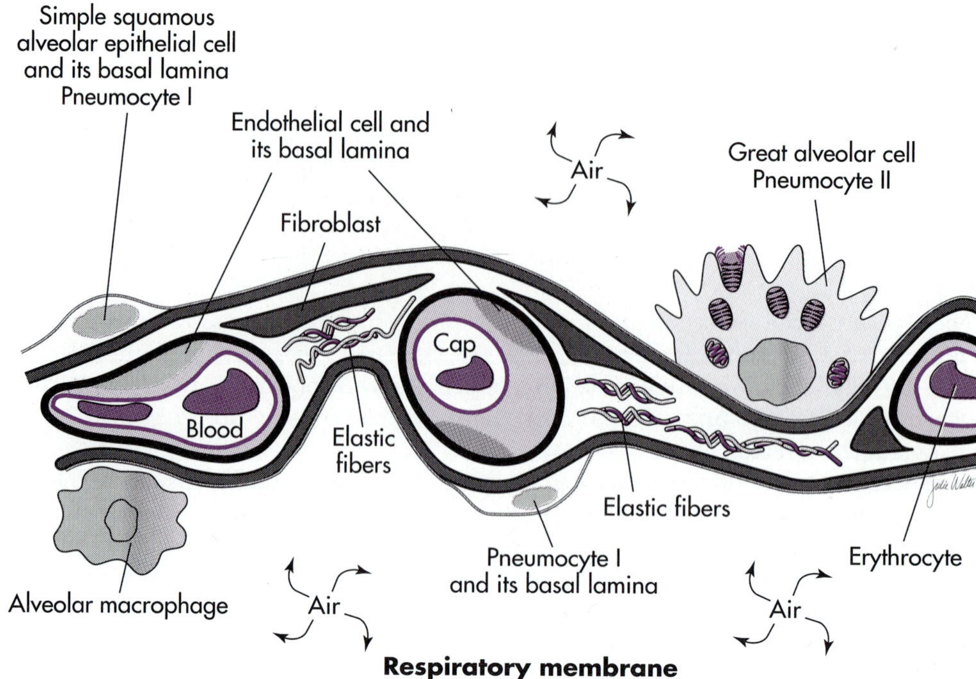

Fig. 10.2 The respiratory membrane or the structures interposed between the blood-air interface in the interalveolar septum. The most efficient region for the transport of gases from air to blood and vice versa is where this membrane is thinnest, i.e., absence of nucleus of pneumonocyte I, great alveolar cell, or alveolar macrophage. The structures involved from air to blood are surfactant, thin strip of pneumonocyte I cytoplasm and its associated cell membrane, basal lamina of pneumonocyte I, basal lamina of endothelial cell, endothelial cell cytoplasm, and its associated cell membrane, blood.

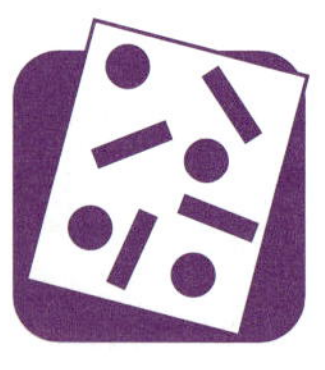

Air→surfactant→plasmalemma of type I pneumonocyte→0.1 to 0.2 micrometers of type I pneumonocyte cytoplasm→plasmalemma of type I pneumonocyte→basal lamina of type I pneumonocyte→basal lamina of endothelium→plasmalemma of endothelium→endothelial cell cytoplasm→plasmalemma of endothelium→blood plasma→plasmalemma of RBC. Carbon dioxide follows the same path but in reverse order.

ALVEOLAR MACROPHAGES

Alveolar macrophages, or **dust cells,** are unique examples of tissue macrophages because instead of wandering around within connective tissue looking for something to eat, in the alveolus they wander over the surface of the alveolus ingesting bacteria and other inhaled particles.

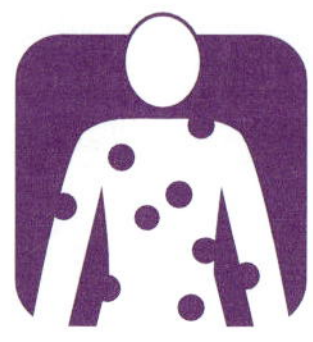

In the smoker's lung the alveolar macrophages ingest the tar or carbon particles associated with smoking. A similar situation exists in the coal miner's lung. However, the alveolar macrophages do not contain "carbonase" (there is no such enzyme) in their lysosomes, and therefore they cannot digest what they ingest. They fill up with this undigested material and give the smoker's lung or the coal miner's lung its permanent black appearance.

In a patient with, e.g., left **heart failure,** the normal amount of blood is not moving through the left side of the heart (defective mitral valve). Blood flow becomes sluggish through the lungs, and the alveolar capillaries become congested, resulting in **chronic passive congestion** or CPC. This results in hypoxia to the endo-thelium, which responds by becoming leaky and leaks tissue fluid into the interal-veolar septum and eventually into the lumen of the alveolus (**pulmonary edema**—the patient actually is drowning in his or her own fluid). RBCs will die in the alveo-lar capillaries in CPC, and the alveolar macrophages will ingest these RBCs. As the macrophage digests the ingested RBC, it demonstrates the presence of a brownish, not black, breakdown product of hemoglobin, or **hemosiderin.** In this situation the alveolar macrophages are **hemosiderinophages,** or "**heart failure**" cells. In fact, a slide of a lung from such a pathophysiologic situation affords an excellent way to demonstrate lung macrophages.

PLEURA

The **visceral** and **parietal** pleura are sheets of mesothelium with an underlying sub-mesothelial connective tissue, which in the visceral pleura is rich in elastic fibers. The two pleura slide over each other.

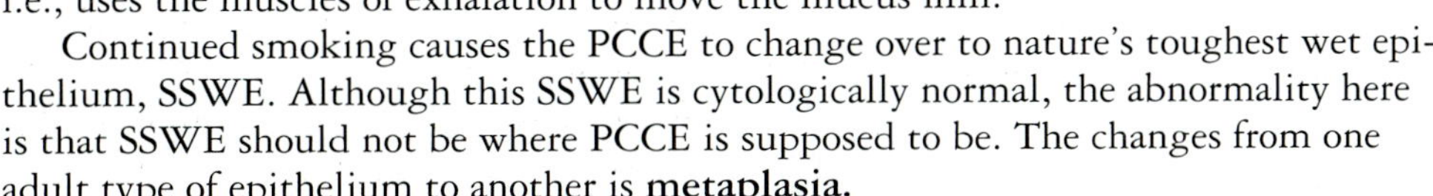

CANCER OF THE LUNG (FIG. 10.1)

There are several different types of cancers of the lung, but the most common (90%) is **squamous cell carcinoma.** The sequence of events goes something like this:

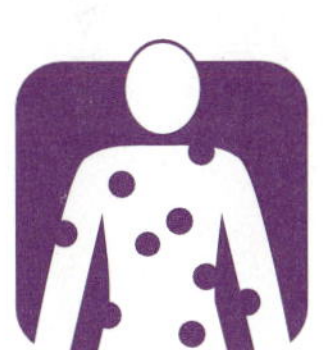

Normal PCCE or its shorter versions farther out the respiratory tree get insulted by cigarette smoke, which is ciliotoxic and stimulates the production of excessive amounts of mucus. Poor ciliary sweeping and more mucus leads to filling of the lungs with too much mucus, especially when sleeping. The smoker coughs a lot, i.e., uses the muscles of exhalation to move the mucus film.

Continued smoking causes the PCCE to change over to nature's toughest wet epi-thelium, SSWE. Although this SSWE is cytologically normal, the abnormality here is that SSWE should not be where PCCE is supposed to be. The changes from one adult type of epithelium to another is **metaplasia.**

If the metaplastic SSWE continues to be traumatized by the presence of cigarette smoke, it undergoes some degenerative changes and becomes cytologically disorga-nized. This is **dysplasia.**

If the dysplastic, metaplastic SSWE continues to be traumatized by the smoke, it can undergo complete cytologic disorganization into an **anaplastic** SSWE, which is squamous cell carcinoma. Once the anaplastic change has occurred the change is irre-versible, and the patient has carcinoma of the lung.

All of the other changes mentioned are reversible if the insult ceases. They are re-versible because the relatively undifferentiated basal cells can genetically "remember" that their daughters should differentiate into the differentiated cell types of PCCE, and they will again do so if the insult of the smoke is removed. In this way cessation of smoking can bring the statistical risk back to near normal over 5 to 10 years.

One other type of lung cancer, the type that killed actor Steve McQueen, is a ma-lignancy of the mesothelial cells on the surface of the visceral or parietal pleura, the malignant mesothelioma. It appears to be caused by exposure to asbestos. Before Steve McQueen became famous as an actor, he worked in a shipyard as a pipefitter.

MULTIPLE CHOICE REVIEW QUESTIONS

1. Which of the following cell types is least likely to be found as part of the alveolar septa of the lung?
   a. Type II cells (great alveolar cells)
   b. Endothelial cells
   c. Type I cells
   d. Ciliated cuboidal cells
   e. Macrophages

2. The true vocal fold can be distinguished from the false vocal fold because the true vocal fold
   a. is lined by stratified squamous wet epithelium.
   b. contains only serous glands.
   c. contains a core of hyaline cartilage.
   d. is located more superior in the larynx.
   e. contains a core of elastic cartilage.

3. Surfactant is produced by
   a. goblet cells.
   b. Type I alveolar cells (small alveolar cell).
   c. dust cells.
   d. Type II alveolar cells (great alveolar cell).
   e. bronchiolar glands.

4. Which of the following is *not* a necessary part of the respiratory membrane?
   a. Pneumonocyte I
   b. Basal lamina of pneumonocyte I
   c. Pulmonary macrophage
   d. Basal lamina of endothelial cell
   e. Endothelial cell

5. In which of the following locations would you find the highest concentration of Clara cells?
   a. Extrapulmonary bronchi
   b. Intrapulmonary bronchi
   c. Terminal bronchioles
   d. Interalveolar septum
   e. Pores of Kohn

Chapter 11

Cardiovascular System

GENERAL

Beginning at the **heart,** blood is distributed through a system of **arteries** to **capillary beds** and returned to the heart by a system of **veins.** In the capillary beds **tissue fluid** is produced and then bathes the cells of the organs and tissues. Some of this tissue fluid is recaptured into the bloodstream on the venous side of the capillary bed. Some of the tissue fluid finds its way into **lymph vessels** and returns to the blood through the lymphatic vessels as **lymph.** Blood can bypass capillary beds by passing through a direct connection between arteries and veins, i.e., the **arteriovenous anastomoses.**

Sometimes capillary beds are connected to other capillary beds by a vein. This is a **portal system.** The best example of a portal system is the capillary bed of the intestines collected into the portal vein for distribution to a second capillary bed in the liver. There is a portal system arrangement connecting capillaries of the median eminence of the hypothalamus to capillaries in the anterior pituitary gland.

The heart and blood vessels, except for the capillaries, in general have walls comprising three subdivisions or layers:

- Innermost layer—**tunica intima** for vessels and **endocardium** for the heart
- Middle layer—**tunica media/myocardium**
- Outer layer—**tunica adventitia/epicardium** (Fig. 11.1)

The inner regions of the vessel or the heart are supplied with oxygen and nutrients from the blood in the lumen. The outer regions are supplied by vessels in the tunica adventitia (**vasa vasorum**) or the epicardium (coronary vessels).

From inside a vessel to outside of it these layers contain

- Tunica intima
  - Endothelium and its basal lamina
  - Subendothelial connective tissue
  - Internal elastic membrane

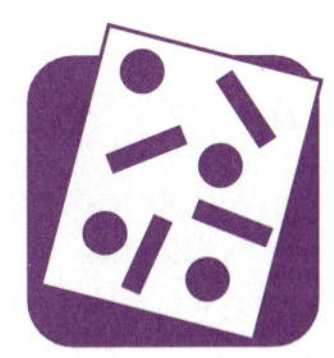

- Tunica media
  - Circular smooth muscle and some fibroblasts, collagen and elastic fibers, and sheets, the outermost one of which is the external elastic membrane

- Tunica adventitia
  - Loose areolar connective tissue, adipose tissue, collagen and elastic fibers, small vessels, and nerves

ARTERIES

■ **Elastic or Conducting Arteries** Examples of elastic arteries are the aorta and pulmonary trunk and their immediate major branches. They contain many **fen-**

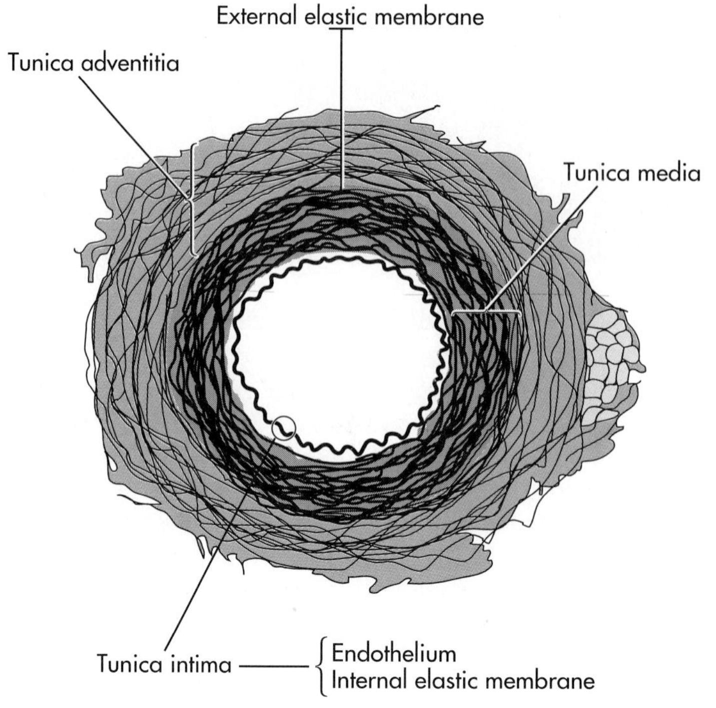

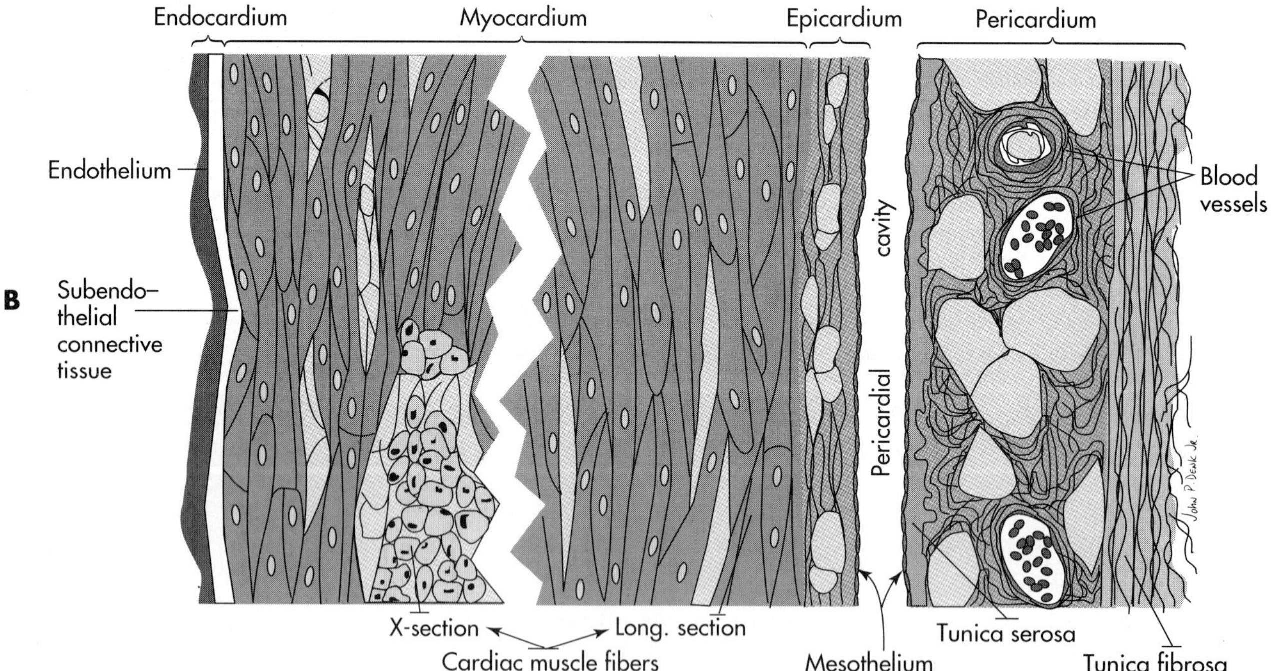

Fig. 11.1 Comparison of the three major layers or tunics composing the wall of a generalized blood vessel (A), and the wall of the heart (B). The tunica intima of the blood vessel is homologous to the endocardium of the heart. Tunica media is myocardium, and tunica adventitia is epicardium.

estrated elastic laminae in the tunica media. These elastic laminae stretch with systole to receive the volume of blood delivered from the respective ventricle. During **diastole,** when the blood in these great vessels attempts to fall back into the ventricle from which it came, the semilunar valves close and the elastic laminae recoil, thereby maintaining pressure in the vessel from the end of one systole to the beginning of the next systole.

■ **Muscular or Distributing Arteries** These include all of the named arteries in gross anatomy other than the elastic arteries. The histologic transition from elastic artery to muscular artery is not abrupt. Immediate branches of the elastic arteries such as the subclavian and the common carotid are also histologic elastic arteries. In muscular arteries the remnants of the many elastic laminae found in the elastic arteries are the **internal** and **external elastic laminae** or membranes. The tunica media is a mass of circular smooth muscle that can contract and relax in response to hormones and the autonomic nervous system, thereby regulating blood flow to an area. An example would be a facial blush.

Muscular arteries are often subdivided by their lumen size or the number of smooth muscle cells in the tunica media, i.e., large, medium, and small muscular arteries. The main point is that as one proceeds out the arterial tree the vessels get progressively smaller and their tunics get thinner.

When the number of smooth muscle cells in the tunica media has dwindled down to 1 or 2, the vessel is called an **arteriole.** The smallest arteriole contains only one smooth muscle cell in its tunica media. This is the **metarteriole.** The amount of **tonus** in these smooth muscle cells plays a significant role in the degree of **peripheral resistance** existing in the arterial tree and therefore contributes to the maintenance of the **mean arterial pressure.**

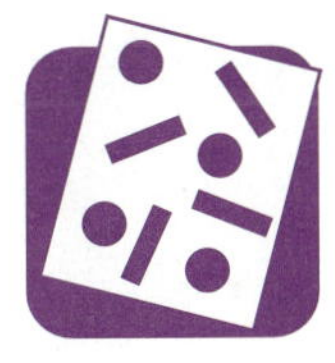

Increased tonus in the arterioles throughout the body would cause the blood pressure to increase. Decreased tonus in the tunica media of the arterioles would cause blood pressure to decrease. Arterioles also "guard" the gateway to the capillary beds. Increased tonus in the arteriolar wall would diminish flow into the capillary bed.

CAPILLARIES

When all the layers of the typical vessel wall disappear and the only thing left is the endothelium and its basal lamina, the vessel is a capillary. The lumen is big enough for one red blood cell (RBC). Some capillary-like vessels have a lumen that is much larger than one RBC wide, and these special vessels are called **sinusoids.** Sinusoids are found in the liver, spleen, bone marrow, and several endocrine glands such as the hypophysis and adrenal cortex.

There are two major types of capillaries.

• **Continuous capillaries** contain endothelial cells that are not fenestrated. Continuous capillaries are found in the CNS, muscle, and the lung. The endothelial cells have between them junctions of the **macula occludens** type, which will allow water and some small hydrophilic molecules (less than 10,000 kDa) to pass. These channels are believed to be the small pores described in functional terms by physiologists. Transport of material across these endothelial cells occurs by **pinocytosis.**

Associated with continuous capillaries there can be an undifferentiated mesenchymal cell called the **pericyte.** Pericytes are enclosed in the basal lamina of the endothelial cell. Pericytes have long cytoplasmic processes and therefore are spindle shaped. They contain actin and myosin and may be contractile. They are devoid of much ultrastructural specialization. However, they can be activated in a variety of situations as in wound healing where they can differentiate into smooth muscle cells or fibroblasts.

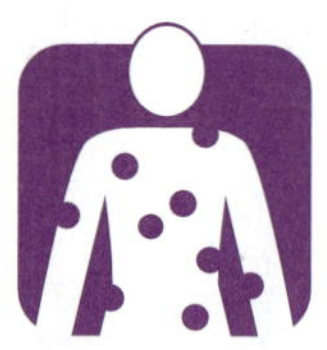

There is an interesting pathologic condition called **traumatic myositis ossificans** in which activated pericytes are believed to play a significant role. First there is a major physically induced injury to a mass of skeletal muscle, such as a football injury to the quadriceps. Then there is an aseptic inflammation of the muscle or myositis. Pericytes, as undifferentiated mesenchymal cells, somehow are stimulated by the trauma or the inflammatory process and differentiate into chondroblasts and osteoblasts as well as fibroblasts. This lesion can then have spicules of cartilage and bone in it, and such spicules eventually will slowly disappear. The danger is that on x-ray films the ossificans component of this lesion can be misdiagnosed as osteogenic sarcoma, when in fact it is a benign condition.

• **Fenestrated capillaries** are composed of endothelial cells that actually have little windows in them. These fenestrations are closed by a nonmembranous diaphragm that is thinner than a unit membrane. Occludens junctions and pinocytotic vesicles are present. Tissue fluid formation is quite rapid from fenestrated capillaries. This type of capillary is found in the gastrointestinal tract, many endocrine organs, and the renal glomerulus.

In addition to lining vessels and the chambers of the heart and participating in the formation of tissue fluid and being the most important factor in the blood-brain barrier, endothelial cells perform some other functions. Endothelial cells produce a protein called **factor VIII–related antigen,** which is one of the blood-clotting factors. In fact this factor is so specific to the endothelial cell that immunochemical staining for this factor is a specific marker for endothelium.

FORMATION OF TISSUE FLUID

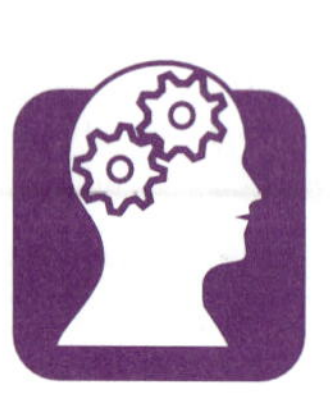

At the arterial side of a capillary bed (Fig. 11.2) the **hydrostatic pressure** tends to force fluid out of the capillary, and **osmotic pressure** exerted by the presence of large molecules in the blood tends to draw fluid into the lumen of the capillary. Since the hydrostatic pressure exceeds the osmotic pressure on this end of the capillary bed, fluid is forced out. This filtrate of blood bathes the cells with water, oxygen, nutrients, etc. It is called **tissue fluid.** It also picks up some waste products of cell metabolism and carbon dioxide before some of it returns to the venous side of the capillary bed. On the venous side of the capillary bed the hydrostatic pressure is lower than the osmotic pressure and fluid is drawn back into the vessel lumen. Not all the tissue fluid produced is returned to the venous side of the capillary bed. The tissue fluid not making it to the lumen of the vessels on the venous side of the capillary bed is eventually collected in blind-ending lymph capillaries as **lymph.**

EDEMA

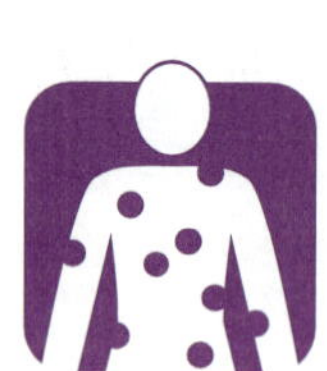

Edema is an excess of tissue fluid in a body region. Edema has many causes, some of which are worth considering in relation to the normal formation of tissue fluid.

An increase in venous hydrostatic pressure to the point that it now exceeds the osmotic pressure on the venous side of the capillary bed would keep fluid from returning to the blood. One can get increased venous hydrostatic pressure by, e.g., heart failure or an enlarging uterus during pregnancy compromising the venous return from the lower extremities (pitting edema).

Any obstruction of the lymphatic drainage would result in the accumulation of excess tissue fluid. Lymphatic obstruction can be caused by surgery as in an axillary node dissection for metastatic breast cancer and subsequent **lymphedema** of the ipsilateral superior extremity. Lymphatic obstruction can also be caused by the presence of parasites (elephantiasis) or cancer cells in the lymph capillaries draining a body region.

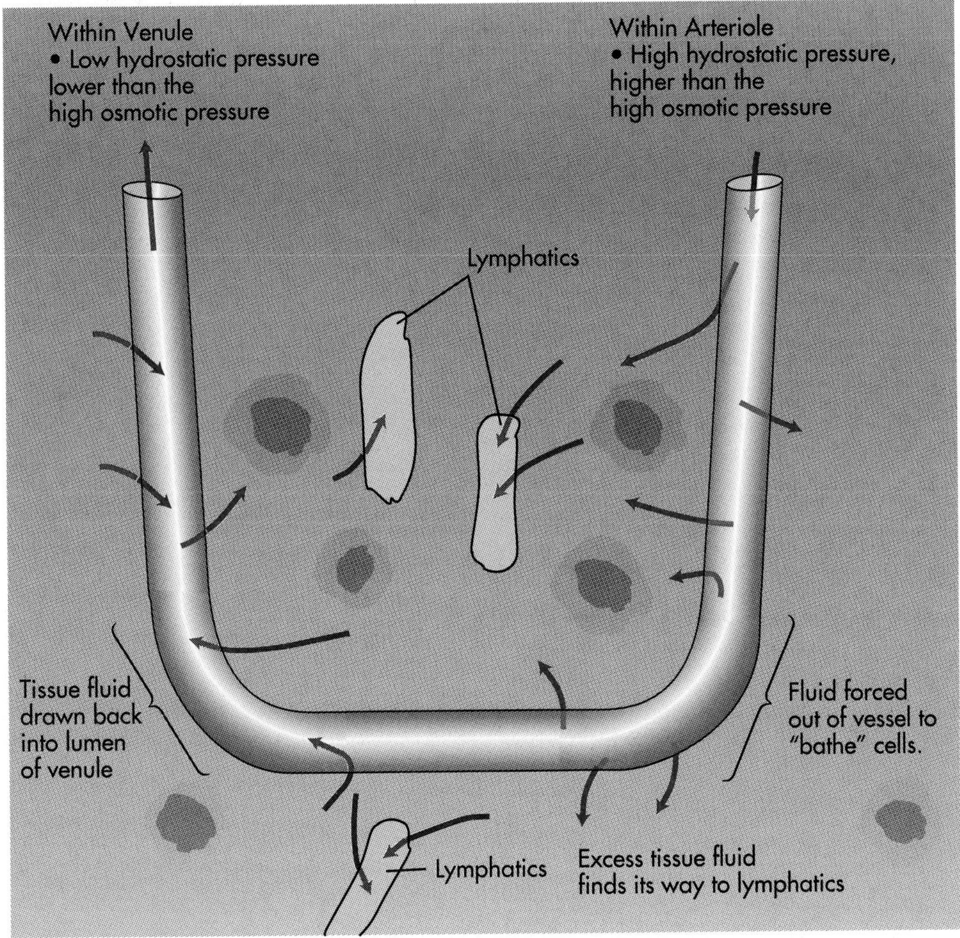

Fig. 11.2 Circulation through a capillary loop and the formation of tissue fluid and its return to the venous side of the capillary loop or as lymph in a lymph capillary.

Injured endothelial cells, as in a crush injury or a burn, can leak an excessive amount of tissue fluid into a region. Malnutrition can result in edema because the person simply does not have enough large molecules to exert enough osmotic pressure to draw fluid back into the blood on the venous side of the capillary bed. This form of edema can be seen as an abdominal ascites, or liters of tissue fluid in the peritoneal cavity.

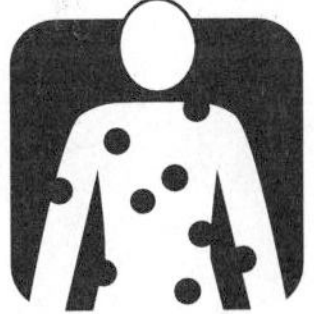

Blood Brain Barrier

The parenchymal of the brain is, in general terms, a pharmacologic sanctuary with few drugs able to readily cross from blood into CNS tissue. The capillaries in the CNS have the **zonula,** not macula, **occludens** type of junctions. Also the basal lamina is thicker than in other capillaries, and pinocytotic vesicles are scarce.

Veins

Because the hydrostatic pressure is higher in the arterial tree than in the venous-drainage tree, the size of the arterial lumen is small relative to the thickness of the arterial wall. In veins, with a low hydrostatic pressure the wall is quite thin relative to the size of the lumen.

Beginning with the postcapillary venules, which have 1 or 2 smooth muscle cells in the tunica media, and increasing in size from venules to the largest veins the wall gets thicker, and the three tunics become increasingly thicker and more apparent. There are venules, and small, medium, and large veins, such as the **superior vena cava.**

The exception to this general histologic plan is found in the inferior vena cava. In this organ the tunica adventitia is the largest tunic because it contains longitudinally arranged smooth muscle fibers in much greater quantity than the circular arranged smooth muscle fibers of the tunica media. Peripheral to the longitudinal smooth muscle, in the inner aspect of the tunica adventitia, is a typical tunica adventitia of loose areolar connective tissue with adipose tissue. The longitudinal smooth muscle of the tunica adventitia in the **inferior vena cava** contracts lengthwise on the column of blood in the vessel lumen and thereby helps squeeze the blood toward the heart.

Since veins have valves, which are simply the tunica intima folded on itself, once the blood passes a valve it cannot flow retrograde beyond the valve. **Varicose veins** occur in the inferior extremity when the venous valves fail to function properly.

Arteriovenous Anastomoses, or AV Shunts

AV shunts are direct connections between arterioles and venules and therefore bypass a capillary bed. The tunica media in the arterioles here is richly innervated by the autonomic nervous system. Relaxation of this muscle will open the shunt and send blood through the shunt, bypassing the capillary bed. Contraction of the smooth muscle in the arterial side of the AV anastomosis will close the shunt and divert blood into the capillary bed. AV anastomoses are common in the lips, ears, toes, nose, and fingertips.

Lymphatic Vessels

Lymphatic drainage begins as blind-ending endothelial capillaries in which the endothelium is very thin and its basal lamina is absent or intermittent. This characteristic allows for easier absorption of fluid and macromolecules. Because the walls of these fine lymph vessels are so thin they would collapse if they were not held open with **anchoring filaments** (5 to 10 nm), which extend from the abluminal plasmalemma of the endothelial cell into the surrounding connective tissue. These anchoring filaments provide for the mechanical maintenance of vessel patency.

The lymph capillaries anastomose with larger and larger lymph vessels, which eventually will have recognizable tunics: intima, media, and adventitia. Eventually the size of the two largest lymph vessels will be reached, the right lymphatic duct and the thoracic duct. Their histologic characteristics are very similar to those of medium to large veins. Lymph vessels, like veins, also have valves.

Because lymph capillaries have such thin walls, fluid can pass from tissue spaces into the lymph capillaries readily. The same is true of absorbed lipid (chyle) in the intestinal villi. In this case the lymph capillary is called a **lacteal vessel.**

Because lymph capillaries and the smaller lymph vessels have such thin walls relative to the comparable venous and arterial vessels, it is easier for invading cancer cells to break into a lymph vessel than it is to break into a vein, with the artery being the most impenetrable. This simple mechanical difference between these three vessels plays a significant role in why cancer cells spread by lymphatic drainage routes.

Heart

The three major layers of the heart are, from inside to outside, the **endocardium, myocardium,** and **epicardium.**

The epicardium is also the **visceral pericardium.** It contains loose areolar connective tissue and adipose tissue. Embedded in this are large arteries, veins (coronary vessels), and nerves. The epicardium is covered by a **mesothelium,** which faces the **pericardial fluid.**

The myocardium is composed of parenchymal elements—the cardiac muscle cells, which have variable sizes depending on the work load, the larger ones found in the ventricles, and the smaller ones found in the atria. Cardiac muscle was described earlier in the chapter on muscle tissue. Within the **atrial myofibers** neuroendocrine granules contain **atrial natriuretic hormone.** When the volume of blood in the atria is larger than normal, these muscle fibers are stretched beyond normal. This causes release of the hormone. The target for the hormone is the distal convoluted tubule in the kidney where it causes an increase in the excretion of sodium and water, thereby decreasing the blood volume.

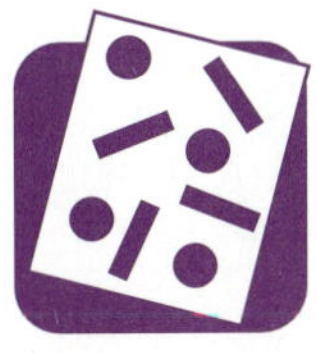

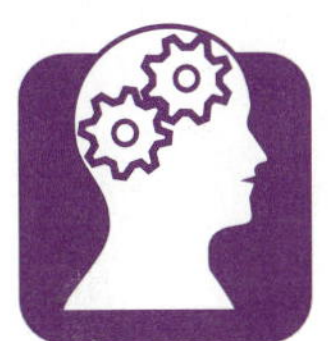

The endocardium has an endothelial lining and some subendothelial connective tissue, which may contain some smooth muscle fibers. Outside this connective tissue layer is another connective tissue layer, which blends in with the connective tissue of the myocardium. This layer of connective tissue at the interface between the endocardium and the myocardium is called the **subendocardial connective tissue.** It is in the subendocardial connective tissue layer, in specific regions of the heart, that the **Purkinje fibers** can be found. Purkinje fibers are specialized cardiac muscle cells that have a perinuclear concentration of glycogen and peripherally displaced myofibrils. The Purkinje fibers are components of the **impulse conduction system** of the heart.

Cardiac Skeleton

The cardiac muscle fibers have an origin and an insertion. They arise and insert into a dense fibrous cardiac skeleton composed of the **fibrous rings** and **trigones** and the **septum membranaceum.**

The cardiac skeleton also forms a strong support base for the attachment of the valves of the heart. The valves of the great vessels and the heart (semilunar, mitral, and tricuspid) in general are folds of endocardium or tunica intima with a thickened fibrous center. The AV valves are attached by tendinous cords (chordae tendineae) to the papillary muscles. In this instance the longitudinally arranged collagen fibers of the **chordae tendineae** become continuous with the connective tissue of the myocardium in the papillary muscle.

Impulse Conducting System
of the Heart

The **sinoatrial,** or **SA, node** is located in the wall of the superior vena cava at the upper end of the sulcus terminalis. It is composed of special nodal fibers that are small cardiac muscle fibers embedded in some dense connective tissue.

- The **atrio-ventricular, or AV, node** is of similar histologic appearance and is located in the inferior end of the interatrial septum.
- The **AV bundle (of His)** is composed of Purkinje fibers.

ARTERIOSCLEROSIS

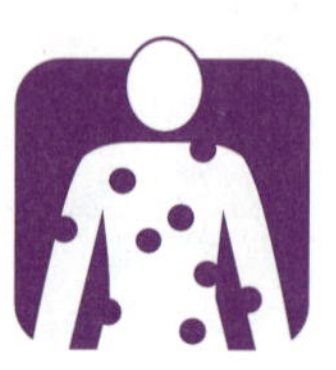

Arteriosclerosis is a term meaning 'hardening and thickening of the arteries'. There are several types of arteriosclerosis. Although it is not the intent of this review to teach pathology, sometimes a little pathology helps the student see the importance of certain terms and concepts of histology, and this is true for vessel histology.

Atherosclerosis is a disease of the tunica intima with intimal thickening and degeneration with fatty streaks and fibrofatty plaques (atheromas) forming and compromising the vessel lumen predisposing to impaired blood flow. Damage to the endothelial cells may expose blood to underlying intimal collagen fibers, and this may cause platelets to aggregate here forming a thrombus.

Medial calcific sclerosis is a disease of the tunica media in which a degenerative process can be followed by calcium deposition in the tunica media.

Hyaline and **hyperplastic arteriolosclerosis** are diseases of the tunica intima. In the first case a hyalinization of the intima occurs. In the second case there is a hyperplasia of cells in the intima resulting in an onionskin appearance.

ANGIOGENESIS IN THE ADULT

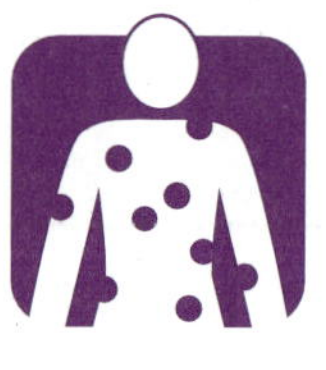

Angiogenesis is a normal process during normal development. However, angiogenesis can occur in the adult also. In the normal situation new vessels are formed in the endometrium during the menstrual cycle and in the connective tissue associated with hair follicles during the hair-growth cycle. New vessels are formed after chemical, physical, and immunologic injury.

Abnormal angiogenesis can occur any place in the body in which a solid neoplasm arises. Tumor cells release a hormone-like substance, called **tumor angiogenesis factor** (TAF), that acts on nearby endothelial cells to sprout new growths, which invade the tumor and supply it with blood and nutrients. Without a blood supply a neoplasm will not grow rapidly. Experimentally, tumor growth has been halted and controlled by administering antibody raised against TAF.

Multiple Choice Review Questions

1. Which of the following is characteristic of an arteriole?
   a. Thick tunica adventitia and large lumen
   b. Thick tunica media in relation to the size of the lumen
   c. Thin tunica media and relatively large lumen
   d. Large blood-filled lumen
   e. Large amounts of elastic fibers in the tunica media

2. Arrange the following in correct sequence for a pin passing from lumen outward through the wall of a medium-size artery: 1, blood; 2, adipose tissue; 3, smooth muscle; 4, most prominent of two elastic membranes; 5, subendothelial fibroblasts.
   a. 1-2-4-3-5
   b. 1-3-2-5-4
   c. 1-4-5-3-2
   d. 1-5-4-3-2

3. All of the following are found in an intercalated disc except:
   a. macula adherens.
   b. fascia adherens.
   c. gap junction.
   d. zonula occludens.

4. All of the following have valves except:
   a. veins.
   b. heart.
   c. lymph vessels.
   d. distributing arteries.

5. Which of the following would be the easiest for invading cancer cells to enter?
   a. Fenestrated capillary
   b. Continuous capillary
   c. Lymph capillary
   d. Venule
   e. Metarteriole

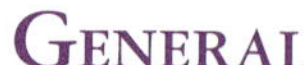

Chapter 12

Blood

GENERAL

Blood is a **specialized connective tissue.** It is of mesodermal origin. It consists of two major components—**formed elements** and **plasma.** If blood is centrifuged, the formed elements are packed to the bottom of the tube leaving the plasma at the top. The percentage by volume of the formed elements relative to the liquid component is a **hematocrit.** A normal hematocrit is about 45. Allowing the plasma to clot and removing the clot leaves **serum.** Blood is a window into the body because no tissue is so accessible and so often examined morphologically, chemically, and immunologically.

FORMED ELEMENTS

■ **Types**

- Red blood cells (RBCs), or erythrocytes (4.5 to 5.5 $\times$ 10^6/mm^3)
- White blood cells (WBCs), or leukocytes (5000 to 9000/mm^3)
  - *Granulocytes*
    - Neutrophils
    - Basophils
    - Eosinophils
  - *Agranulocytes*
    - Lymphocytes
    - Monocytes
- Platelets or thrombocytes (250,000/mm^3)

■ **Numerical Abnormalities (more than normal vs less than normal)**

- Leukocytosis versus leukopenia
- Thrombocytosis versus thrombocytopenia
- Polycythemia versus anemia

ERYTHROCYTES

- 7.2 microns in diameter (since present everywhere, it is a histologic ruler)
- No nucleus and no organelles
- Life-span of 120 days; constantly aging, dying; thus constantly replaced
- Highly deformable biconcave disks
  - Poikilocytes (RBCs of abnormal shape)

- Sickle cell anemia
- Spherocytosis

- Biconcave shape increases surface area; 4000 square meters total for all RBCs in body

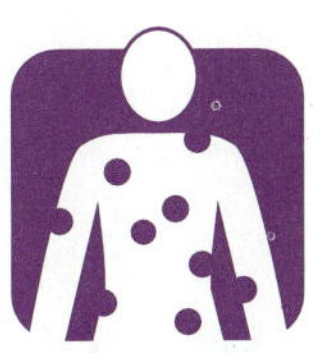

- Plasmalemma-bound bags of water (60%) and hemoglobin (35%)
  - HbA: adult normal hemoglobin
  - Decrease in amount of oxyhemoglobin (cyanosis)
  - HbS: sickle cell anemia
  - HbF: normal fetal type

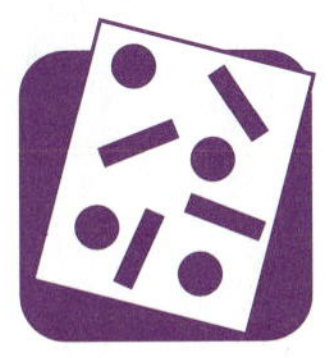

- Tonicity
  - Isotonic with 0.9% NaCl (normal saline solution); i.e., RBCs in saline retain normal size and shape.
  - NaCl higher than 0.9%—hypertonic to RBC; water leaves, RBC shrinks, wrinkled—crenates
  - NaCl lower than 0.9%—hypotonic to RBC; water enters, RBC swells, bursts—hemolysis

- Cytoskeleton
  - Interaction between cytoskeleton and plasmalemma is well studied
  - **Spectrin**—large, long cytoskeletal protein microfilament with actin-binding sites at each end; forms dense meshwork under P surface of plasmalemma; hereditary spherocytosis involves a defect in spectrin

PLATELETS (THROMBOCYTES)

- Pieces of megakaryocyte cytoplasm
- Live for 10 to 12 days; must be constantly replaced
- Two morphological regions

  1. **Granulomere**. Central area with granules containing serotonin and other granules, alpha granules, containing platelet-derived growth factor; a few other organelles.
  2. **Hyalomere**. Peripheral light area containing microtubules. Open canalicular system. Communicates with surface.

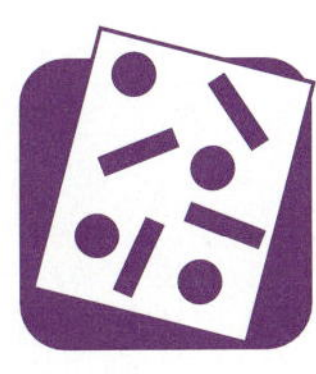

- Plug microdefects in endothelial lining of blood vessels
- Role in hemostasis or blood clotting

  - Release **thromboplastin**
  - Thromboplastin converts **prothrombin** to **thrombin**
  - Thrombin converts **fibrinogen** to **fibrin** monomers
  - Fibrin monomers polymerize forming fibrin threads
    - like synthesizing a fishing net in the water around a fish you want to catch
  - Fibrin threads "catch" formed elements and other platelets that aggregate resulting in a thrombus; aspirin helps prevent blood clots by blocking a

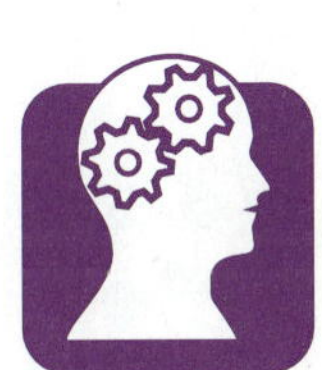

factor platelets need to aggregate; daily aspirin useful in lessening risk of myocardial infarction and stroke.

- Thrombus

  - Ante mortem—above events utilized while person is alive; clot is whorls of trapped, formed elements in fibrin strands.
  - Post mortem—blood simply settles out forming three layers.
      Heaviest—deoxygenated RBCs (currant jelly layer)
      Middle—zone of WBCs (chicken fat layer)
      Top—serum

- Embolus—piece of thrombus breaks off and travels in blood, can plug lumen of vessel resulting in infarction or loss of blood supply beyond plug: myocardial, pulmonary, cerebral, renal, etc., infarctions.

LEUKOCYTES

- Leave the blood, function in loose connective tissue areas
- Short life-span for all, except some lymphocytes, means constant cell loss, constant cell replacement
- Two major kinds:

  1. Granulocytes
     - Neutrophils
     - Basophils
     - Eosinophils
  2. Agranulocytes
     - Monocytes
     - Lymphocytes

- Differential count—normal percentage of each type in peripheral blood

  - 70% neutrophils
  - 20% lymphocytes
  - 6% monocytes
  - 3% eosinophils
  - 1% basophils

- Cytosis or philia—above normal percentage
  - Monocytosis, eosinophilia

- Penia—below normal percentage
  - Neutropenia

NEUTROPHILS, OR POLYMORPHONUCLEAR LEUKOCYTES (PMNs)

Three to 5-lobed nucleus; the more mature, the higher the number of lobes. Most immature—bean-shaped nucleus—"band" or "stab"; 1% band or stab count is normal; higher % would indicate immature PMNs released from bone marrow.

- Drumstick, or heterochromatinized, X chromosome in 3% of PMNs in female
- Nonreplicating or fixed postmitotics
- Cytoplasmic granules
  - Neutrophilic, or flesh toned, are difficult to see on LM
  - EM
  - 400 nm—contain bactericidal substances or phagocytins
  - 700 nm—lysosomes containing peroxidases and other hydrolytic enzymes

■ Phagocytes

- It is their job to ingest and destroy bacteria routinely.
- Major role in inflammation. Phagocytosis of bacteria, specific granules fuse
with phagosome first, and then larger granules add their contents—dead bug.
  - Chronic granulomatous disease of childhood. Phagocytosis of bacteria is
    OK, but certain gram-negative bacteria are not killed. They survive in-
    side the cell, are released when PMN normally dies, but reinfect child.
    Defect is genetic absence of hydrogen peroxide.

EOSINOPHILS

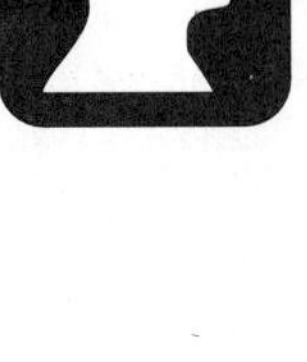

- Bilobed nucleus
- Eosinophilic granules in cytoplasm—lysosomes rich in **peroxidase**. These ly-
  sosomes contain crystalline core of **major basic protein.**
- Phagocytosis of antigen-antibody complexes—defense system role
- Eosinophilia—higher than normal percentage of eosinophils in differential
  count is associated with allergic reactions and parasitic infections

BASOPHILS

- Bilobed to irregular-shaped nucleus
- Large basophilic granules
  - **Heparin, histamine, SRS** (slow reactive substance of anaphylaxis)
  - Metachromatic when stained with toluidine blue
- IgE on plasmalemma
  - Originally secreted by a type of plasma cell
  - Allergen combines with IgE—cell degranulates, participates in
    hypersensitivity reactions

LYMPHOCYTES

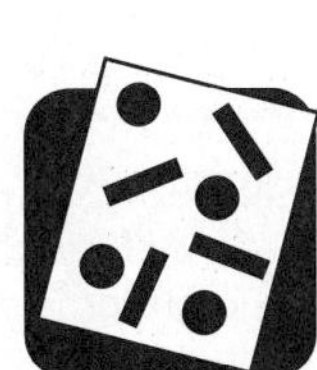

Round, pyknotic (heterochromatinized) nucleus; small rim of cytoplasm

- Few organelles
- Major role in defense system
- Types
  - **B cells** or lymphocytes originally derived from bone marrow
  - **T cells** or lymphocytes originally derived from the thymus gland
  - **Null cells**, which carry neither B-cell nor T-cell surface antigens and
    therefore are not classifiable as B or T cells

MONOCYTES

Relatively large; characteristic **bean-shaped nucleus** with clumpy-stringy chromatin pattern

- Cytoplasmic granules—lysosomes
- Phagocytes, which travel in blood, leave it to function in connective tissue.
- Also called histiocytes, or tissue macrophages

INFLAMMATION

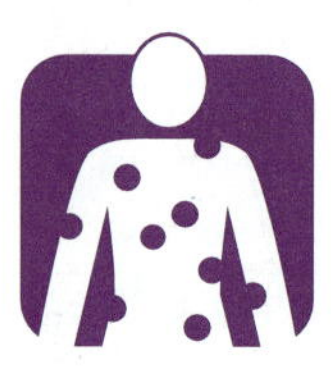

- Aseptic if damaged tissue but no bacteria involved
- Septic if bacteria involved
- A connective tissue phenomenon

  - Ground substance depolymerizes, becoming more liquid
  - Area vessels dilate—increased blood flow to region—**rubor**; when this increases heat in area—**calor**
  - Vessels increase permeability—excess tissue fluid accumulates—edema, which causes region to swell—**tumor**
  - Swelling (tumor)—pressure on nerve endings—pain, or **dolor**
  - Rubor, calor, tumor, dolor—4 cardinal signs of inflammation
  - PMNs emigrate from bloodstream, migrate to connective tissue area, eat bacteria. Endothelial cells express large amounts of an adhesion molecule, the platelet-endothelial cell adhesion molecule, or PECAM-1 (also known as endo-CAM), especially at intercellular junctions. PECAM-1 is necessary for PMN emigration. Antibody against PECAM-1 can prevent PMN emigration.

- PMNs—first cell type to arrive on scene of "bacterial accident"—acute phase of inflammatory process; in subacute phase—lymphocytes, monocytes, plasma cells begin to arrive and mix with PMNs; when lymphocytes, monocytes, and plasma cells predominate—chronic phase
- Suffix -itis is added to organ name to indicate inflammation of that organ. For example, appendicitis, cystitis, myocarditis, pericarditis, nephritis, hepatitis. The type or history of the inflammation can be indicated by the adjective acute, subacute, or chronic, e.g., acute appendicitis, chronic gastritis, subacute cystitis.

Table 12.1   *Types of Peripheral Blood Cells*

	RBC	PLATELET	LYMPHOCYTE	MONOCYTE	PMN	EOSINOPHIL	BASOPHIL
No/mm³ or percent in differential count	$4.5\text{-}5 \times 10^6$	$1.5\text{-}4 \times 10^5$	20%-25%	4%-8%	60%-70%	1%-4%	0.5%-1%
Diameter (μm)	7-8	2-5	7-12	9-12	10-12	10-12	10-12
Nuclear shape	——— Anucleate ———		—— Mononuclear ——			—— Lobulated ——	
					2-5 lobes	2-3 lobes	2-3 lobes
Cytoplasmic granules							
Azure	–	–	+	+	+	+	+
Specific	–	–	–	–	+	+	+
Life-span (days)	120	7-12	Months-years	Months	Hours-days	8-12 days	?

RBC, Red blood cell; *PMN*, polymorphonuclear neutrophil leukocyte.

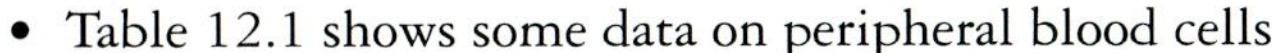

• Severe infections result in release of immature PMNs, bands or stabs, from bone marrow; thus the percentage of band count will increase—**"shift to the left"**; as inflammation subsides, the percentage of band count decreases toward normal— **"shift to the right."**

• **Lazy leukocyte syndrome**. Contractile actin microfilaments in normal PMN participate in ameboid motion; some people have a genetic defect in this microfilament system. Their PMNs show normal development in bone marrow, but their mobility is severely impaired; they cannot leave the bone marrow. Clinically one sees severe neutropenia and recurrent infections such as sinusitis, stomatitis, and otitis media.

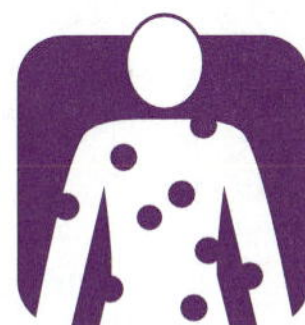

• Table 12.1 shows some data on peripheral blood cells.

MULTIPLE CHOICE
REVIEW QUESTIONS

1. Some staphylococci are phagocytosed by a PMN. Thirteen hours later when the PMN dies, viable and healthy staphylococci are liberated from this PMN. The disease state indicated by these findings is
    a. Chediak-Higashi disease.
    b. chronic inflammation.
    c. chronic granulomatous disease of childhood.
    d. macrocytic hypochromic anemia.
    e. chronic myelogenous leukemia.

2. The specific granules in the neutrophils of the peripheral blood are actually
    a. pigment granules.
    b. rough endoplasmic reticulum.
    c. mitochondria.
    d. plasma globulin precursors.
    e. lysosomes.

3. What percent of a normal differential count is contributed by eosinophils?
    a. 70%
    b. 20%
    c. 6%
    d. 3%
    e. 1%

4. Which of the following is a molecule that plays an important role in maintaining the biconcave shape of the normal RBC?
    a. Lysosomal enzymes
    b. Hemoglobin A
    c. Hemoglobin F
    d. Spectrin
    e. Glycocalyx

5. Which of the following is known to contain IgE antibody on its cell surface?
    a. Neutrophil
    b. Basophil
    c. Eosinophil
    d. Lymphocyte
    e. Monocyte

Chapter 13

Bone Marrow

GENERAL

The formed elements of blood are continuously lost and therefore must be continuously replaced. Replacement of blood cells occurs in **hematopoietic tissue,** which has two major divisions:

- **Bone marrow, or myeloid tissue**
- **Lymphoid tissue** (Lymphoid tissue is covered in greater detail in Chapter 14.)

HEMATOPOIESIS

- Begins in the embryo in **blood islands,** or **angiogenic cell clusters,** in the wall of the yolk sac during the second week of embryonic life.
- From second to sixth month of intrauterine life the liver and the spleen become the main hematopoietic organs. Thereafter the red bone marrow assumes this role.

During the fetal period of hematopoiesis the type of hemoglobin produced is **HbF.** At the end of the fetal period the type changes to the adult type of **HbA.**

- In the late fetal stage and early childhood red bone marrow is found in the skull, ribs, sternum, vertebrae, clavicles, pelvis, and long bones. After puberty the major sites are the ribs, sternum, vertebrae, skull, clavicles, and pelvis. The iliac crest is the primary site for bone marrow biopsy, with the sternum being the secondary site.
- Adult bone marrow accounts for about 5% of the total body weight or about 3000 grams.
- There are 100 times more cells in the bone marrow than there are people in the world.

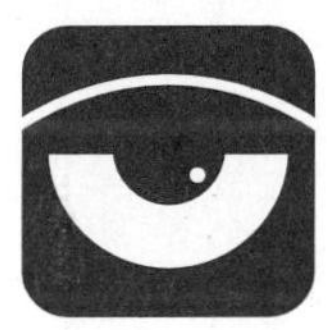

- Because the liver and the spleen were major hematopoietic organs during fetal life, they can become hematopoietic again during adult life in certain disease-related situations (**extramedullary hematopoiesis** or **myeloid metaplasia,** meaning that they have undergone a change to a new formation not normally characteristic of these organs).

HISTOLOGIC ORGANIZATION
OF RED BONE MARROW

- **Stroma** of fibroblasts, collagen, and reticular fibers, and reticular cells in a three-dimensional meshwork with sinusoids and vascular channels
- **Sinusoids** connect the arterial and venous sides of the circulation and form a vascular compartment within the red bone marrow.

Walls of sinusoids contain many mature and some slightly immature bone marrow cells passing from the hematopoietic tissue to gain access to the circulating blood.

- **Hematopoietic cord**—region located between sinusoids

Large numbers of adipose cells are present.

- Stromal cells produce a variety of **growth factors** that act in a paracrine mode on the myeloid parenchyma (see Fig. 13.1).
- Cells undergoing cytodifferentiation in RBC and WBC lines

The easiest to see are **megakaryocytes** and **megakaryocytoblasts.** Huge multilo-bated nucleus, lots of cytoplasm, preferentially located in the hematopoietic cord adjacent to the sinusoidal wall. The most mature forms have skinny cytoplasmic extensions that pass through the wall of the sinusoid and stretch along the luminal wall of the sinusoid. When these filamentous extensions "shatter," platelets are released.

- Red bone marrow is a dynamic, highly proliferating tissue producing millions of cells per day because millions of mature blood cells die every day, e.g.:
  - RBCs: **erythrocytopoiesis**
  - Neutrophils, basophils, eosinophils: **granulocytopoiesis**
- Monocytes: **monocytopoiesis**
  - Platelets: **thrombocytopoiesis**
  - B lymphocytes: **lymphocytopoiesis**

- For example, with respect to erythrocytopoiesis, it is instructive to consider the following amazing situation:
- There are 5×10^6 RBCs/mm^3, 5×10^9 RBCs/cm^3, 5 trillion RBCs/liter = 25 trillion RBCs/5 liters of blood. The average RBC lives for about 120 days, and so every 120 days 25 trillion RBCs must be produced! 10,368,000 seconds in 120 days = 2,400,000 RBCs produced by your red bone marrow every second, or 18 lb. of RBCs/year!

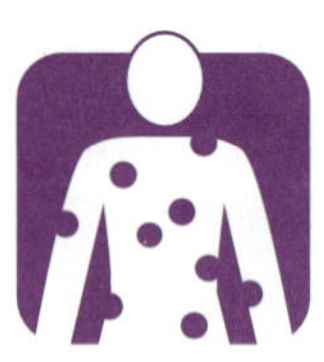

There are few if any cancers that grow to 18 lb. in 1 year. It has been calculated that the human adult contains about 10^{14} cells, 1% to 2% of which are lost every day (think of the normal cell loss from bone marrow, skin, and the gastrointestinal tract). If this cell loss did not occur but the rate of replacement remained the same, you would double your body weight every 100 days and in 50 years you would weigh 122,000 lbs!

The dynamic balance between cell loss and cell production in the hematopoietic system is of extreme importance relative to many abnormal situations, and these can serve as very instructive lessons. In a patient with **chronic** or long-standing **hemorrhage,** as in the case of a bleeding ulcer in the GI tract, all the formed elements of blood are being abnormally dumped into the lumen of the GI tract. This continued, abnormal loss of all the formed elements of blood is detected by the bone marrow, and the myeloid tissue responds with **enhanced granulocytopoiesis, erythrocytopoiesis,** and **thrombocytopoiesis** to meet the demand for normal levels of these cells in blood.

In a patient with a **severe septicemia** it is the neutrophil population that suffers significant loss fighting with the bacteria, not the RBC or platelet populations. In this situation there is a greater demand for PMNs, and so the bone marrow responds with an **increased rate of granulocytopoiesis** but no increase in erythrocytopoiesis or thrombocytopoiesis. In fact, the demand for PMNs can be so great that not only is there enhanced granulocytopoiesis but the bone marrow also allows slightly immature PMNs, the band or stab stages of PMN cytodifferentiation, to gain access to the circulation. In this case the percentage band or stab count will increase (called a "**shift to the left**").

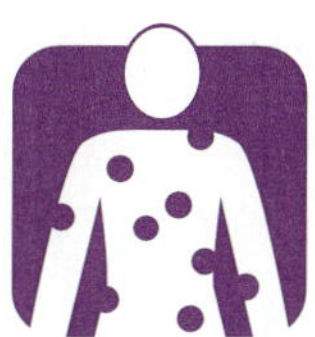

If an infusion of a large number of RBCs is given to a normal person as part of an experiment, the RBC count will have been artificially increased, i.e., experimental **polycythemia.** In this case the abnormally high number of RBCs in the peripheral blood negatively feeds back to the myeloid tissue and **suppresses erythrocytopoiesis.**

In a child with the congenital heart anomaly, tetralogy of Fallot, the defect results in **hypoxia** because not enough deoxygenated blood is being routed to the lungs where it can be oxygenated. Even at rest, but certainly after mild exercise, such a child will be **cyanotic** (bluish lips, bluish capillary beds under the finger nails). This generalized hypoxia is detected by the kidney, which responds by releasing the hormone **erythropoietin.** The target for erythropoietin is the red cell line of cytodifferentiation; i.e., **erythrocytopoiesis is increased,** and clinically apparent **polycythemia** is present.

Another example of the dynamic nature of the hematopoietic system is offered by the heavy **cigarette smoker.** The **carbon monoxide** in the cigarette smoke binds to hemoglobin with 240 times more affinity than oxygen does. Such a person would be chronically hypoxic, have increased levels of erythropoietin, and be polycythemic.

Cell Kinetics of Hematopoiesis

The parenchymal cells in the red bone marrow can be divided into three major **cell kinetic** compartments.

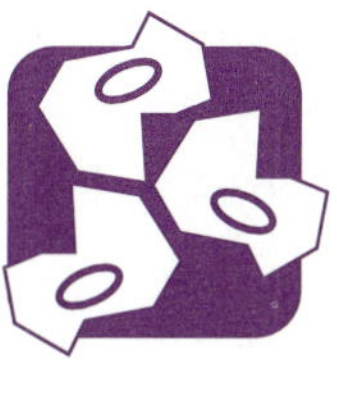

■ **Stem Cell Compartment**

- Composed of **vegetative intermitotics (VIM)**
- Self-replicating and self-sustaining
- Some cells destined to remain in the compartment as true **stem** cells

Other daughter cells begin to differentiate and by doing so move out of this kinetic compartment into the next compartment where they continue to divide, but while doing so they also undergo cytodifferentiation.

Even though cells in the stem cell compartment are VIMs, not all of them are running the cell cycle at any one point in time. Many of them are resting, or are out of cycle in the G_0 phase of the cell cycle. The cells classified as members of the stem cell compartment are indicated with the superscript 1 in Fig. 13.1.

■ **Differentiating Intermitotic (DIM) Compartment (Differentiating-Multiplicative Compartment)** DIM cells run the cell cycle and divide forming daughter cells, which also run the cell cycle producing daughters of their own. Every cell in the compartment is also undergoing cytodifferentiation. This kinetic compartment is not self-sustaining because all the daughter cells produced in this compartment are destined to differentiate out of the compartment by eventually becoming fixed postmitotics. If influx from the stem cell compartment was stopped, eventually all the DIMs would differentiate into fixed postmitotics and the differentiating-multiplicative compartment would "dry up." Cells belonging to this compartment are given the superscript 2 in Fig. 13.1.

■ **Functional Compartment: Fixed Postmitotic (FPM) Cells**

- The most mature cells at the end of each line of cytodifferentiation and their immediate 2 precursor cells in each line.
- Cells in this compartment function, age, and die.
- This compartment is not self-sustaining. Thus there is continual cell loss from this compartment, which is continuously replaced by cell production in the DIM and VIM cell compartments.

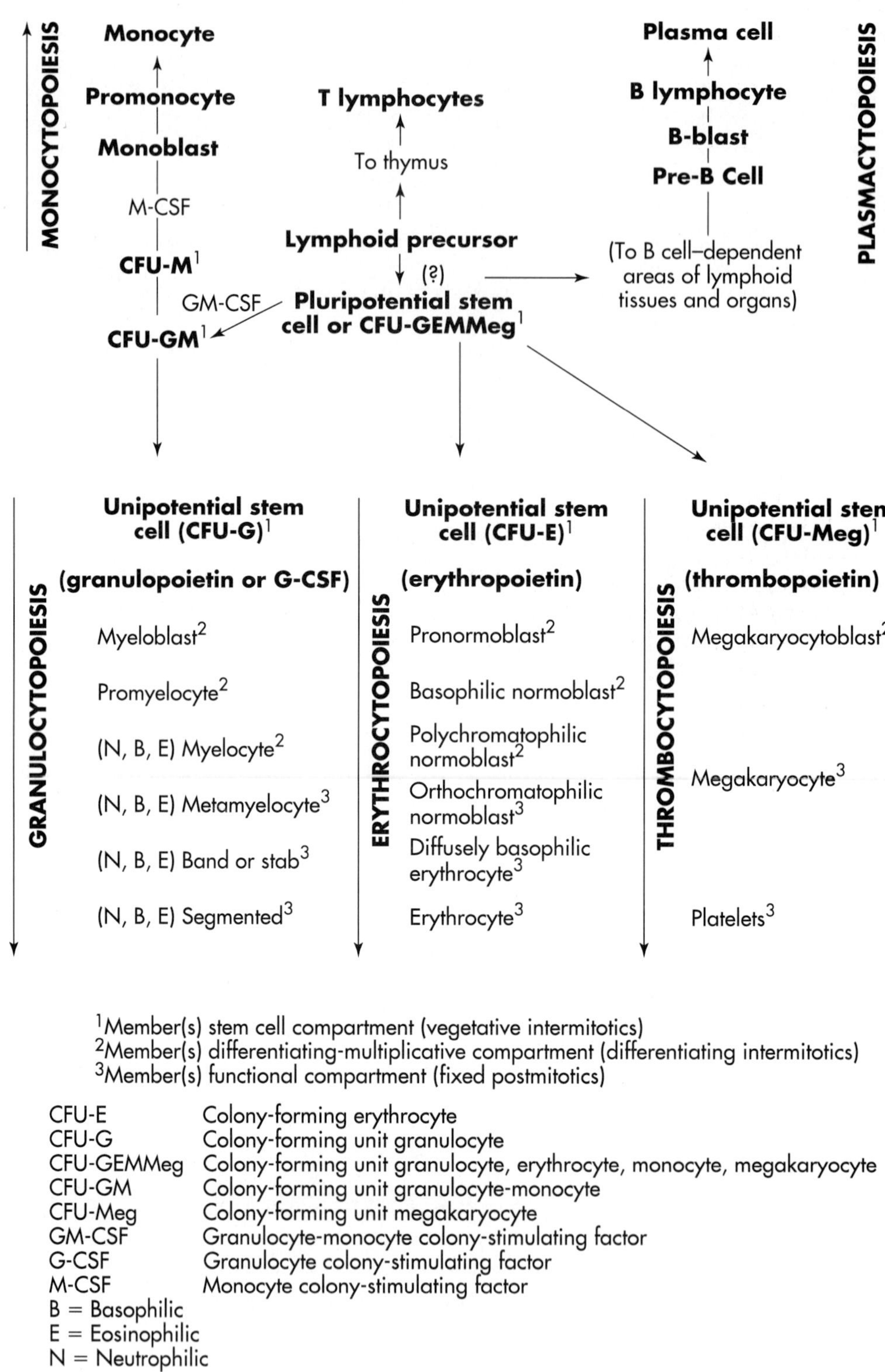

Fig. 13.1 Summary flow chart of hematopoiesis including named stages of cytodifferentiation, appropriate stimulating factors and cell kinetic compartments.

- For both the erythroid and granulocyte lines of cytodifferentiation in the FPM compartment the red bone marrow holds large numbers of completely or near-completely fully differentiated cells in reserve, which can be released into the circulation when necessary. The storage pool of mature granulocytes held in reserve in the red bone marrow contains about 16 times the number of circulating granulocytes. A similar reserve pool of slightly immature RBCs also exists in the red bone marrow.
- The cells belonging to this compartment are indicated with a superscript 3 in Fig. 13.1.

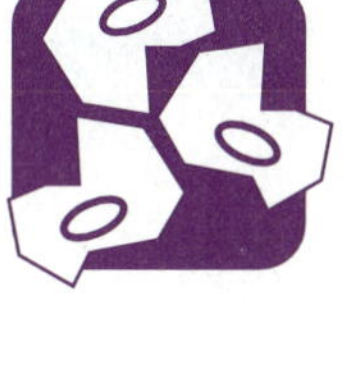

CYTODIFFERENTIATION DURING HEMATOPOIESIS

■ **Colony-Forming Unit, or CFU—A True Stem Cell**

- **Pluripotential**
- **Daughter cells of CFU**
  - *More CFUs*
  - *Cells that enter*
    - Granulocytopoiesis (G)—CFU - G cell
    - Erythrocytopoiesis (E)—CFU - E cell
    - Monocytopoiesis (M)—CFU - M cell
    - Megakaryocytopoiesis (Meg)—CFU-Meg cell

    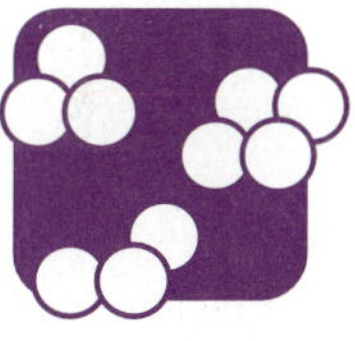

    Thus CFU-GEMMeg cell gives rise to daughter cells

    - **CFU-E,** or the colony-forming unit committed to the erythroid line
    - **CFU-Meg,** or the colony-forming unit committed to megakaryocytopoiesis
    - Before granulocytopoiesis and monocytopoiesis begin there is an intermediate step:
      - **CFU-GM,** which then gives rise to
        - **CFU-G,** or the colony forming unit committed to the granulocyte line
        - **CFU-M,** or the colony forming unit committed to the monocyte line

    There are many growth factors and differentiation factors operating in this system, and they are named and positioned in Fig. 13.1. The factor stimulating the CFU-GEMMeg to differentiate into the CFU-GM is **GM-CSF,** or **granulocyte/monocyte colony-stimulating factor.**

GRANULOCYTOPOIESIS

The morphologically distinct and named stages in granulocytopoiesis are myeloblast→promyelocyte→myelocyte→metamyelocyte→band or stab→mature cell:

■ **Myeloblast**

- **Relatively large**

- Prominent nucleoli
- Delicate chromatin pattern in round/oval nucleus
- No specific cytoplasmic granules

■ **Promyelocyte, or Progranulocyte**

- Myeloblast differentiates
- Forms small immature cytoplasmic granules, azurophilic
- Round/oval nucleus, prominent nucleoli

■ **Myelocyte**

- Promyelocyte differentiates
- Forms more mature or specific granules
    - *Neutrophilic (N) myelocyte*
    - *Basophilic (B) myelocyte*
    - *Eosinophilic (E) myelocyte*
- Round nucleus, nucleoli not readily apparent

■ **Metamyelocyte**

- Nuclear indentation begins and progresses
- Specific cytoplasmic granules
    - *Neutrophilic metamyelocyte*
    - *Basophilic metamyelocyte*
    - *Eosinophilic metamyelocyte*

■ **Band, or Stab**

- Metamyelocyte continues to differentiate
- Nuclear indentation 50% complete
    - *Neutrophilic band*
    - *Basophilic band*
    - *Eosinophilic band*
      Some of these very young or not quite completely differentiated granulocytes normally gain access to the circulation. About 1% to 3% bands or stabs is considered normal. If the band or stab count increases, it can indicate an abnormal loss of the more mature granulocytes, and the bone marrow responds by allowing more bands or stabs to gain access to the circulation.

■ **Mature Neutrophil, Eosinophil, Basophil** In general, as cells differentiate during granulocytopoiesis, the number of granules increases, the size of the entire cell decreases, the lobation of the nucleus increases, cell deformability increases, cell motility increases, adhesiveness increases, and the capability of phagocytosis increases. Total time from stem cell to segmented PMN is 12 days!

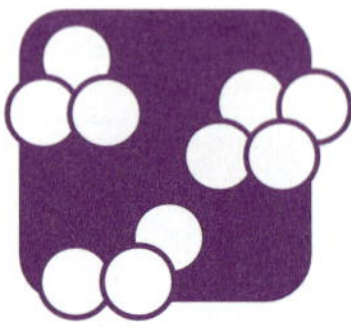

ERYTHROCYTOPOIESIS

As cells mature within the erythroid line of cytodifferentiation (erythrocytopoiesis), they will end up with no granules, lots of hemoglobin, almost no organelles, and no nucleus. A pluripotential CFU, the CFU-GEMMeg cell differentiates into a **uni-**

potential **CFU-E** cell, which then differentiates into the first morphologically recognizable cell in the red cell line.

■ **Normoblast**

- Similar in appearance to myeloblast except:
- Agranular basophilic cytoplasm
    - *Caused by presence of free polysomes*
    - *Future site of synthesis of hemoglobin*

■ **Basophilic normoblast**

- Pyknotic change in nucleus apparent i.e., formerly vesicular chromatin pattern becomes clumpy or stringy.
- Nucleoli are still present but not so easy to distinguish.
- Tremendous increase in free polysomes results in intense cytoplasmic basophilia.

■ **Polychromatophilic normoblast**

- Hemoglobin synthesized on free polysomes
- Cytoplasm, a mixture of areas containing eosinophilic hemoglobin and basophilic areas containing free polysomes. This red and blue mottled cytoplasm—polychromatophilic. More pyknosis and heterochromatinization of nucleus. As more and more hemoglobin is manufactured at the expense of the polysomes, the cytoplasm slowly takes on an eosinophilic cast on top of a diffusely basophilic background.

■ **Orthochromatophilic normoblast**

- Eventual complete heterochromatinization of nucleus
- Cytoplasm is one color: eosinophilic with basophilic background When hemoglobin concentration reaches certain level **nuclear extrusion** occurs.

    - Takes 10 minutes, cell undergoes active, convulsive movements, nucleus exocytosed surrounded by thin rim of cytoplasm, becomes "dinner" for nearby macrophage. Sometimes a small piece of nucleus remains in the RBC—**Howell-Jolly body** which are found in certain types of anemias such as megaloblastic and hemolytic anemia and after splenectomy.

■ **Diffusely basophilic erythrocyte**

- Newly produced, immature RBC
- Eosinophilic cytoplasm, but since some polysomes still present—diffuse basophilia
- Polysomes can be precipitated with special stains—**reticulocytes**
    - Constitute 1% to 3% of RBCs
    - Increased in chronic bleeding as bone marrow allows more immature RBCs out into circulation

Erythropoiesis is regulated in part by **erythropoietin,** a glycoprotein hormone of about 46,000 daltons. EP stimulates the CFU-E to proliferate and differentiate and causes the transcription of mRNAs specific for erythroid maturation. However, once the maturation sequence is initiated the maturation process proceeds on its own. Total time from stem cell to mature RBC is 7 days!

THROMBOCYTOPOIESIS

As cells mature in the megakaryocyte line of cytodifferentiation, they become **polyploid** giant cells with huge, multilobated nuclei.

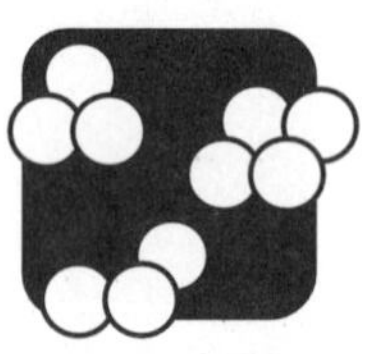

- DNA replication without an accompanying cytokinetic event leads to **endoreduplication.**
- Nucleus becomes increasingly polyploid (2N to 4N to 8N to 16N to 32N to 64N).
- The relative percentage of each ploidy class of megakaryocytes is known: 4N = 3%, 8N = 25%, 16N = 50%, 32N = 20%, 64N = 2%
- The larger the nucleus, the larger the cell and the more platelets are produced.

As the ploidy increases during maturation of the megakaryocyte, the cytoplasm begins to fill with dense membrane-bound granules and channels of SER called **platelet demarcation membranes.** The cell extends a thin pseudopod, actually a **filopod,** through the wall of the sinusoid. Filopods, also known as **proplatelets,** extend along the luminal wall of the sinusoid and then "shatter," releasing platelets directly into the circulation. There are about 35,000 platelets produced per day per microliter of blood.

Monocytopoiesis also occurs in red bone marrow (Fig. 13.1). Young monocytes leave the hematopoietic cords and enter the peripheral circulation for 1 or 2 days and then migrate into connective tissue areas and body cavities, where they carry out their role as tissue macrophages. As tissue macrophages they live for about 60 days and do not reenter the blood.

Lymphocytopoiesis also occurs in red bone marrow. In this situation the type of lymphocyte produced is a **B lymphocyte** (see Chapter 14). In intact bone marrow lymphocytes can be found dispersed throughout the tissue and are also found in discrete lymph nodules.

In general:

- Granulocytopoiesis accounts for 60% (12 days to make a granulocyte) of the cells in the marrow.

- Erythrocytopoiesis accounts for about 30% (7 days to make an erythrocyte). Remaining 10% is accounted for by lymphocytopoiesis, monocytopoiesis, and megakaryocytopoiesis.

- Given the average number of days it takes to make a mature granulocyte or RBC and the relative volumes of cells in granulocytopoiesis and erythrocytopoiesis, it is important to note what is meant by the **myeloid/erythroid** (ME) ratio.

- A normal M/E ratio is 3:1 (2:1 to 4:1). Thus an ME ratio of 3:1 reflects normal granulocytopoiesis and erythrocytopoiesis. An ME ratio of 8:1 could indicate **erythroblastopenia,** or a decrease in the number of cells participating in erythrocytopoiesis. An ME ratio of 1:5 would indicate an abnormal expansion of the erythropoietic mass.

LEUKEMIA

Leukemia represents an abnormal proliferation of one or more of the immature cells of the red bone marrow; i.e., it is a neoplasm of red bone marrow. Many of the leukemias are named according to the type of marrow precursor cell that is proliferating abnormally. This is one reason why you should know the names of the stages of granulocytopoiesis, erythrocytopoiesis, etc. and what they look like.

■ Acute leukemia

- Short, severe disease found mostly in children and young adults
- **Acute myeloblastic leukemia (AML)**

Peripheral blood and marrow contains large numbers of mostly myeloblasts and some promyelocytes. The defect is that maturation has been stopped at the myeloblast-to-promyelocyte stage, but growth continues.

- **Acute monocytic leukemia**
- Peripheral blood and bone marrow filled with monocytoblasts

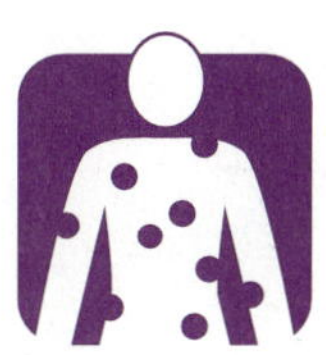

■ Chronic leukemia

- Much slower onset than acute leukemia. The patient is usually an adult. The person may feel well, and the disease sometimes is diagnosed on a routine physical examination. Again the leukemia is named for the immature cell type that is present in abnormal numbers.
- **Chronic myelogenous leukemia (CML)**

Blood and bone marrow will contain a high number of myeloblasts, promyelocytes, myelocytes, metamyelocytes, and even mature granulocytes and sometimes several of the immature cells of the red blood cell series. CML is the leukemia associated with the **Philadelphia chromosome,** which is a translocation of the distal segment of the long arm of no. 22 to the distal portion of the long arm of no. 9.

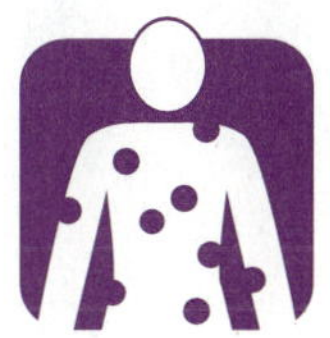

- To emphasize the use of the normal terminology for the different precursor cells in the naming of many of the leukemias it is worth looking at the names of some other leukemias:
  - **Stem cell leukemia**
  - **Myelomonocytic leukemia**
  - **Erythroleukemia**
  - **Eosinophilic leukemia**

    Immature cells from just the eosinophil subdivision of granulocytopoiesis fill up the marrow and circulate in peripheral blood.

- **Basophilic leukemia**

  Immature cells from the basophil subdivision of granulocytopoiesis are involved.

- Promyelocytic leukemia
  - Peripheral blood has only the promyelocyte stage of differentiation circulating.

Clinical Application of Bone Marrow Stem Cell Knowledge and Bone Marrow Transplantation

- Stem cells have the capacity for self-renewal; they are the VIM cells.
- Because of this it is possible to harvest stem cells from bone marrow and use them for autologous or homologous transplantation.

- In a typical situation a patient has inoperable cancer and needs aggressive chemotherapy.
- Before the even lethal doses of chemotherapy, bone marrow is harvested and cryopreserved.
- Then the patient is treated with high doses of chemotherapy agents and even total body irradiation. This eventually would kill the patient because it kills all bone marrow stem cells. But since some bone marrow stem cells were harvested before lethal treatment, they can be transplanted back to the patient and "rescue" the patient from death.

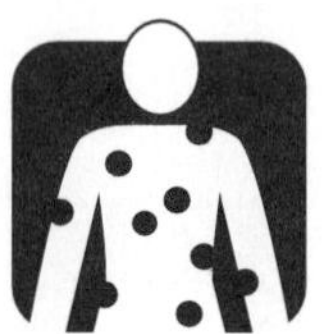

- While the untreated marrow cells are outside of the patient, they can be "purified" of any metastatic cancer cells by tagging the tumor cells with monoclonal antibodies and sorting them away from the normal, nonneoplastic cells in a cell sorter using the technique called **flow cytometry.**
- Tumor cells are tagged by fluorescein-labeled monoclonal antibodies to tumor-specific antigens. These antibodies attach only to tumor cells. When activated by passing through a laser beam, the fluorescein fluoresces, and that tagged cell can be electronically removed (sorted) away from the normal, nonlabeled cells.

CLINICAL USE OF GROWTH FACTORS

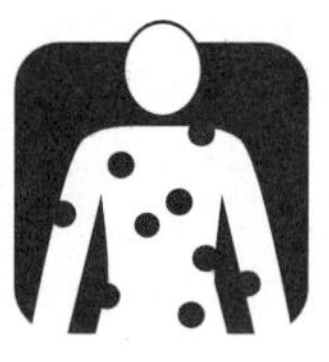

Many of the stimulating factors have been purified and even manufactured using recombinant DNA technology. For example, **GM-CSF** has been produced by recombinant techniques to form **rhGM-CSF** (rh = recombinant human). It has been used to ameliorate the neutropenia associated with myelosuppressive chemotherapy; i.e., clinicians can use treatment with rhGM-CSF to significantly shorten the time of the neutropenia by stimulating granulocytopoiesis and monocytopoiesis with GM-CSF. The gene for human GM-CSF has been mapped and it is located on the long arm of chromosome no. 5.

G-CSF, or **granulocyte colony-stimulating factor** stimulates the CFU-G. **rhG-CSF** crosses species boundaries and works in mice, hamsters, and monkeys as well as in humans. The response to treatment with G-CSF is a dose-dependent neutrophilia. G-CSF has been used clinically to accelerate hematologic recovery after high-dose chemotherapy or radiation therapy–induced myelosuppression and to shorten the duration of neutropenia.

A **rhM-CSF** has been produced. Treatment with it results in a substantial monocytosis.

ALTERNATIVE TERMINOLOGY

Some authors use a nomenclature for the stages of erythrocytopoiesis different from the one used here. It is an attempt to match the names of the stages in the erythroid line with the more familiar nomenclature for the stages of granulocytopoiesis. This alternative terminology is presented here to prevent possible confusion.

- Pronormoblast = **Rubriblast**
- Basophilic normoblast = **Prorubricyte**
- Polychromatophilic normoblast = **Rubricyte**
- Orthochromatophilic normoblast = **Metarubricyte**

MULTIPLE CHOICE
REVIEW QUESTIONS

1. Which of the cells listed below is the most immature?

    a. Myelocyte
    b. Pronormoblast
    c. Metamyelocyte
    d. Polychromatophilic normoblast
    e. Reticulocyte

2. Arrange the following in proper sequence for cytodifferentiation: 1, thrombopoietin acts on a unipotential stem cell; 2, many channels of SER can be found in the cytoplasm; 3, ploidy increases from 2N to 4N; 4, filopod explodes in the lumen of a sinusoid; 5, individual membrane-bound structures containing granules are formed.

    a. 1-3-2-4-5
    b. 2-3-1-4-5
    c. 3-4-2-1-5
    d. 4-1-3-2-5

3. The following statement describes which of the kinetic compartments in the bone marrow: "not self-sustaining, continual cell loss occurs, cell aging and cell death occurs":

    a. Stem cell compartment (VIM)
    b. Differentiating-multiplicative compartment (DIM)
    c. Functional compartment (FPM)
    d. Reverting postmitotic compartment (RPM)

4. Arrange the following in proper sequence for cytodifferentiation in granulocytopoiesis: 1, cell with 2 or 3 prominent nucleoli; 2, nuclear indentation first apparent; 3, specific neutrophilic, basophilic, or eosinophilic granules first appear; 4, cell migrates from hematopoietic cord to vessel lumen; 5, cell migrates from capillary lumen to connective tissue space.

    a. 1-3-2-4-5
    b. 2-3-4-1-5
    c. 4-2-1-3-5
    d. 3-2-4-1-5
    e. 3-4-2-1-5

5. A patient in your care has leukemia. You look at a smear of peripheral blood from this patient and the most common cell type that you see is large cell with a round nucleus that has several prominent nucleoli in it and the cytoplasm is filled with small azurophilic granules. What is your diagnosis?

    a. Lymphoblastic leukemia
    b. Basophil leukemia
    c. Monoblastic leukemia
    d. Promyelocytic leukemia
    e. Stem cell leukemia

Chapter 14

The Defense System

GENERAL

The defense system protects the individual from exogenous or "nonself" antigenic insults and is involved in cleaning up modified, defective, worn-out "self" antigens.

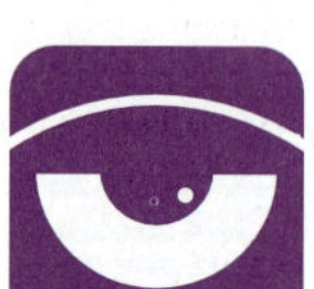

Nonself antigens introduced into or onto the body as macromolecules in, e.g., viruses, bacteria, environmental toxins such as poison ivy, spontaneously arising neoplasms (tumor-specific antigens), and cells, tissues, or organs from other individuals:

- **autograft:** self to self
- **isograft:** between genetically identical individuals such as identical twins or highly inbred research animals
- **allograft:** from one individual to another within the same species
- **xenograft:** across species boundaries (baboon to human)

Distinguishes between self antigens and nonself antigens, reacts against nonself and thereby protects self from threat imposed by nonself.

- **Natural immunologic tolerance:** You are tolerant of your own macromolecules, which would not be immunologically tolerated by someone else.

- **Acquired immunologic tolerance:** You will be tolerant of any nonself antigens if they are introduced during fetal life. As the defense system differentiates, it must become tolerant of all self antigens; exogenous antigens (graft) introduced while this process is going on will be considered as self. However, if the graft contains immunologically competent cells, they will consider their new immunologically incompetent host to be nonself and a **graft versus host reaction** can occur as is the case when an adult spleen is transplanted into an embryo or an allograft of bone marrow is placed into a person rendered immunologically incompetent by anticancer radiation and chemotherapy.

- Immunologically competent cells continuously **recirculate** from blood to lymphoid tissues or organs back to blood and are widely distributed (big toe today but ear lobe tomorrow).

- Immunologically competent cells are **programmed** during their differentiation to respond to only one kind of antigen; the cells display antigenic specificity. Once activated by exposure to the appropriate antigen these immunologically competent cells proliferate or undergo **clonal expansion** forming many copies of themselves. During this clonal expansion some cells become **effector cells,** and some become **memory cells,** which are long-lived cells in a sense waiting for a second exposure to the antigen they have been programmed against. If this antigen shows up again, the second response, because of memory, occurs more rapidly.

- Removal of worn-out, defective self antigens, e.g., RBCs over 120 days old, defective RBCs, aged connective tissue fibers, megakaryocyte nuclei after platelet release, by macrophages throughout the body.

- Includes the lymphoid organs: thymus, lymph nodes, spleen, and tonsils; aggregates of lymphoid tissue wherever it is found (Peyer's patches in the small intestine); diffuse lymphatic tissue (lymphocytes, plasma cells, macrophages) wherever it is found, as in the lamina propria under all wet epithelia.

CELL-MEDIATED IMMUNOLOGIC RESPONSE

- A property of the lymphocytes derived from the **thymus,** i.e., the **T-cell system,** no matter where T cells are found after their relocation from the thymus throughout the body.

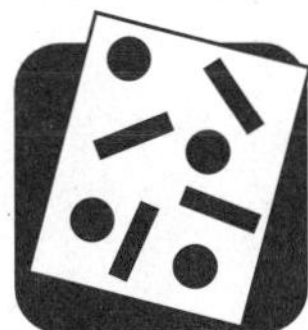

- Primary host defense against fungi, viruses, protozoa, mycobacteria, allografts, and neoplasms.
- Involves T cell–to–target cell contact for destruction of the target by **killer,** or **cytotoxic, T cells (Tk).** Tk cells physically move, migrate, and search for their specific target, but when the target is found, the destruction of the target is a nonspecific killing by a protein, **perforin,** which causes holes to form in the plasmalemma of the target cell.

■ Other Subsets of T Cells

- **T helper (Th) cells** upregulate antibody production and also "help" many other immune responses so much so that the Th cell has been referred to as the conductor of the immune symphony. Most of this help or modulation of the immune response by the Th cell is mediated through hormone like substances called **cytokines** or **lymphokines.** The AIDS virus specifically kills Th cells.

- **T suppresser (Ts) cells** downregulate antibody production.

- T delayed type hypersensitivity (Tdth) cells produce the biological mediators **MAF (macrophage activating factor)** and **MIF (migration inhibitory factor).** MIF was the first cytokine discovered (1966) and has been produced by recombinant DNA technology (1989). It immobilizes macrophages and thereby keeps them at the site of insult. MAF activates the "stopped" macrophages to perform their function.

> **CD antigens** are found only on T cells, not B cells.
> Two major classes of CD antigens (CD from 'cluster of differentiation'):
> **CD8** is expressed by Ts and Tk cells, and **CD4** is expressed by Th cells.

- 70% of blood lymphocytes are classifiable as T cells, and the same is probably true of diffuse lymphatic tissue (lamina propria).
- Histologically found in **thymus-dependent areas,** or zones in lymphoid organs: midcortex to deep cortex of lymph nodes, marginal zone and around artery of white pulp in spleen, internodal areas between adjacent lymph nodules in the gut.

■ T-Cell Activation

- Surface **receptor** binds with the antigen for which it is specific. This causes a calcium-binding protein to bind **calcineurin,** which activates calcineurin's enzymatic activity, which turns on **interleukin-2,** an intracellular signaling molecule that causes **blast transformation** and **clonal expansion.**

Antibody (Humoral)-Mediated Immunologic Response

This is a property of the lymphocytes derived from the bone marrow, i.e., the **B-cell system.** B cells must differentiate into **plasma cells,** which then synthesize and release **antibodies,** which circulate and specifically combine with the antigen initiating the response. **Antibodies** are glycoproteins found in the globulin fraction of the blood plasma, i.e., the **immunoglobulins IgA, IgD, IgG, IgM, IgE.** Antibodies serve to recognize and help destroy nonself antigens.

Once a B cell is programmed to respond to its specific antigen it produces receptors for that antigen, which become integral membrane proteins in the plasmalemma of the B cell, providing the molecular basis for recognition of that antigen if that specific antigen ever shows up. When that antigen shows up, it is recognized by the receptor, and such recognition activates this B cell or set of B cells to differentiate into **plasma cells,** which synthesize and release antibody specific to the activating antigen. Only one type of specific antibody can be produced by a plasma cell, i.e., **monoclonal antibody.**

Successful B-cell activation requires the presence of

• Factors (**cytokines** or **lymphokines,** e.g., the **interleukins**) produced by a subset of T lymphocytes, the helper T cells. Another subset of T cells affects B cell activity in a fashion opposite to the Th cell, and these are the T suppresser, or Ts, cells which cause a downregulation of antibody production.

  • **Antigen-presenting cells**

    1. **Macrophage,** which phagocytoses the antigen, internally **processes** it and then brings a purified form of the antigen to its surface for **presentation** to a B cell
    2. **Antigen trapping and presenting cells,** such as the **dendritic reticular cells** in lymph nodes, which do not have to phagocytize the antigen to process and present it

      • 20% of blood lymphocytes are B cells, and the same is probably true of diffuse lymphatic tissue. Histologically found in lymph nodules wherever they are found.

Null Cell System

  • Lymphocytes not identifiable as either a B cell or a T cell by surface markers
  • **Natural killer cells (Nk),** which are particularly sensitive to the presence of any kind of transformed cell such as a neoplastic cell
  • **K cells,** or killer cells (not Tk or Nk), which require the presence of antibody to carry out their cytotoxic role; 10% of blood lymphocytes are null cells

Cells or Parenchyma of the Defense System

■ **Macrophages**

  • Remarkable capability for phagocytosis
  • **Fixed** in position or attached to reticular fibers such as Kupfer cells of the liver, reticular cells in the spleen, bone marrow, and lymph nodes. Structure is elongated because of attachment to reticular fiber, vesicular nucleus with prominent nucleolus, e.g. the reticular cells in spleen, bone marrow, lymph nodes, and thymus.

• **Free** (not attached to a reticular fiber) such as all wandering tissue macrophages or **histiocytes,** which really are blood monocytes that have emigrated from the vascular system into connective tissue areas; same cell—two names depending on where located. Structure consists of a large cell with abundant amount of cytoplasm containing large numbers of lysosomes (depends on time since its last meal); typically a bean-shaped nucleus with a clumpy-stringy (spaghetti and meatball) chromatin pattern; pseudopods at cell surface and surface invaginations. May fuse with one another to form **multinucleated giant cells,** such as foreign-body giant cells, Langhans' giant cells (pathognomonic for TB lesion), osteoclasts.

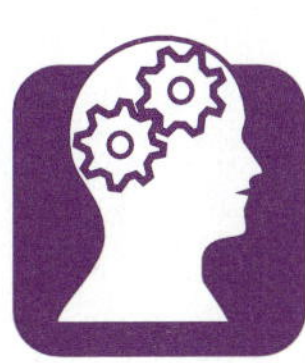

• Phagocytosis of worn-out, defective, dead, and dying self cells

• Phagocytosis of nonself antigens or cells

• During cellular digestion phase, macrophage processes and then presents on its surface a purified, modified form of the original nonself antigen (**antigen presentation**), which can be available for lymphocyte activation. Some cells such as the **dendritic reticular cells** in the germinal centers of lymph nodules do not need to phagocytize foreign antigen before presenting it; i.e., they trap it on their surface and process it there.

▪ Lymphocytes

• Free, round, and very mobile; thin rim of cytoplasm with little ultrastructural specialization; heterochromatinized nucleus

• Three kinds: T, B, or null

• Undergo **blast transformation** when activated by antigen they are programmed against: enhanced endocytosis, increased RNA synthesis, nuclear hypertrophy, euchromatinization of previous pyknotic nucleus, severalfold increase in cell size. The resulting morphology is of a blast stage of differentiation, i.e., **lymphoblasts.** DNA synthesis and mitosis occurs which results in a **clonal expansion;** clinical karyotyping takes advantage of this: expose blood lymphocytes to a foreign antigen (mitogen such as phytohemagglutinin), cause clonal expansion, i.e., DNA synthesis and mitosis; use vincristine to arrest progress around the cell cycle at metaphase; study metaphase chromosomes.

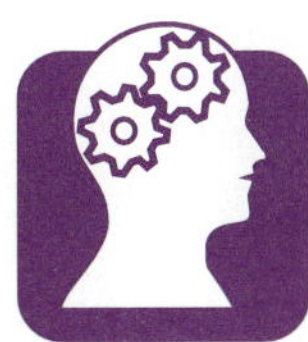

• If **T cell**, some products of the clonal expansion become **cytotoxic effector cells** and some become **memory T cells,** which can run through a second blast transformation much faster than the first.

• If **B cell,** some of the products of the blast transformation and clonal expansion differentiate into **plasma cells,** and some redifferentiate into **memory B cells,** which can run through a second blast transformation more quickly (Fig. 14.1).

▪ Plasma Cells

• Eccentric nucleus with clock-faced chromatin pattern, intense basophilia of the cytoplasm caused by well-developed RER; light area between cytoplasm and nucleus is where the well-developed Golgi apparatus is located.

• Terminally differentiated, fixed postmitotic cell with a life-span of about 2 to 3 weeks

• Free cells, which wander around in connective tissue areas

• Synthesis and release of **immunoglobulins**

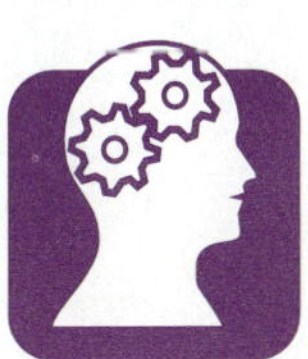

1. IgG, most abundant
2. **IgA,** primarily found in tears, saliva, and mucus of gastrointestinal and respiratory tracts
3. **IgM** and **IgD,** circulate but are also membrane bound on the surface of B cells, where they function as B-cell antigen receptors

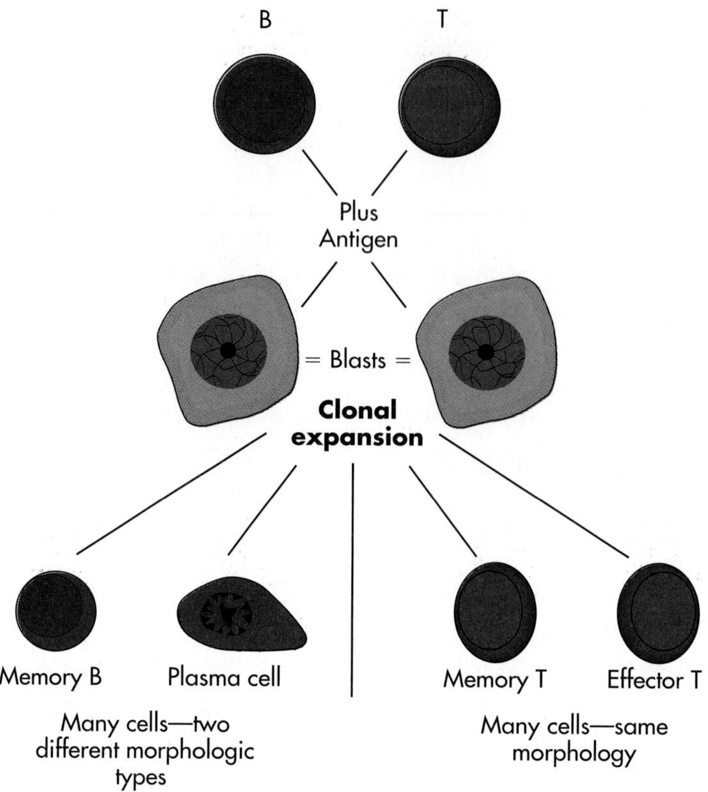

Fig. 14.1 T-cell and B-cell clonal expansion in response to activation by exposure to an appropriate antigen. Virgin T and B cells and appropriate antigen become mitotically active "blasts" producing many daughter cells, some of which differentiate into effector cells or memory cells.

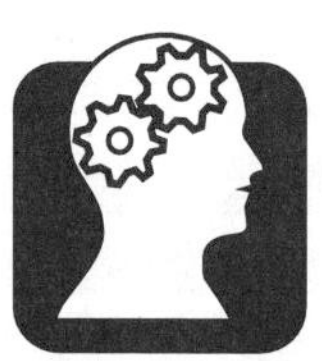

4. **IgE,** found on the surface of **basophils** and **mast cells** and plays a role in **immediate hypersensitivity reactions;** i.e., cell surface has receptors for IgE, which is bound at the cell surface with the antigen-recognition site exposed; when antigen specific for this recognition site binds to the IgE, the cell **degranulates,** releasing a variety of biological mediators such as **histamine, heparin, eosinophil chemotactic factors of anaphylaxis, neutrophil chemotactic factor, prostaglandins, platelet-activating factor,** and **slow-reacting substance of anaphylaxis.** These compounds cause the runny nose, itchy eyes, and sneezing episodes characteristic of an attack of hay fever. Even more severe and serious reactions can occur in response to an IgE buildup after a bee sting or first exposure to penicillin, i.e., **severe immediate hypersensitivity** and even **anaphylatic shock.**

• Only one specific type of antibody (e.g., IgG against antigen X) from one plasma cell (e.g., IgG against antigen W would come from a different clone of plasma cells); in other words, plasma cells derived from one type of B lymphocyte are little factories of **monoclonal antibody production.** Since plasma cells are **terminally differentiated** and do not divide (fixed postmitotics), it was frustrating to see these factories die off at the end of their 2 to 3-week life-span. The Nobel prize was given for the discovery that a terminally differentiated plasma cell could be fused with a neoplastic plasma cell (plasmacytoma) and the

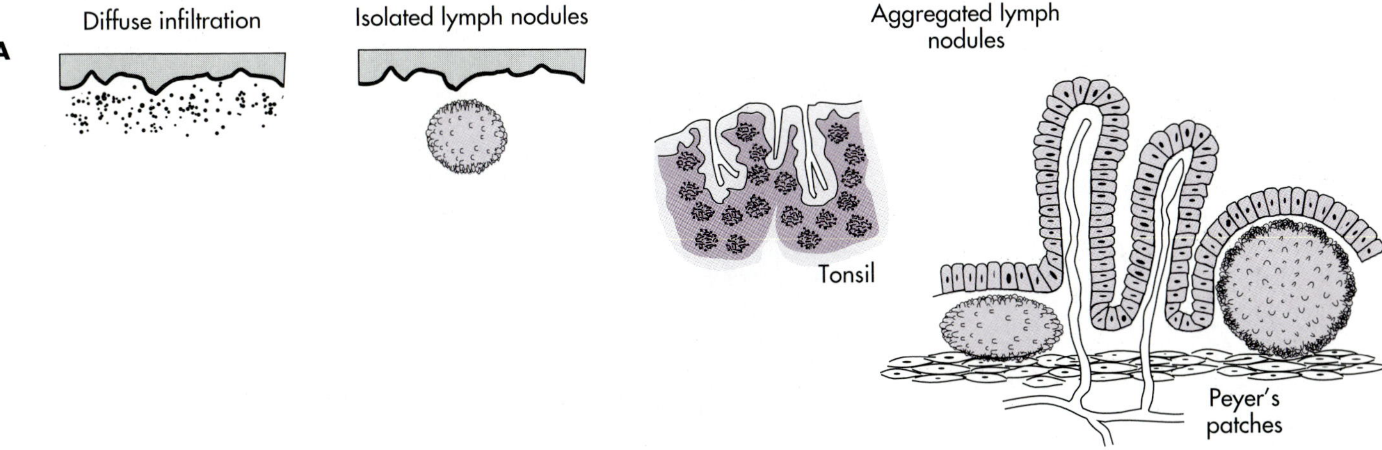

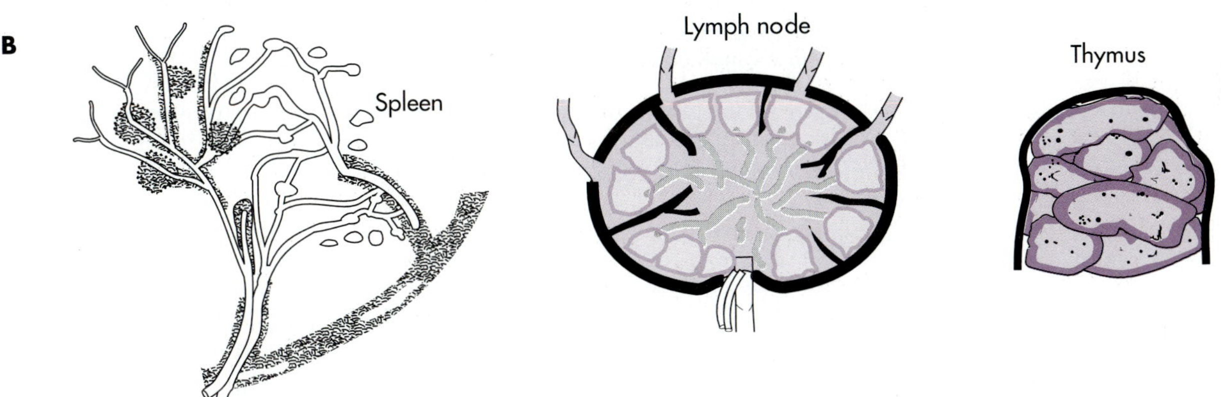

Fig. 14.2 Overview of the different levels of organization of lymphoid tissues and organs.

resulting heterokaryon would retain the capability to divide, which means it could then be used as a single cell starter for the development of a clone of its descendants *and* continue to make monoclonal antibody.

- All plasma cells come from B lymphocytes.

LYMPHATIC TISSUE (FIG. 14.2)

■ Diffuse Lymphatic Tissue

- Lymphocytes, plasma cells, and histiocytes in the loose areolar connective tissue under all epithelial surfaces except endothelium. For wet epithelia this is the **lamina propria**. In the integument this is the **papillary layer** of the **dermis**.

■ Lymph Nodules (Not Nodes)

- Nonencapsulated, single or in groups; examples of aggregates of lymph nodules, **tonsils, appendix, Peyer's patches**
- Round, tightly packed accumulation of lymphocytes (mostly B) with or without a lighter central region; the germinal center

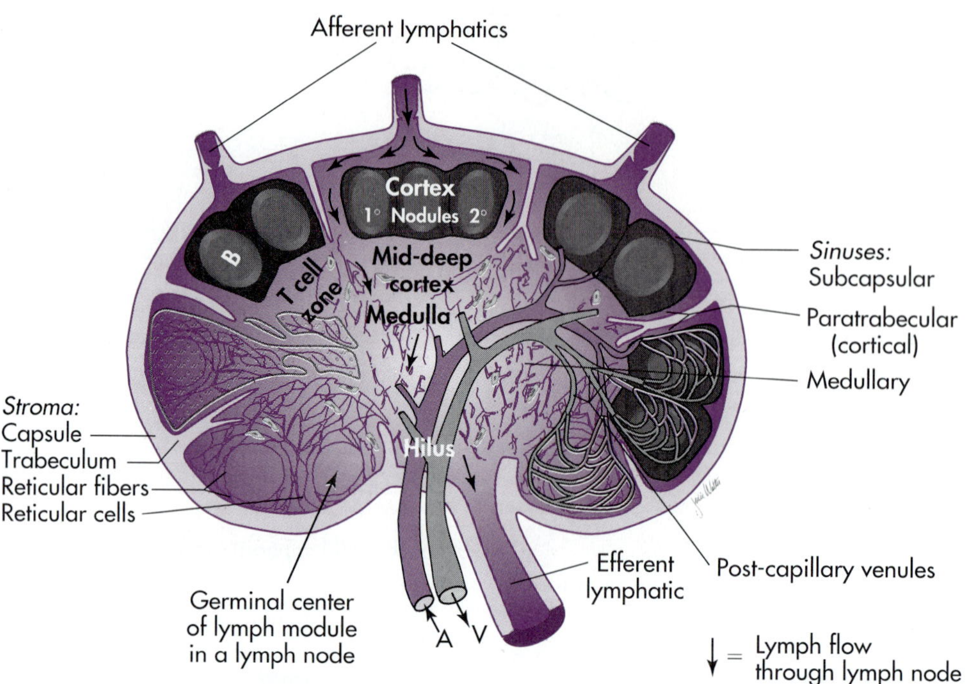

Fig. 14.3 Histophysiologic sketch of a lymph node as a filter of lymph. Lymph enters afferent lymphatics, which pierce the capsule and drain into the subcapsular sinus→ paratrabecular sinus→medullary sinus→efferent lymph vessels.

■ Germinal Center

- Not present before birth

- Evidence for exposure to nonself and **clonal expansion** of **mostly B cells** (germinating). If an animal is born into a sterile environment by C-section and kept there, no germinal centers would arise because no exposure to foreign antigens would occur.

- Surrounded by a rim or corona of densely packed small lymphocytes, which were born in the germinal center and are in the process of leaving

- Many mitotic figures

- B lymphocytes undergoing clonal expansion and then redifferentiation into memory B cells *or* into plasma cells. Presence of **lymphoblasts-prolymphocytes-lymphocytes; plasmablasts-proplasmacytes-plasma cells**

- **Dendritic reticular cells** with oval nucleus and prominent nucleolus associated with reticular fibers; function as antigen trapping-processing-presenting cells to virgin or memory B cells

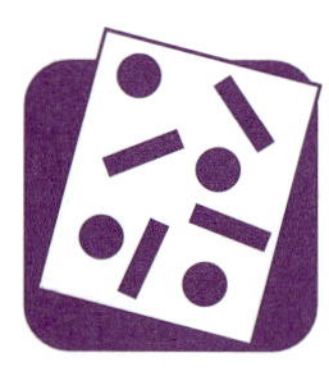

LYMPHOID ORGANS

■ Lymph Node

- Capsule of connective tissue pierced by **afferent lymphatics** bringing lymph into the organ

- **Cortex (Fig. 14.3). Outer** is composed of many **lymph nodules,** i.e., mostly a **B-cell area. Deeper cortex** has **no lymph nodules** but lots of lymphocytes; this is mostly a **T-cell area. Thymus-dependent** zone contains special venules that are lined not by squamous endothelium but by cuboidal to low columnar endothelium, i.e., **high endothelium venules (HEVs).** Both B cells

and T cells recirculating through a lymph node recognize this special epithelium and stick to it and leave the blood vascular system here to enter parenchymal regions of the lymph node.

• **Medulla** is a lighter area than cortex; it contains medullary sinuses and cords; probably half and half T cells and B cells.

• **Hilum.** Arteries enter, veins leave, and efferent **lymph vessels** leave.

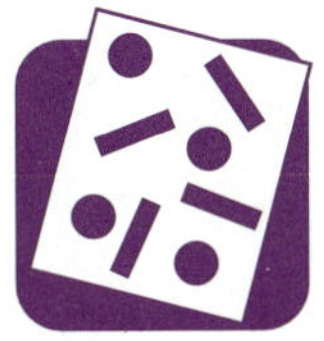

• Stroma of **reticular fibers,** which may have reticular cells, dendritic cells, or fixed macrophages attached. Collagenous trabeculae extend in from capsule.

• Circulation and **filtration of lymph. Afferent lymphatic** to **subcapsular sinus** to **paratrabecular sinus** to **medullar sinus** to **efferent lymph vessel.** All sinuses bridged or lined by fixed macrophages, reticular cells. Performs filtration function of organ. Same "circulatory" path taken by malignant cells as they drain through lymph nodes.

• **Neonatal thymectomy** or **agenesis of the thymus (DiGeorge's syndrome)** results in no T cell–dependent zones in lymph nodes and spleen, inability to reject allografts, and some compromise of Th function to the B-cell system.

▪ Spleen

• Capsule surfaced by mesothelium, some smooth muscle fibers

• Trabeculae extend from capsule into organ.

● Red pulp

• 80% of parenchyma of the organ

• **Venous sinusoids** with longitudinally arranged **nonphagocytic endothelial cells** with relatively large spaces between them for ease of cell movement between them.

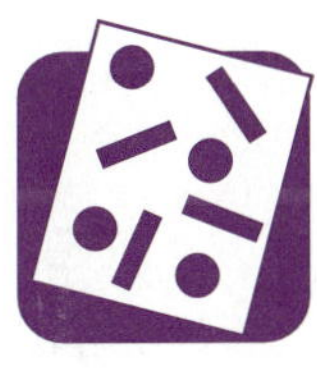

• Pulp between adjacent sinusoids is geometrically arranged into cords (the **cords of Billroth**). Terminal capillaries open into cords of Billroth. Cord composed of fixed and free macrophages, reticular fibers, and all formed elements of blood. Cords serve as a **blood filter.** Macrophages phagocytose, process, and present nonself, blood-borne antigens. They also phagocytose defective, aged, blood-born self antigen; e.g., 142-day-old RBC arrives in capillary terminating in cord but never makes it out (is eaten by macrophage in cord). Iron is conserved for reutilization. Nondefective formed elements of blood are "inspected" by these macrophages and allowed to pass between endothelial cells of sinusoid wall and return to circulation (Fig. 14.4).

● White pulp (two types)

• **Lymph nodules** with germinal centers—**B cell areas.** Unlike in lymph node, here they contain an arteriole obviously off center in the germinal center but referred to as the central artery or arteriole.

• Accumulations, or **collars, of lymphocytes** around arterial vessels, which leave trabeculae to enter splenic pulp, i.e., mostly a **thymus-dependent zone.**

● Marginal zone

• Interface between red pulp and white pulp where lymphocytes are moving from a T-cell or B-cell area into red pulp.

• Many antigen-presenting cells presenting antigen to T cells and B cells

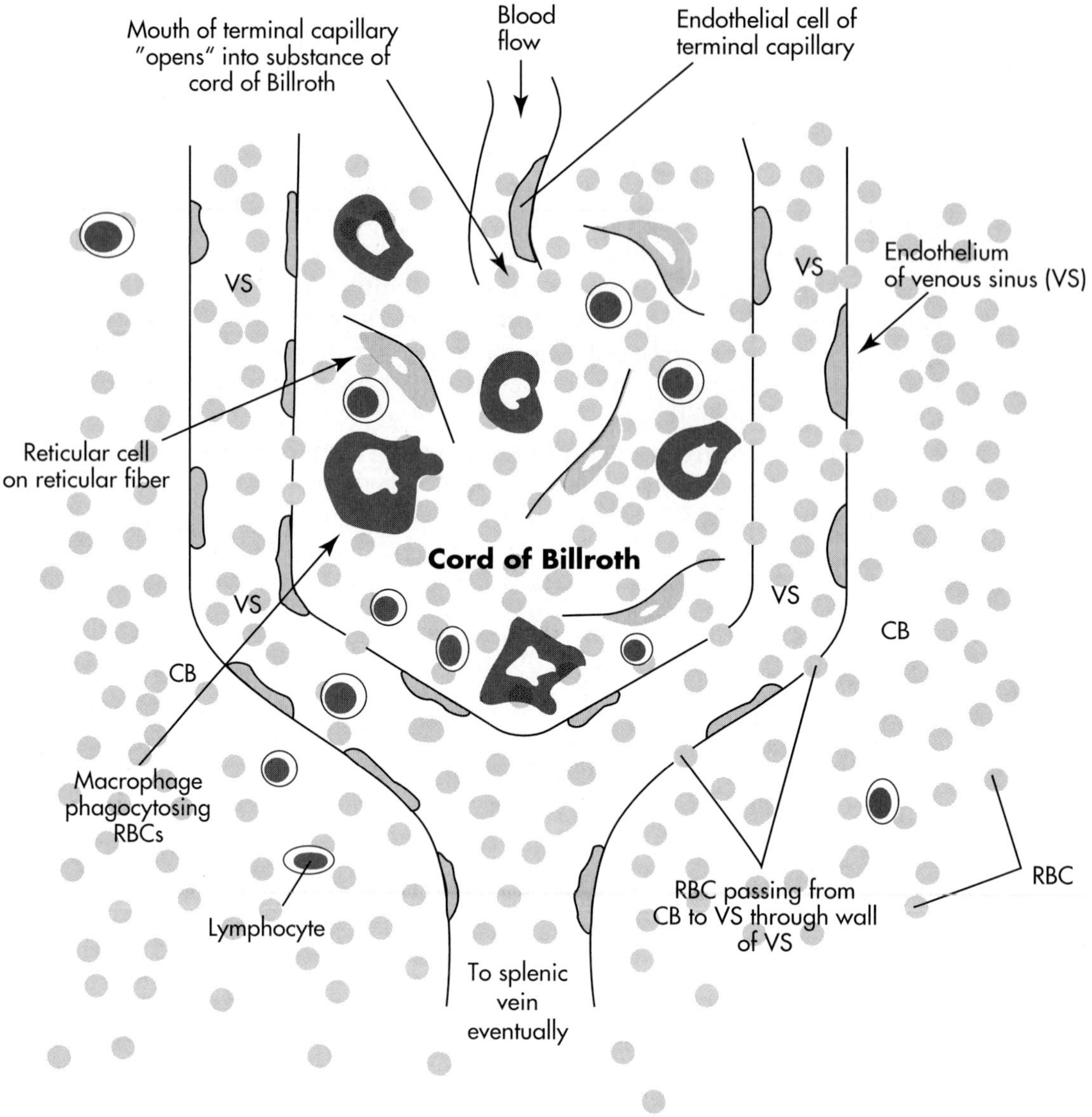

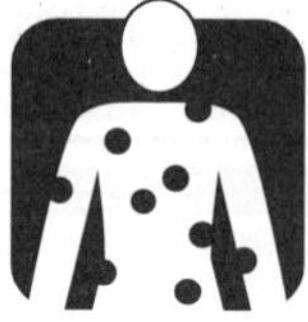

Fig. 14.4 Histophysiologic sketch of the spleen as a filter of blood. Blood is delivered into the substance of a cord of Billroth by a terminal capillary. The blood and its formed elements must pass around the parenchymal cells of the cord, such as fixed and free macrophages, before regaining access to the bloodstream by passing from the cord through the wall of the venous sinus. Defective and aged RBCs are phagocytosed by the phagocytes in the interstices of the cord.

- Production of both T cell and B cell clones
- Th and Ts interaction with B cells

● **Circulation of blood (for filtration)**

- Splenic artery→trabecular artery→artery of white pulp (with collar of mostly T cells)→central arteriole in lymph nodule (B cell area→arteriole leaves white pulp area and enters red pulp→branches like a painter's brush→penicillar arterioles→terminal vessel terminates into interstices of cord of Billroth (**open circulation** because here blood not enclosed in endothelium-lined tube but just dumped into cord of Billroth), where it gets filtered or inspected→passes through staves (elongated endothelial cells) of the barrel (venous sinusoid walls at outer edges of cords of Billroth)→returns to "normal" circulation.

■ Thymus

- Capsule and its extensions divide organ into obvious but incomplete lobules.
- **No afferent lymphatics** enter, but organ does produce lymph, and efferent lymphatics leave organ.
- **No lymph nodules**
- Dense cellular area—outer aspect of each lobule—**cortex.** The outer cortex is mostly composed of lymphoblasts. The inner cortex is mostly of more mature lymphocytes. Lymphocyte cytodifferentiation (anti-antigen programming) occurs from outer cortex→inner cortex→medulla.
- Lighter, less cellular area—center of each lobule—**medulla**

Contains programmed, immunologically competent T cells, which migrate through walls of postcapillary venules to gain access to blood to be distributed throughout body and to all thymus-dependent zones.

- ● Hassall's corpuscles
  - Squamous cells wrapped around each other forming little balls
  - These cells contain desmosomes and keratohyaline granules.
  - Remnants of branchial, ectodermal-groove epithelium that get caught up in development and migration of gland during fetal life.

  Reticular cells on reticular fibers in both cortex and medulla are of **endodermal origin** (epithelium of pharyngeal pouch), not mesodermal origin as all other reticular cells are. They are an important component of the blood-thymus barrier. They produce **thymosin,** a factor important for normal development of T cells.

  Programming of differentiating T cells involves survival of cells programmed against nonself, but **clonal ablation** or **inactivation** of cells programmed against self. Those programmed against self die in large numbers with the result that the particular individual is **naturally immunologically tolerant** to his or her own antigens. This occurs during fetal period. If a nonself antigen is introduced during this process, it will be considered by the thymus as "self" and that clone of T cells will be ablated or inactivated, resulting in acquired immunologic tolerance to that specific antigen (Fig. 14.5).

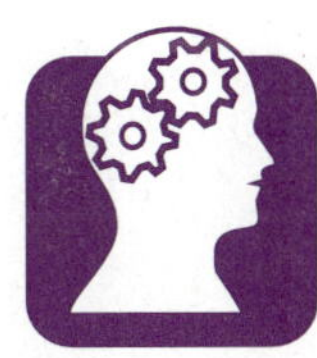

- ● Blood-thymus barrier
  - **Leaky during fetal life,** allowing for development of **natural immunologic tolerance**
  - Not leaky at about the **time of birth** and therefore no more tolerance is generated, i.e., from birth on only **immunologic *in*tolerance** or competence
    - Structure from blood outward to thymic parenchyma
      - **Endothelium**
      - Endothelial basal lamina

        Pericyte may sit in this basal lamina.

      - **Perivascular space**

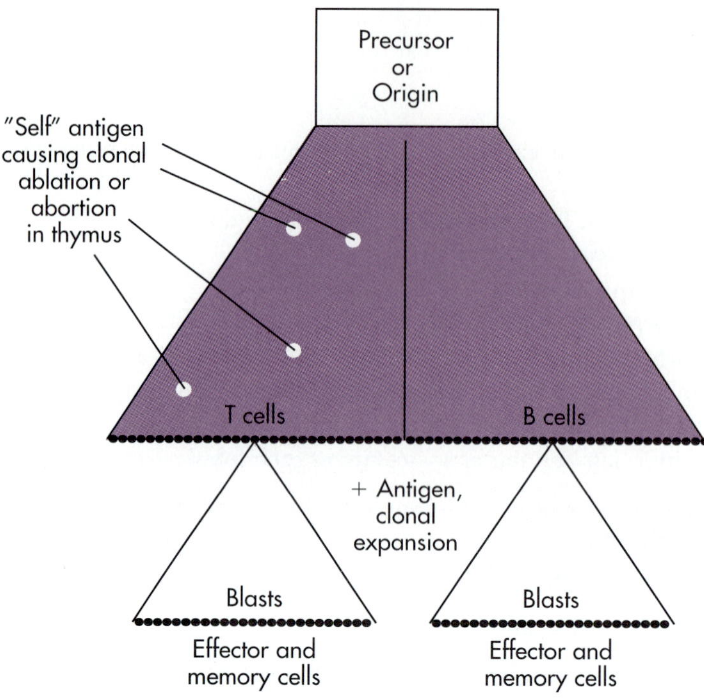

Fig. 14.5 Diagram of clonal expansion in both T- and B-cell lineages relative to the numbers of these cells derived from precursor cells. A special situation exists for T-cell formation in which self antigen can ablate or abort or inactivate T cells being designed against self antigen.

- Basal lamina of reticular cell
- Cytoplasm of reticular cell

Reticular cells form tunnels in which the capillaries and arterioles course. Outside of the epithelially derived reticular cell would be T lymphocytes.

DEFENSE SYSTEM AND CANCER

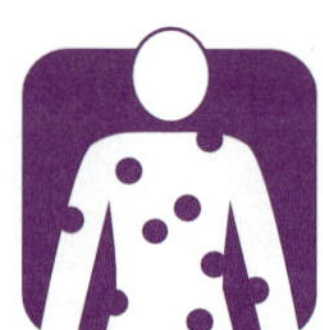

- **Tumor-specific antigens (TSA)** are found on all neoplastic cells.
- Nk cells are particularly sensitive to TSAs, Tk cells to a lesser degree.
- Neoplastic cells killed probably daily by Nk and Tk activity.
- Patients **immunosuppressed** (depression of cell-mediated immunity for continued survival of an allograft as in the case of a kidney transplant) have a seventyfold increase in the incidence of cancer over the normal, nonimmunosuppressed population.

DEFENSE SYSTEM AND PREGNANCY

- Mother will reject allograft from her newborn but does not reject same tissue while she is pregnant.
- Fetus is **histoincompatible** with mother.
- Fetus and mother have successful immunologic coexistence.

Anatomical separation or barrier between maternal-fetal tissue interface in placenta—Nitabuch's membrane (or layer), a sialic acid coating or masking of fetal antigens from maternal lymphocytes.

• Fetal tissue is hypoantigenic.

• Maternal **serum alpha macroglobulin** functions as an immune blocking factor during pregnancy by blocking cell-mediated immunity (actually binds to T cells) but not humoral immunity in mother.

• Transient involution of maternal thymus during pregnancy. Allografts survive for exceptionally long times.

Fig. 14.6 provides an overall summary of the immune system cells.

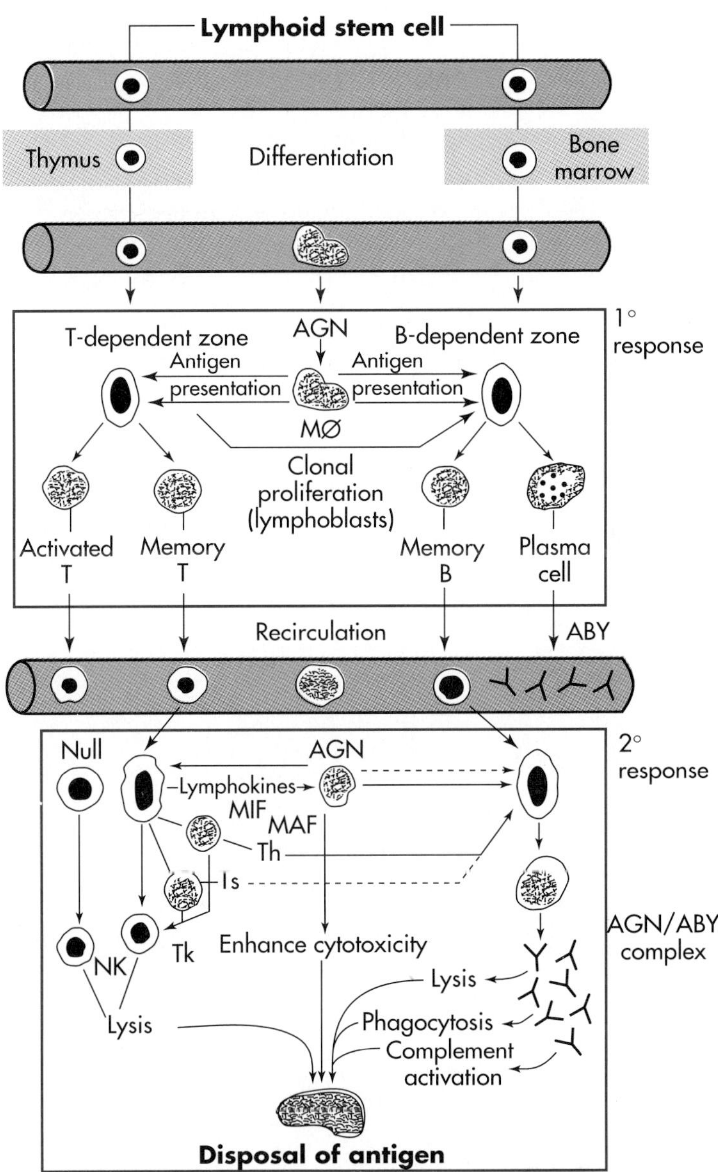

Fig. 14.6 Overview of the cells of the immune system and their interactions with foreign antigen and other cells of the immune system and their traffic patterns from blood to lymphoid tissues and organs to blood again.

MULTIPLE CHOICE REVIEW QUESTIONS

1. Where in the body of a normal, healthy young man would you expect most erythrophagocytosis to be occurring?

    a. Marginal zone in spleen
    b. Medulla of thymus
    c. Hematopoietic cord in bone marrow
    d. Cord of Billroth in spleen
    e. Paratrabecular sinus in lymph node

2. Arrange the following in proper sequence for a pin passing from a thymocyte through the thymic barrier to an intravascular position: 1, thymocyte; 2, endothelium; 3, thrombocyte; 4, perivascular space; 5, reticular cells.

    a. 1-2-3-4-5
    b. 1-5-4-3-2
    c. 1-5-4-2-3
    d. 1-4-5-3-2
    e. 1-3-5-2-4

3. All the following could correctly describe any lymphocyte you see on a peripheral blood smear except

    a. T effector cell.
    b. B effector cell.
    c. T virgin (without antigenic experience) cell.
    d. B cell ready for a "second-set" reaction to an antigen.
    e. T cell with "memory" of a prior antigenic experience.

4. Which of the following produces thymosin?

    a. Dendritic reticular cell in germinal center
    b. Th cell in blood
    c. Tdth cell in a lamina propria
    d. Epithelially derived reticular cell in a medulla
    e. Hassall's corpuscle

5. All of the following cells can process and present antigen *except*

    a. histiocyte.
    b. Kupffer cell.
    c. dendritic reticular cell.
    d. Langerhans' cell in epidermis.
    e. CD8 lymphocyte.

Chapter 15

Digestive System

General

The digestive organ system includes a) the gut tube, beginning at the lips and ending at the anus, and b) the extramural glands associated with the tube such as the liver, gallbladder, pancreas, and salivary glands. The GI tract not only is designed to function in its well-known nutritional role, but also is a major endocrine organ, and it plays a role in the defense system as well.

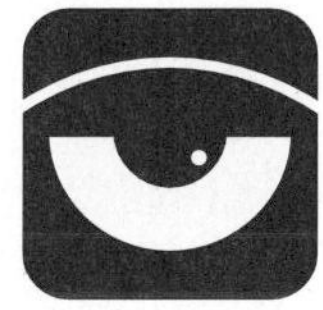

Basic Plan of the Gut Tube

■ **Three Major Tunics**

● Inner mucosa

- **Luminal epithelium** can be secretory, absorptive, protective; contains **enteroendocrine** cells, which secrete hormone toward capillaries in adjacent connective tissue (lamina propria); enteroendocrine—**APUD** cell (amine precursor uptake and decarboxylation)
  - Subepithelial **lamina propria** of loose areolar connective tissue
  - **Muscularis mucosae** of smooth muscle (Fig. 15.1)

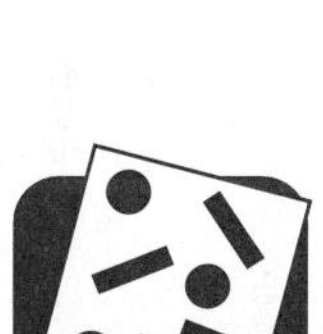

● Middle submucosa

- Loose areolar connective tissue

● Outer muscular layer, the muscularis externa

- Usually inner circular
- Outer longitudinal

■ **Outside of the Muscularis Externa Layer**

● Serosa

- **Mesothelial** cell surface with some submesothelial connective tissue; **visceral peritoneum** (slippery surface, slides over adjacent visceral peritoneum and **parietal peritoneum**)

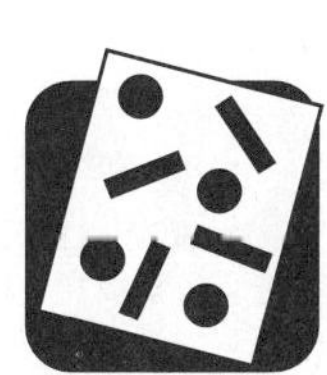

● Fibrosa or adventitia

- Loose areolar and adipose connective tissue blending with same tissue of surrounding organs

● Examples

- Surface of gallbladder exposed to peritoneal cavity (serosa)
- Surface of gallbladder imbedded in liver (fibrosa or adventitia)
- Surface of ascending colon facing peritoneal cavity is covered by a serosa even though it is retroperitoneal
- Surface of ascending colon facing posterior body wall is an adventitia or fibrosa

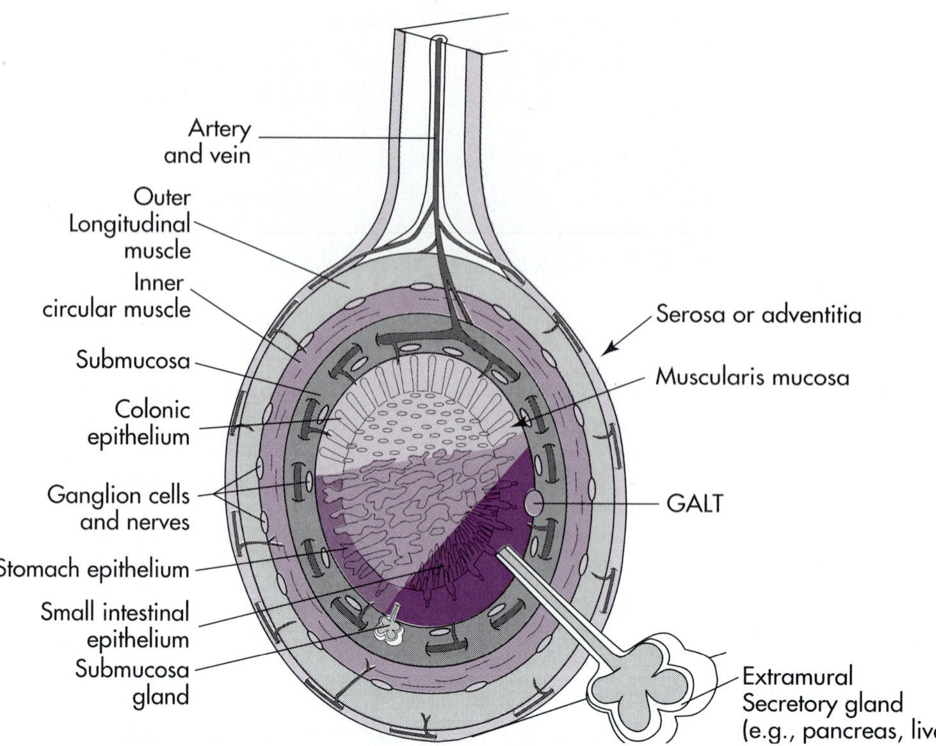

Fig. 15.1 General plan of the gastrointestinal tract. From lumen outward: mucosa (lining epithelium→lamina propria→muscularis mucosa), submucosa (with autonomic nerve plexus), muscularis externa (inner circular to outer longitudinal smooth muscle (with myenteric nerve plexus)→outer covering of serosa (visceral peritoneum) or fibrosa with adventitia (connective tissue). *GALT,* Gut-associated lymphatic tissue, such as isolated lymph nodules and aggregates of lymph nodules (Peyer's patches).

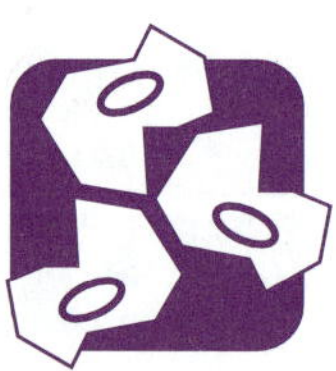

- ■ **Surface Area Increased**

  - **Microvilli** on each absorptive cell of mucosa
  - Folds of inner two layers of mucosa (but not muscularis mucosae) forming **villi**
  - Folds of submucosa forming valves of Kerkring, or **plicae circulares**

- ■ **Cell Turnover**

  - Luminal epithelium **desquamated** or **sloughed** constantly
  - Must be replaced constantly by cell birth and cell migration from birth site to site of desquamation. High rate of cell loss, high rate of cell renewal, high susceptibility to drugs designed to stop cell division, GI toxicity in patients receiving cancer chemotherapy.
  - Desquamated cells can be captured and used for **Pap smear cytology,** e.g., gastric lavage.

- ■ **Innervation (Necessary for Peristalsis)**

  - Sympathetic postganglionic fibers
  - **Parasympathetic preganglionic fibers** to neuron cell bodies in ganglia in wall of tube to **postganglionic fibers** to glands and smooth muscle
  - Two plexuses
    - **Submucosal (Meissner's)**

- **Myenteric (Auerbach's),** or typically between inner circular and outer longitudinal layers of smooth muscle
- **Aganglionosis,** or absence of autonomic ganglia in segment of colon leading to paralysis of this region. Gut tube proximal (closest to stomach) to aganglionic segment becomes distended (**megacolon**). Grossly, the aganglionic segment looks normal but is nonmobile, and histologically one notes the absence of Meissner's and Auerbach's plexuses.

GALT

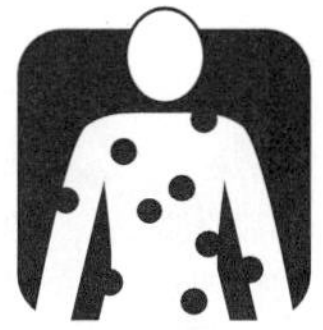

- **Gut-associated lymphatic tissue;** diffuse lymphatic tissue of lamina propria along with isolated or grouped lymphatic nodules (**Peyer's patches**). Surface epithelial cells over lymph nodules are squamous and have microfolds (**M cells**) instead of microvilli, take up macromolecules from lumen, and present these "dietary" antigens to immunologically competent cells in the underlying lymph nodules.
- Diffuse lymphatic tissue of lamina propria includes lymphocytes, macrophages, plasma cells. Plasma cells secrete **IgA,** which coats surface lining of GI tract.

ORGANS OF THE GASTROINTESTINAL TRACT

■ **Lip**

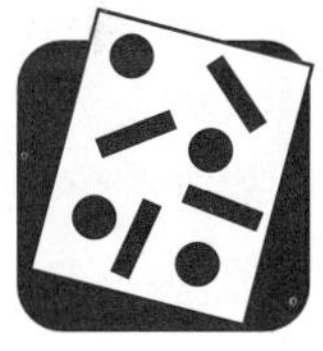

- Core of skeletal muscle, the **orbicularis oris**
- Surfaced on one side by **dermis** and **epidermis**
- Surfaced on the opposite side by a **mucosa** (stratified squamous wet epithelium and lamina propria but no muscularis mucosae)

■ **Tooth (From Inside to Outside)**

● Pulp

- A connective tissue–filled area with many blood vessels and nerves

● Dentin

- Surrounds the pulp cavity
- Produced by **odontoblasts,** which form a cellular layer at the interface between the pulp and the dentin itself
- Lots of **hydroxyapatite:** more than in bone but less than in enamel

● Enamel

- Produced by **ameloblasts**
- Hardest substance in the body, 98% hydroxyapatite
- Covers the **crown** of the tooth
- Cementum
- Cementum covers the **root** of the tooth or that part of the tooth located in the socket of bone. Unlike enamel, cementum is much like bone with 45% hydroxyapatite.

■ **Tongue**

- **Body**—anterior two thirds; **root**—posterior third; V-shaped groove between body and root is the **sulcus terminalis.**
- Core is composed of skeletal muscle fibers, which run in 3 geometric planes; this is diagnostic for the tongue.

- Both surfaces are covered by a mucosa that has stratified squamous wet epithelium, which contains keratin (parakeratinized), but this amount of keratinization does not result in calling this epithelium stratified squamous dry type.
- Mucosa on the dorsum does not have an underlying submucosa; no muscularis mucosae in tongue.

● **Lingual papillae on dorsum of body only**

— *Filiform* Most numerous, elongated projections, the tips of which point posteriorily; no taste buds

— *Fungiform* Plump or mushroom shaped, scattered among the filiform papillae; taste buds present

— *Circumvallate* About a dozen dome-shaped mounds just anterior to the sulcus terminalis, surrounded by a trench; highest concentration of taste buds, **Minor salivary glands** of the serous type (von Ebner) secrete into trench continuously washing and rinsing the trench out so that any change in ingested food can be detected quickly.

● **Taste bud**

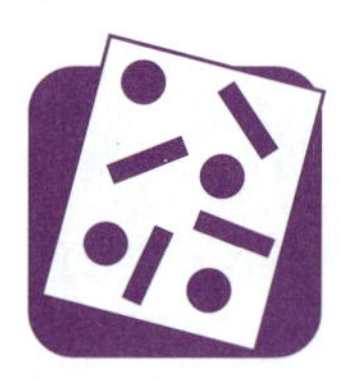

- Oval structures extending across the mucosal epithelium, detect **bitter, acid, sweet,** or **salt**

— *Three cell types*
Receptor or neuroepithelial cell

- Elongated cells with microvilli that extend to the **taste pore,** which is a small opening at the surface of the taste bud. These cells have nerve fibers terminating around their bases and are stimulated by direct contact of dissolved substances touching microvilli.

Sustentacular, or supporting, cell

- Elongated like the receptor cells, intermingled with them

Basal cell

- Located at the end of the taste bud opposite the taste pore are stem cells for both the supporting and receptor cells, which are completely replaced about every 10 days.

■ **Palate**

● **Hard**

- Core of bone
- Superior, or **nasal, mucosa** is respiratory mucosa with seromucous glands
- Lingual side is **oral mucosa** with parakeratinized stratified squamous wet epithelium. The lamina propria is firmly attached to the periosteum of the palatine bone and contains purely mucous glands.

● **Soft**

- Same as above, except core is not bone but skeletal muscle, which when contracted raises the soft palate against the wall of the pharynx closing off the **choanae** and preventing food from entering the nasal cavity during swallowing.
- Posterior tail, or **uvula,** is surfaced by stratified squamous wet epithelium on all sides.

Pharynx

- Common chamber for food and air
- Where air only—respiratory mucosa
- Where food can be present—oral mucosa
- Under mucosa—skeletal muscle of pharyngeal constrictors
- Ring of lymphatic tissue (Waldeyer's ring) surrounds and protects entranceway to both respiratory and digestive tubes: **lingual, pharyngeal,** and **palatine tonsils.**

Esophagus

- Contains all layers of common plan of GI tube; most well developed muscularis mucosae between lamina propria and submucosa
- Stratified squamous nonkeratinized epithelium
- Mucosal folds when no food is passing.

● Muscularis externa

- Only skeletal muscle in upper third
- Only smooth muscle, the muscle of the GI tube, in lower third
- Middle third has mixture of smooth and skeletal muscle types because of transition between the two types.
- Mucous glands in its submucosa—**esophageal glands proper**
- Mucous glands in its lamina propria, especially inferior end—**esophageal cardiac glands**

Stomach

- General histologic plan of GI tube, except that muscularis externa has an additional layer of obliquely arranged smooth muscle and the mucosa has **gastric glands** invaginated from surface.
- Surface epithelium—simple columnar but every cell secretes mucus, i.e., **mucous columnar cells.** Type of mucus produced here is **insoluble mucus,** which protects the surface lining from being digested.
- Surface lining is punctuated by epithelial recesses, or **gastric pits,** which are also lined by mucous columnar cells.
- Several gastric glands open into each gastric pit.

● Gastric gland

— *Isthmus region*

- Necks of glands communicate with pits; mucous columnar cells; several necks communicate with one pit

— *Neck region*

- The part of the gastric gland between the isthmus and the base
- **Mucous neck cells** are shorter than mucous columnar cells of the surface, and the mucus they secrete is soluble as opposed to the insoluble mucus from the mucous columnar cells.
- **Stem cell region** containing undifferentiated, dividing cells, the daughters of which migrate and differentiate into two directions: upward to become mucous columnar cells of the pit and surface lining and downward to become **parietal, enteroendocrine,** or **zymogenic (chief)** cells of the fundic region of the gastric gland

— *Base or fundic region* Deep extension of gastric gland into lamina propria of mucosa

— *Other parenchymal cells of gastric gland*

Zymogenic, or chief, cell

- Typical protein-secreting cells with basal RER and apical secretory granules; secrete **pepsinogen,** which when exposed to the low environmental pH is converted into the proteolytic enzyme **pepsin.**

Parietal cell

- Large and somewhat triangular cells with eosinophilic cytoplasm
- Extensive **intracellular canalicular system**
- Many microvilli at surface and many mitochondria
- Manufacture **intrinsic factor,** which is necessary for absorption of **vitamin B_{12}** by the small intestine; if little or no intrinsic factor produced **pernicious anemia** results.
- Manufacture **HCl** by transporting hydrogen and chloride ions across the canalicular membranes

Enteroendocrine (APUD) cell

- Hormone-producing cells; secrete toward capillaries in lamina propria; apex of cell faces basal lamina; nucleus close to free surface
  - Manufacture and release hormones or hormone-like substances:

    SEROTONIN
    - A vasoactive substance

    GASTRIN
    - Stimulates gastric secretion, especially of HCl

    MOTILIN
    - Regulates smooth muscle activity in small intestine

    CHOLECYSTOKININ-PANCREOZYMIN (CCK)
    - Stimulates pancreatic enzyme secretion and gallbladder contraction; inhibits gastric emptying

    SECRETIN
    - Stimulates pancreatic bicarbonate ion secretion

— *Miscellaneous*

- Gastric glands in cardiac portion of stomach (near entrance of esophagus) are purely mucous glands.
- Gastric glands in the pyloric region are also mostly mucus producing; here the pit forms about a half of the mucosa, and the gland proper forms the other half.
- Gastric glands in the fundic region of the stomach produce most of the gastric pepsin and HCl; pit forms about a fifth and the gland proper forms about four fifths of the mucosa; all different cell types are located here.

Chyme

- The final, low pH product leaving the pyloris and entering the duodenum

■ **Small Intestine**

● **General histologic plan present with some additions**

- **Plicae circulares (valves of Kerkring)** are permanent folds of mucosa and submucosa; begin in lower duodenum; most are found in jejunum; decrease in size and amount in ileum.

- **Submucosal mucous glands** (of **Brunner**) found in duodenum only; mucus for lubrication

- Extramural glands empty secretions into duodenum (pancreas, gallbladder, liver)

- Lubrication also provided by **unicellular glands,** the **goblet cells**

- Absorption provided by **enterocytes,** or **columnar absorptive cells,** with microvilli

- Mucosa is folded into **villi;** lamina propria core contains diffuse lymphatic tissue (macrophages, lymphocytes, plasma cells) and blind-ending lymphatic capillaries, the **lacteals**

- Intestinal glands (of **Lieberkühn**)

  - Base is near muscularis mucosae; straight tubular gland extends from there to opening between adjacent villi.

  - **Stem cells** near base divide; daughter cells remain as stem cells or migrate up length of gland and differentiate into goblet cells or enterocytes while migrating; they reach tip if villus and desquamate, taking about 4 days. Constant loss is replenished by constant cell production. GI tract therefore is very susceptible to anti–cell division drugs resulting in GI toxicity during cancer chemotherapy.

  - Daughters of stem cells also differentiate into Paneth cells and enteroendocrine cells.

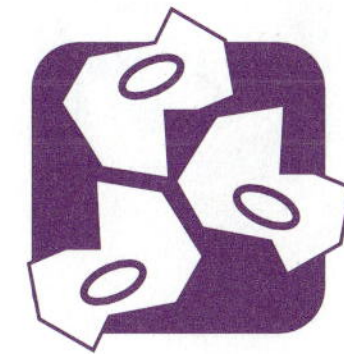

- Cells 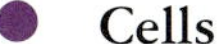

  — *Paneth cells*

    - Eosinophilic cells near fundus of intestinal gland, many granules, secrete variety of digestive enzymes, secrete an **antibacterial lysozyme** that can digest cell walls of certain kinds of bacteria; also phagocytosis of some protozoa, probably involved in regulation of intestinal flora

  — *Enteroendocrine cells (see above)*

  — *Goblet cells*

    - Interspersed with enterocytes; increase in number as one proceeds down small intestine to rectum; apical half of cell filled with **mucigen granules;** lubrication of luminal contents

  — *Enterocytes*

    - Absorptive cells; many microvilli, carbohydrates, and amino acids, i.e., the breakdown products of intraluminal digestion caused by digestive enzymes, absorbed by enterocytes and passed to capillaries

    - At lateral surface near apex of cell, adjacent enterocytes joined together by **junctional complexes** that consist of three components from lumen inward

      1. Zonula occludens (ZO)
      2. Zonula adherens (ZA)
      3. Macula adherens (MA)

    This complex, but especially the ZO, prevents material from passing between enterocytes; i.e., it must pass through them.

> - **Micelles** (very small particles) produced by bile salt breakdown of dietary lipids, taken in by endocytosis after a chemical modification at the cell surface, move to SER and RER, and then Golgi apparatus in a process of rebuilding into chylomicrons.
> - **Chylomicrons** are released at the lateral cell membrane below or "behind" the junctional complex. They pass between cells, across the basal lamina, and enter the **lacteals,** eventually being collected in the thoracic duct and "dumped" into the bloodstream.
>
> — *M cells* Squamous epithelial cells in surface lining over adjacent lymph nodules; act as antigen presenting cells to lymphocytes of lymph nodules

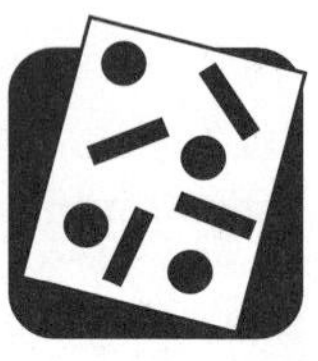

■ **Large Intestine** General histologic plan intact except:

- Few if any Paneth cells
- Enterocytes decrease in number as goblet cells increase in number from cecum to anal canal.
- Muscularis externa, outer longitudinal layer robust in three strips, the **taeniae coli;** between taeniae coli and subjacent circular smooth muscle is an excellent place for surgical pathologist to look for presence or absence of myenteric autonomic ganglia during surgical resection of an aganglionic segment of colon.
- No villi; no plicae circulares
- Function is **absorption** of **water** and **electrolytes, lubrication** of feces with mucus.

● **Appendix**

  - Large number of **lymph nodules** in lamina propria extending into submucosa
  - Outer longitudinal layer of smooth muscle intact

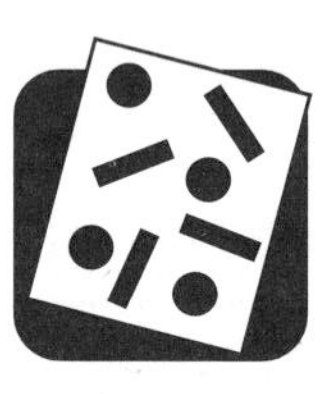

■ **Anal canal**

- Upper portion continuous histologically and grossly with rectum contains longitudinal folds, or **anal columns** (of **Morgagni**), between which are troughs, the **anal sinuses;** anal columns connected by small transverse folds at lower end **(anal valves),** forming the pectinate line, which can be seen in the cadaver.
- Lower portion surfaced by stratified squamous nonkeratinizing epithelium, which becomes continuous with skin of anus
- **Internal anal sphincter** formed by circular smooth muscle of muscularis externa
- **External anal sphincter** formed by skeletal muscle
- Mucosal and submucosal veins may become varicosed forming **hemorrhoids**
- Mucus-producing anal glands

LIVER

■ **General**

- Largest gland in the body

● **Exocrine**

  - Synthesis and release of **bile**
    - Bile moves in direction opposite to blood flow

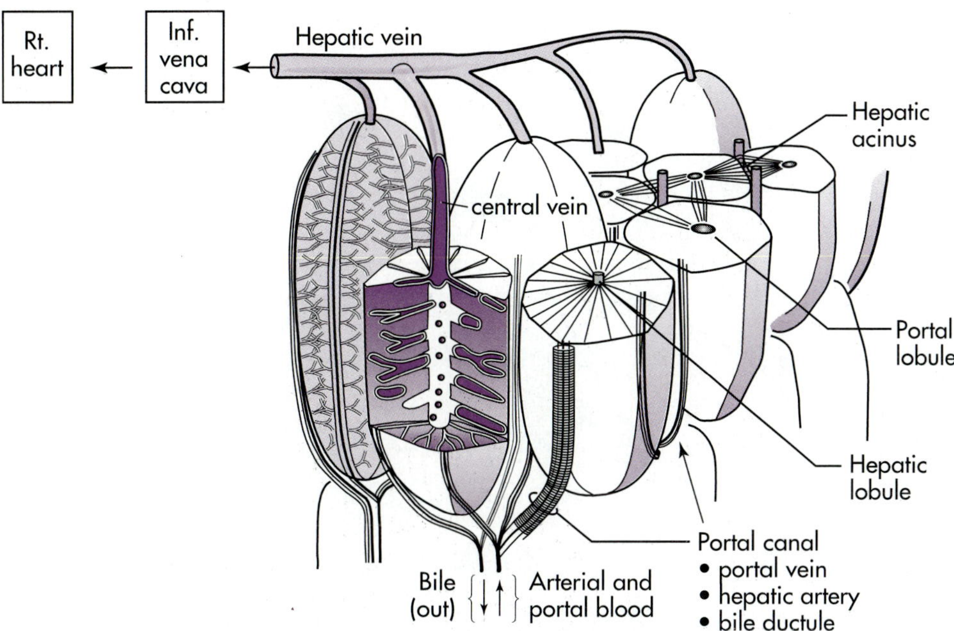

Fig. 15.2 Three-dimensional organization of the liver emphasizing arterial and venous blood flow and the flow of bile.

- Bile transported first in a **canalicular system** between hepatocytes and then in smaller to progressively larger bile ductules and ducts

- Endocrine

  - Synthesis and release of substances directly into the bloodstream
    - **Albumin**
    - **Prothrombin** and **fibrinogen**
    - **Glucose**
    - **Lipoproteins**
  - Storehouse for **glycogen**

  - Degradation of toxic substances, e.g., phenobarbital and ethanol, and of endogenous substances, e.g., some steroid hormones (estrogen)

  - Metabolic **transformation** (activation) of some drugs, e.g., the cancer-chemotherapeutic drug cytoxan or cyclophosphamide is not toxic in the bottle; it must pass through the liver to be changed into the active metabolite.

  - Sits between two veins: portal vein from small intestine, spleen, pancreas: and hepatic vein from liver to inferior vena cava (Fig. 15.2)

  - Receives arterial blood from common hepatic artery

  - Arterial and venous blood mixed in **sinusoids** lined by endothelial cells and fixed macrophages, the Kupffer cells

  - Stroma consists of a capsule and connective tissue packing around all branches of the **hepatic triad** (bile duct, hepatic artery, portal vein); servicing these parenchymal elements, the hepatocytes, are reticular fibers.

- **Histophysiologic Organization (Figs. 15.2; 15.3)**

  - **Classical or hepatic lobule**
    - Stresses endocrine role

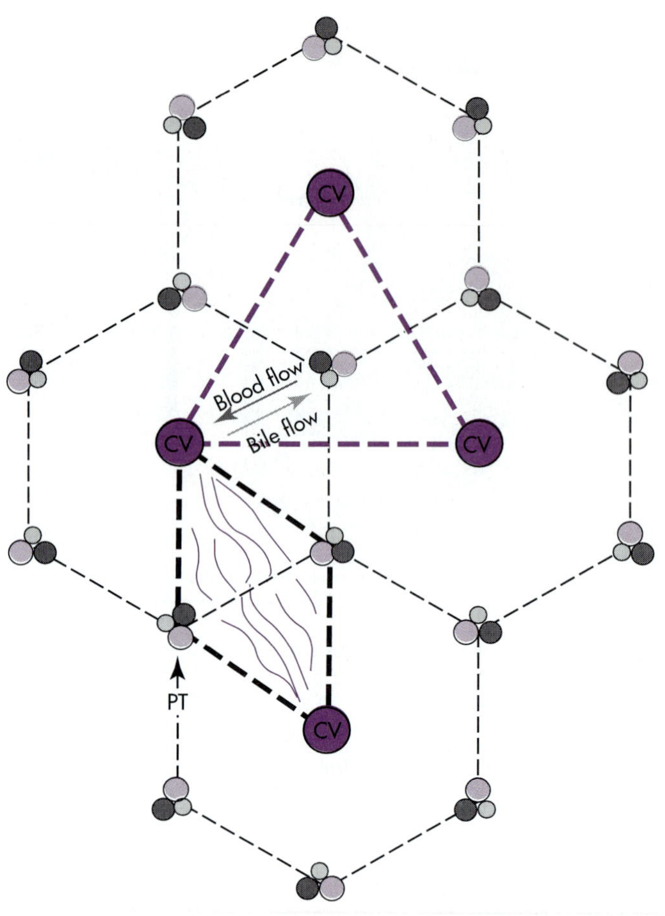

PT = Portal tract or triad (branch of hepatic artery, portal vein, bile duct)

CV = Central vein

⬡ = Classical hepatic lobule (CV at center)

△ = Portal hepatic lobule (Portal triad at center)

◇ = Acinus

Fig. 15.3 Comparison of the classical lobule, portal lobule, and the acinus of the liver.

- Hexagonal (like a benzene ring—6 sides and 6 points)
- Center is a vein—central vein
- Periphery (points of benzene ring)—portal tracts (trinity) or canal
  - Branch of hepatic artery
  - Branch of portal vein
  - Branch of bile duct
  - All held together by connective tissue, which contains lymph vessels
- **Portal lobule**
  - Stresses exocrine role
  - Triangle

- Center is portal tract or canal.
- Periphery—3 points of triangle—the 3 "surrounding" central veins

● **Acinus (modern functional unit)**

- Diamond shape: 2 central veins at each end with 2 portal tracts at the other 2 ends; many more acini than lobules
- Center is vascular backbone with contributions from the vessels in each of the 2 portal tracts.
- Arterial blood in branches of hepatic artery at backbone or center of acinus supply oxygenated blood from backbone to the 2 adjacent central veins—parts of hepatic lobules. This arterial blood loses oxygen as it flows out from backbone to central veins dividing the 2 halves of the acinus (diamond) into 3 zones:

— *Zone 1* Closest to the vascular backbone or center of the acinus; highest oxygen saturation and nutrient level; most metabolically active, most resistant to insult, first to regenerate after partial hepatectomy

— *Zone 2* Between zones 1 and 3; intermediate oxygen saturation, etc.

— *Zone 3* Closest to the central veins, lowest oxygen saturation, etc.

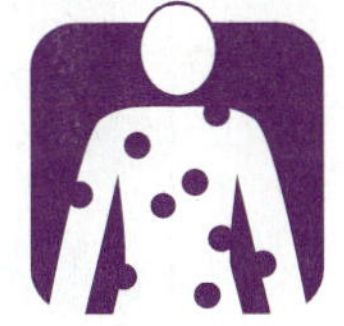

- In a patient with heart failure caused by a bad valve, the heart cannot pump off all the blood delivered to it. Eventually blood will dam up into the superior and inferior venae cavae, in effect waiting its turn to go through the heart.

These people have throbbing neck veins and sluggish blood flow in the inferior vena cava, hepatic vein, central veins, and sinusoids.

In this situation hepatocytes in zone 3 of the acinus get less oxygen than normal, and normal was barely enough to begin with.

They die as a result and are replaced by fibroblasts and collagen fibers (scarring)—**cirrhosis,** but in a very specific location—**cardiac cirrhosis.**

- In a patient with an obstruction to the flow of bile out of the liver, bile will back up the biliary tree to the small branches of the bile duct in the portal tracts and even into the bile canaliculi. Bile pigment spills into bloodstream and can color mucous membranes yellow **(jaundice).** Bile is quite caustic and irritates the connective tissue in the portal tracts, forming scar tissue—cirrhosis, but in a specific location—**biliary cirrhosis.**

■ **Ultrastructure**

● **Sinusoid**

- Lined by discontinuous or **fenestrated endothelial cells** and stellate fixed macrophages, the **Kupffer cells**
- Peripheral to the endothelial–Kupffer cell lining, and between this lining and the hepatocytes is a space that, because of the fenestrations in the endothelium, contains blood plasma without the formed elements of blood. This **perisinusoidal space** is the **space of Disse.**

Hepatocyte microvilli project into the space of Disse. Hepatocytes take material from and give material to the plasma in this space. Eventually some of this plasma finds its way into the lymphatics in the portal tracts (Fig. 15.4).

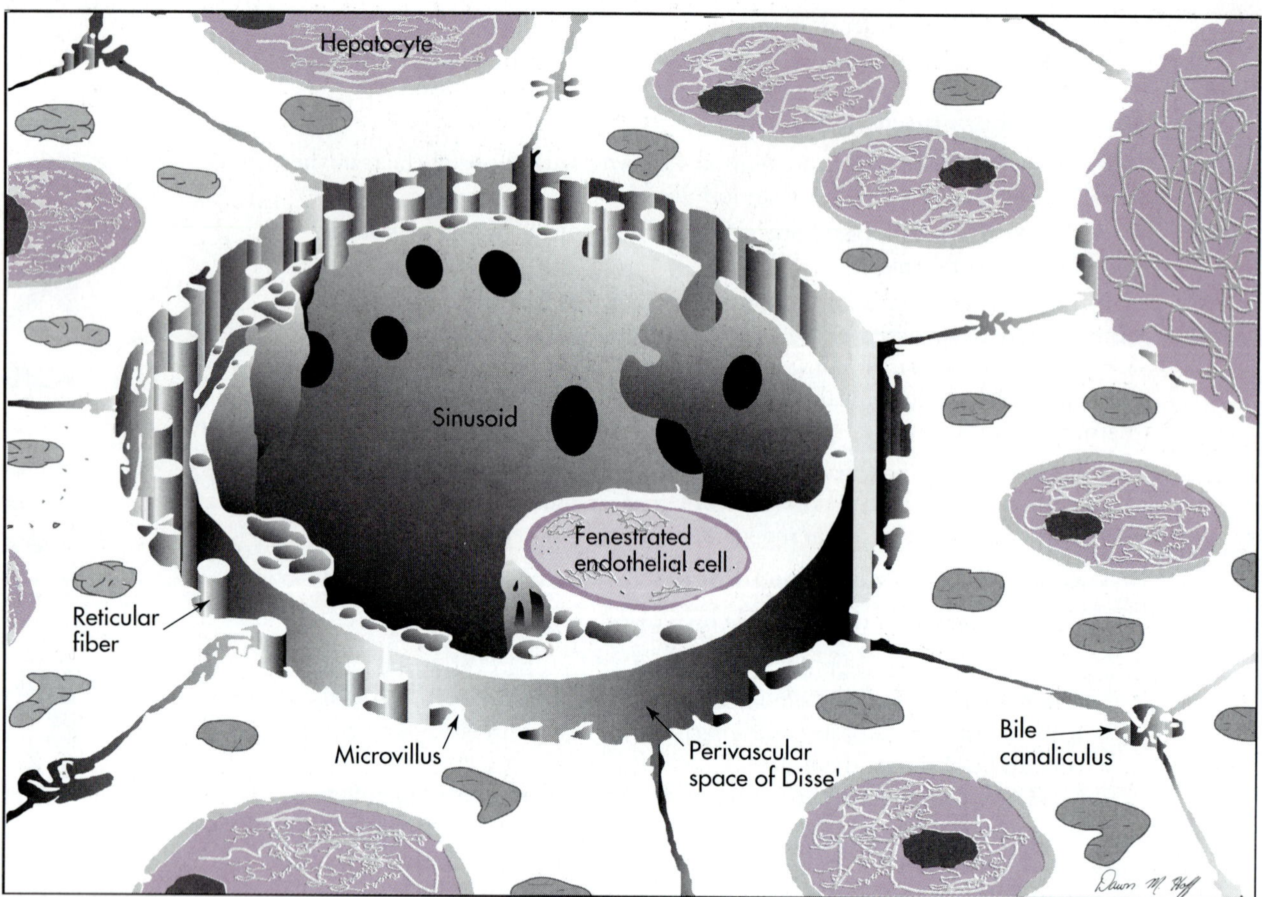

Fig. 15.4 Three-dimensional morphology of liver parenchymal cells (hepatocytes) and their relations to each other (bile canaliculi) and to the blood sinusoid with its fenestrated endothelium. Between the outside of the sinusoid and the body of the hepatocyte lies the perivascular space of Disse.

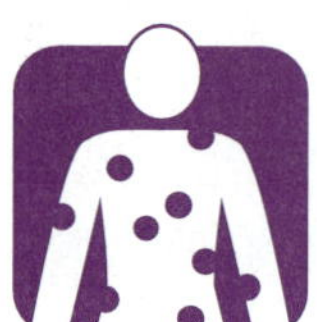

- **Lipocytes,** or storage cells for vitamin A, are found in the space of Disse; they release it into the blood for its trip to the retina.

In fetal liver the perisinusoidal space contains hematopoietic cells, since the liver and spleen are hematopoietic organs from the second to sixth fetal months.

- Apparently the hematopoietic stem cells are retained in the adult liver but are not normally used. In certain clinical conditions such as chronic anemia these stem cells can be reactivated and the liver can once again become hematopoietic. This condition is known as **myeloid metaplasia** of the liver, or **extramedullary hematopoiesis** relative to the bone marrow.

- **Hepatocyte**

  - Large polygonal cells with central nuclei
  - Several surfaces face spaces of Disse.
  - Several other surfaces face adjacent hepatocytes; **bile canaliculi** formed on these surfaces as tiny grooves are sealed laterally by **zonulae occludentes.**
  - Arranged "back to back" to form anastomosing cords or plates

- Basophilic cytoplasmic regions contain RER and free polysomes.
- Acidophilic cytoplasmic regions contain mitochondria and **peroxisomes,** which break down hydrogen peroxide produced by normal metabolic activity. They also contain **catalase** and **alcohol dehydrogenase.**
- Unstained cytoplasmic regions contain multiple (up to 50 per hepatocyte) Golgi bodies, SER glycogen inclusions (PAS positive), and lipid droplets.

GALLBLADDER

- Sac that **stores bile** made in the liver and **concentrates bile** by removing water
- Releases bile in response to presence of fat in duodenum

Enteroendocrine cells in duodenum release CCK, which causes smooth muscle in wall of gallbladder to contract.

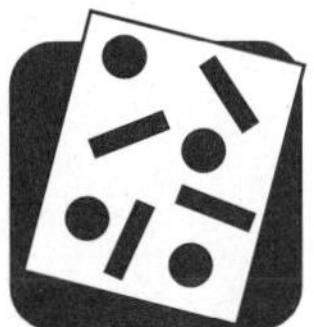

■ **Structure**

● **Simple columnar epithelium**

- Junctional complexes force material through instead of between cells
- **Microvilli**
- Salt is pumped from cytoplasm into intercellular space proximal to the junctional complex by a **sodium/potassium-activated ATPase pump** located in lateral plasmalemma.
- Water follows, and the intercellular space becomes distended with fluid, which eventually passes through the BM into the capillaries of the lamina propria.

As salt and water are removed from the cytoplasm into the intercellular spaces, more water and salt are absorbed by the apical surface.

- No muscularis mucosae in mucosa: no submucosa
- Muscularis externa is thin with 3 indistinct layers
- Surface facing peritoneal cavity—**serosa**
- Surface facing liver—**adventitia** or **fibrosa**
- Emptied gallbladder has mucosa thrown into large folds.

PANCREAS

- Exocrine component
- Serous acini at beginning of branched duct system
- Unique in that duct system begins inside the acinus
- Duct cells inside of acinus—**centroacinar cells**
- Typical serous cells: basal nuclei and RER with prominent Golgi and apical secretory granules

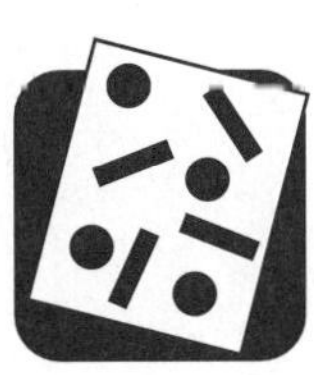

- Synthesize **lipase, amylase, trypsinogen, pepsinogen, DNAse,** and **RNAse**
- For transport down duct system to duodenum
- CCK causes release of these enzymes.

- Ductal epithelial cells release **sodium bicarbonate buffer** in response to **se-**

cretin from enteroendocrine cells in duodenum; the buffer raises pH of chyme to optimum level for pancreatic enzyme function.

■ **Endocrine Component (See Chapter 19)**

● Islets of Langerhans

- Beta cells—insulin
- Alpha cells—glucagon
- Delta cells—somatostatin

SALIVARY GLANDS

■ **Parotid Gland**

- Serous acini (100%)
- Branched or compound duct system

■ **Submandibular Gland**

- Mixed: ⅔ serous acini + ⅓ mucous acini
- Some mucous acini have serous demilunes.
- Compound duct system

■ **Sublingual Gland**

- 90% mucous acini
- Compound duct system

Multiple Choice
Review Questions

1. All the following are components of the digestive tube (tract), *except*

    a. autonomic ganglia in a submucosa.
    b. antigen-presenting cells.
    c. diffuse lymphatic tissue in a lamina propria.
    d. muscularis mucosae composed of skeletal or smooth muscle depending on what region.
    e. blood and lymphatic vessels.

2. Where in the gastrointestinal tube is there an abrupt transition between simple columnar epithelium and stratified squamous nonkeratinized or parakeratinized epithelium?

    a. Gastroesophageal junction
    b. Lower anal canal and skin
    c. Lip
    d. Oropharynx and esophagus
    e. Gastro-duodenal junction

3. In which organ do all of the surface cells secrete mucus?

    a. Esophagus
    b. Stomach
    c. Duodenum
    d. Transverse colon
    e. Lower anal canal

4. Junctional complexes (ZO-ZA-MA) are found in surface epithelial cells in all of the following *except*

    a. gallbladder.
    b. duodenum.
    c. ileum.
    d. lower anal canal.
    e. jejunum.

5. All of the following absorb significant amounts of water and electrolytes *except*

    a. gallbladder.
    b. colon.
    c. ileum.
    d. rectum.
    e. esophagus.

Chapter 16

Urinary System

GENERAL

The urinary system is composed of

- kidneys
- ureters
- bladder
- urethra

FUNCTIONS OF THE KIDNEY

- The kidney is a bifunctional glandular organ. It is a compound tubular exocrine gland for urine production. It is an endocrine gland for production of renin (blood-pressure regulation) and erythropoietin (erythrocyte production).
- Rids body of waste products of metabolism (e.g., Urea, NH_3 [ammonia], creatinine)
- Maintains constant internal milieu
  - Regulates volume of blood and tissue fluid (water)
  - Regulates composition of blood and tissue fluid
    - pH
    - Blood pressure and osmotic pressure
    - Water
    - Electrolytes

ANATOMY OF THE KIDNEY

- The kidney is a bean-shaped organ with little stroma (mostly parenchyma) (Fig. 16.1).
- It is covered by a fibrous capsule.
  - The capsule is discontinuous at hilum (entrance blood vessels and ureter).
  - The hilum expands into interior to form renal sinus, which houses an expansion of the ureter (renal pelvis), which branches to form the major calyces and the minor calyces.

On gross section, the kidney divides into

- cortex (surface), which contains mostly secretory units having a granular appearance

- medulla (interior), which contains mostly ducts, giving it a striate appearance
  - The cortex runs down into medulla forming renal columns and dividing medulla into pyramidal structures (medullary pyramids). Tips of two or three pyramids extend into minor calyx as papilla.

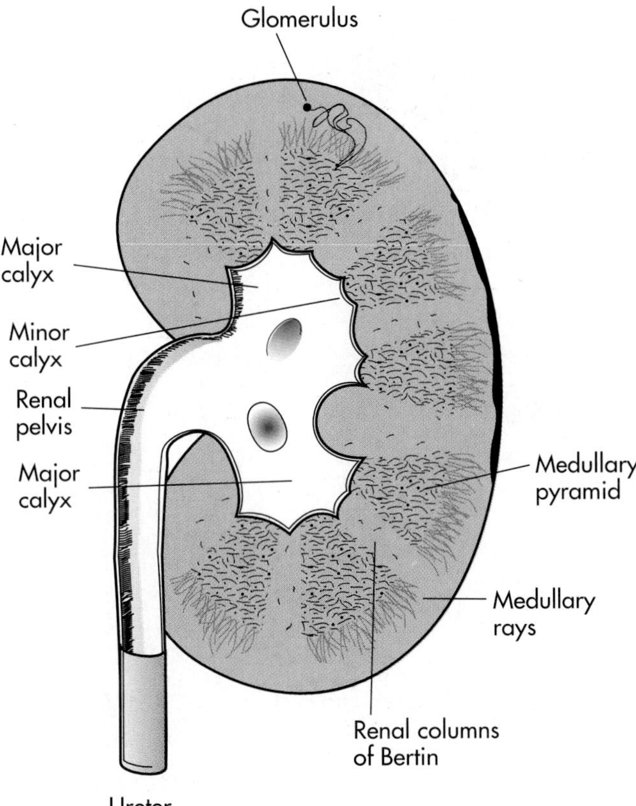

Fig. 16.1 General organization of the kidney.

- The cortex is divided by medullary rays, which extend from medulla into cortex.

In this manner the kidney is divided into

- renal lobe, which is composed of the medullary pyramid and its overlying cortex
- renal lobules, which are composed of the medullary ray and nephrons (Fig. 16.2) draining into that ray
  - The medullary ray is at the core of the lobule.
  - The boundaries of lobules are imaginary lines drawn midway between medullary rays. The interlobular arteries and veins aid in defining the boundaries of the renal lobule.

The functional unit of the kidney is the uriniferous tubule.

- Uriniferous tubule = nephron + collecting tubules
- The nephron extends from the malpighian (renal) corpuscle to the distal convoluted tubule.
  - Cortical nephrons are most numerous (85% of nephrons).
  - Juxtamedullary nephrons (15% of nephrons) maintain hypertonicity of medulla.
  - Collecting tubules extend from the arched collecting tubule to the papillary duct.

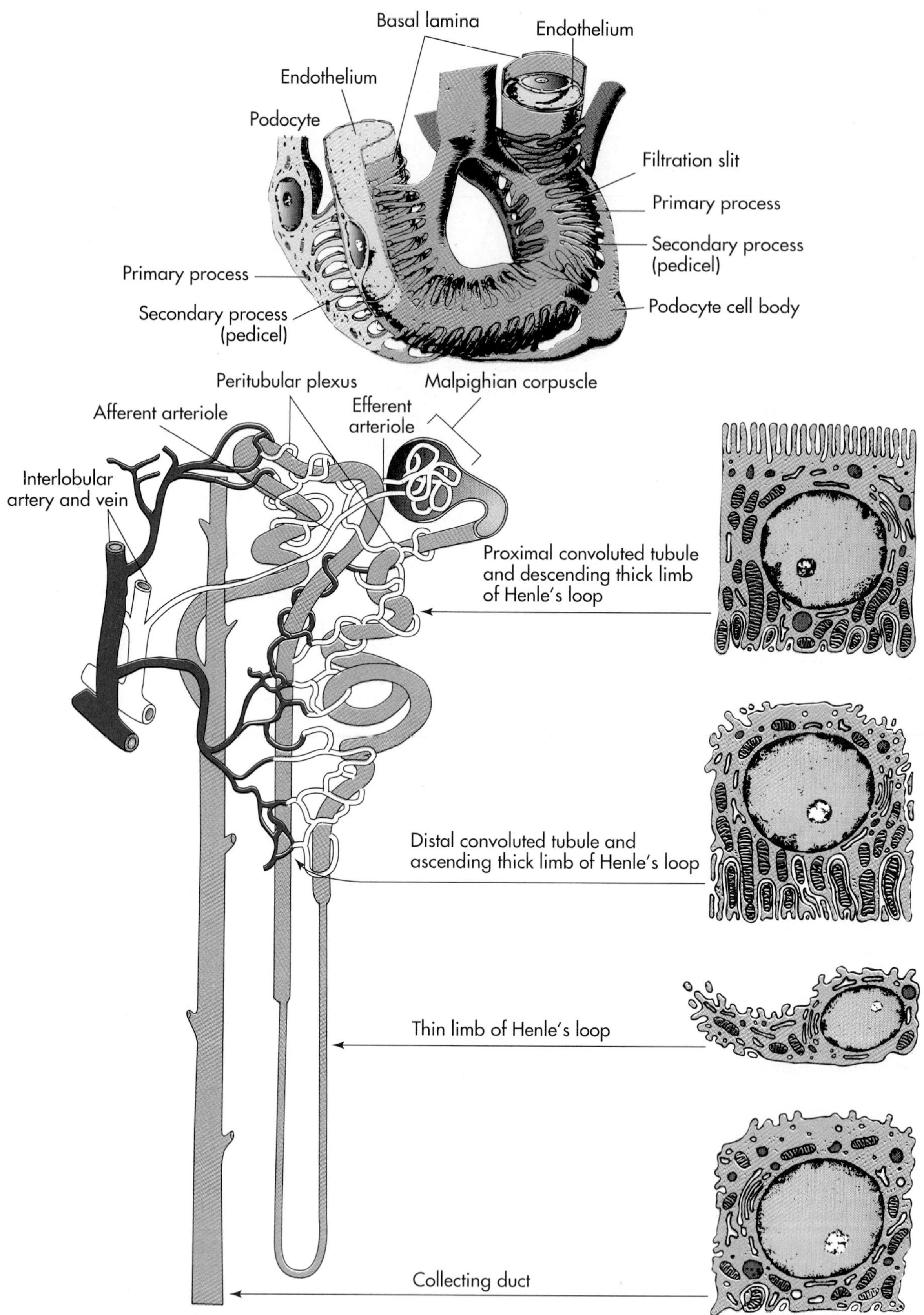

Fig. 16.2 Ultrastructure of the cells of the nephron–uriniferous tubule and the distribution of blood vessels. The ultrastructure of the glomerulus is demonstrated in a three-dimensional reconstruction showing the relationship of the podocytes to the glomerulus. The ultrastructure of the cells of the uriniferous tubule is demonstrated in thin-section transmission electron microscopy. *(Modified from Junqueira LC, Carneiro J:* Basic histology, *East Norwalk, Conn., 1992, Appleton & Lange.)*

■ Malpighian (Renal) Corpuscle = Glomerulus + Bowman's Capsule

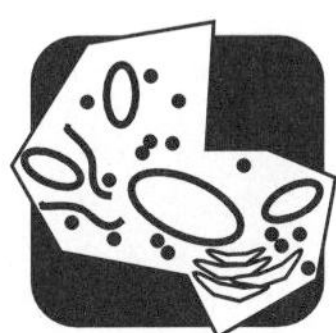

- Glomerulus
  - Afferent arteriole→capillary network→efferent arteriole
- Bowman's capsule extends from
  - visceral layer to Bowman's space to parietal layer
- Visceral layer—podocytes
- Each podocyte has several processes from which extend the foot processes or pedicels.
  - Interdigitation of pedicels
  - Slits covered by a diaphragm (slit membrane)
- Fenestrated endothelial cells (lack diaphragm)
- Basal lamina of capillary and podocytes is the only continuous structure separating the podocyte and endothelial cell.
  - Total cross-sectional area of the efferent arteriole is less than total cross-sectional area of the afferent arteriole. (This leads to an increased blood pressure in the glomerulus.)
  - Total hydrostatic pressure in the capillary is 19 mm higher than in Bowman's space.
  - Fluid filtered through basal lamina and slit membrane
    - Molecules with molecular weight greater than 60,000 daltons are retained in capillary.
    - Molecules with molecular weight less than 60,000 daltons are filtered into space in Bowman's capsule (glomerular filtrate).
  - Glomerular filtrate has the same composition as blood, minus the high-molecular-weight material.
  - The basal lamina is also charge selective, restricting passage of negatively charged ions.
  - Flow of fluid from capillary (urinary membrane)
    - Capillary lumen → fenestrated endothelium → basal lamina (endothelium + podocyte) → slit membrane (diaphragm of podocytes) → Bowman's capsule space
  - Mesangial cells are similar to pericytes but are phagocytic and are believed to support capillary loops.
  - Parietal layer is composed of simple squamous epithelium.
  - There are about 170 liters of glomerular filtrate formed per day. This is approximately 10% of the blood that passes through the glomeruli each day. Of the 170 liters of glomerular filtrate produced, 1.5 liters of urine are concentrated by **reabsorption and secretion.**

- **Reabsorption** is transport across tubal epithelium from lumen of tubule (tubular fluid) into capillary lumen (blood) by means of tissue (peritubular) fluid. The fluid is taken up by capillaries of peritubular plexus.
- **Secretion** is transport across tubal epithelium from blood in capillary (by means of tissue fluid) into the lumen of the tubule.

■ Proximal Convoluted Tubule (PCT) Measures Approximately 14 mm in Length (Fig. 16.3)

Lumen continuous with Bowman's space

- Proximal three fourths is convoluted.

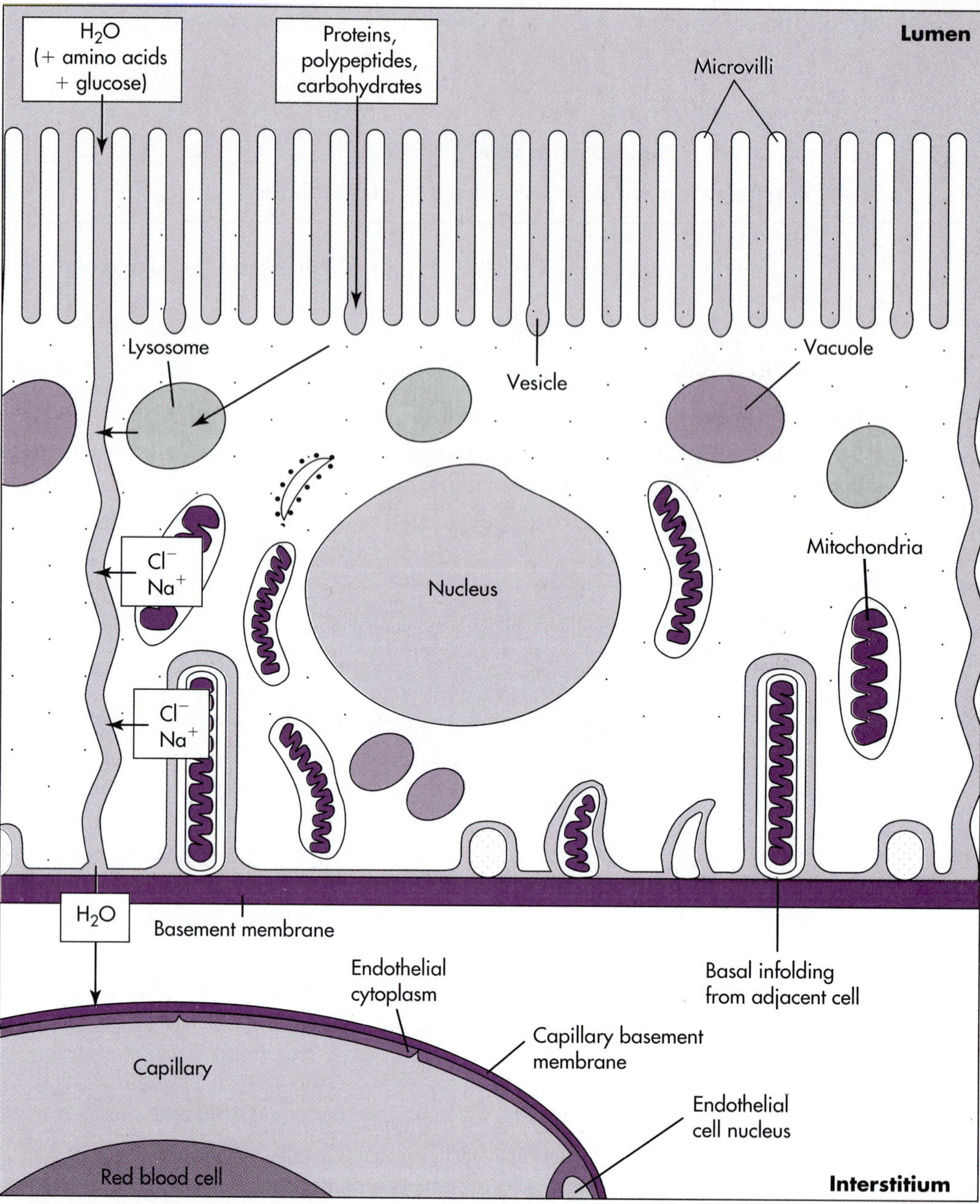

Fig. 16.3 Resorption in the proximal convoluted tubule. Na^+ ions are actively transported into the spaces between adjacent tubule cells by the Na^+, K^+ ATPase pump. Cl^- ions passively follow. Water reabsorption is a consequence of osmotic draw caused by the active transport of Na^+ into the spaces. Proteins and polypeptides are taken up by endocytosis. *(Modified from Stevens A, Lowe JS:* Histology, *1992, Gower Medical {London}.)*

- Distal fourth is straight.

Specialized organelles in cuboidal epithelial cells

- Mitochondria in basal portion of cells are aligned and compartmentalized.
- Interdigitations of the basal plasma membrane increase surface area.
- Brush border on apical portion of cell (microvilli)

- Tubular invaginations
- Vacuoles and granules

Changes in glomerular filtrate as it passes through proximal convoluted tubule

- Unchanged—uric acid, PO_4
- Resorbed from lumen—Na^+, Cl^-, H_2O, glucose
- Secreted into lumen—creatinine
- Tubular fluid in PCT—isotonic
- Role of pinocytosis in resorption—water resorption

■ The Thin Segment of Henle's Loop Measures 2 to 10 mm in Length

- Lumen continuous with that of proximal convoluted tubule
- Composed of simple squamous epithelial cells
- Specialized cellular organelles
  - Many intermingled infoldings
  - Slits for passage of molecules
  - Microvilli sparse
  - Thin segment freely permeable to H_2O and Na^+
  - Fluid in lumen hypertonic

■ The Thick Ascending Segment of Henle's Loop Measures 9 mm in Length

- Lumen continuous with that of thin segment of Henle's loop
- Cuboidal epithelial cells
  - Sparse microvilli
  - Basal striations (active transport of Na^+)
  - Mitochondria
- Impermeable to free movement of H_2O and Na^+
  - Carrier-mediated (active) transport pumps Na^+ from lumen into stroma.
  - This increases the osmotic pressure of the stroma causing
    - H_2O to be drawn out of thin segment by diffusion
    - Na^+ to enter descending limb by diffusion
  - Fluid in lumen, less hypertonic

■ The Distal Convoluted Tubule (DCT) Measures 5 mm in Length (Fig. 16.4)

- Lumen continuous with that of thick ascending portion of Henle's loop
- Actively secretes K^+ and NH_3^+
- Scattered microvilli
- Extensive basal infoldings
- Many mitochondria
- Fluid hypotonic
- The DCT is the target organ for hormones that regulate osmolarity of blood.
  - Aldosterone (adrenol corticosteroid) acts on PCT, loop of Henle, but principally on DCT.
    - Increased aldosterone release causes increased Na^+ reabsorption.

- Decreased aldosterone release causes decreased Na^+ reabsorption.

Antidiuretic hormone secreted by the pars nervosa of pituitary increases permeability DCT to H_2O (also acts on collecting tubules the same way).

- Increased tonicity blood (hypertonic)→increased ADH release→increased H_2O reabsorption (increases tonicity of urine→decreases tonicity of blood).
- Decreased tonicity (hypotonic) blood→decreased ADH release→decreased H_2O reabsorption (decreases tonicity of urine→increases tonicity of blood).

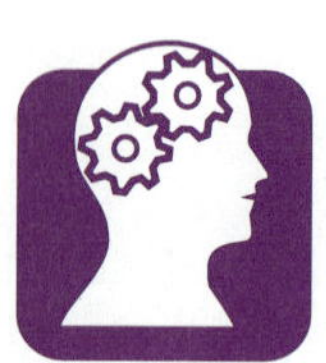

■ The Juxtaglomerular Apparatus is Related to Blood Pressure (Fig. 16.5)

DCT contacts malpighian corpuscle at interval between afferent and efferent arteriole. At the point of contact one distinguishes

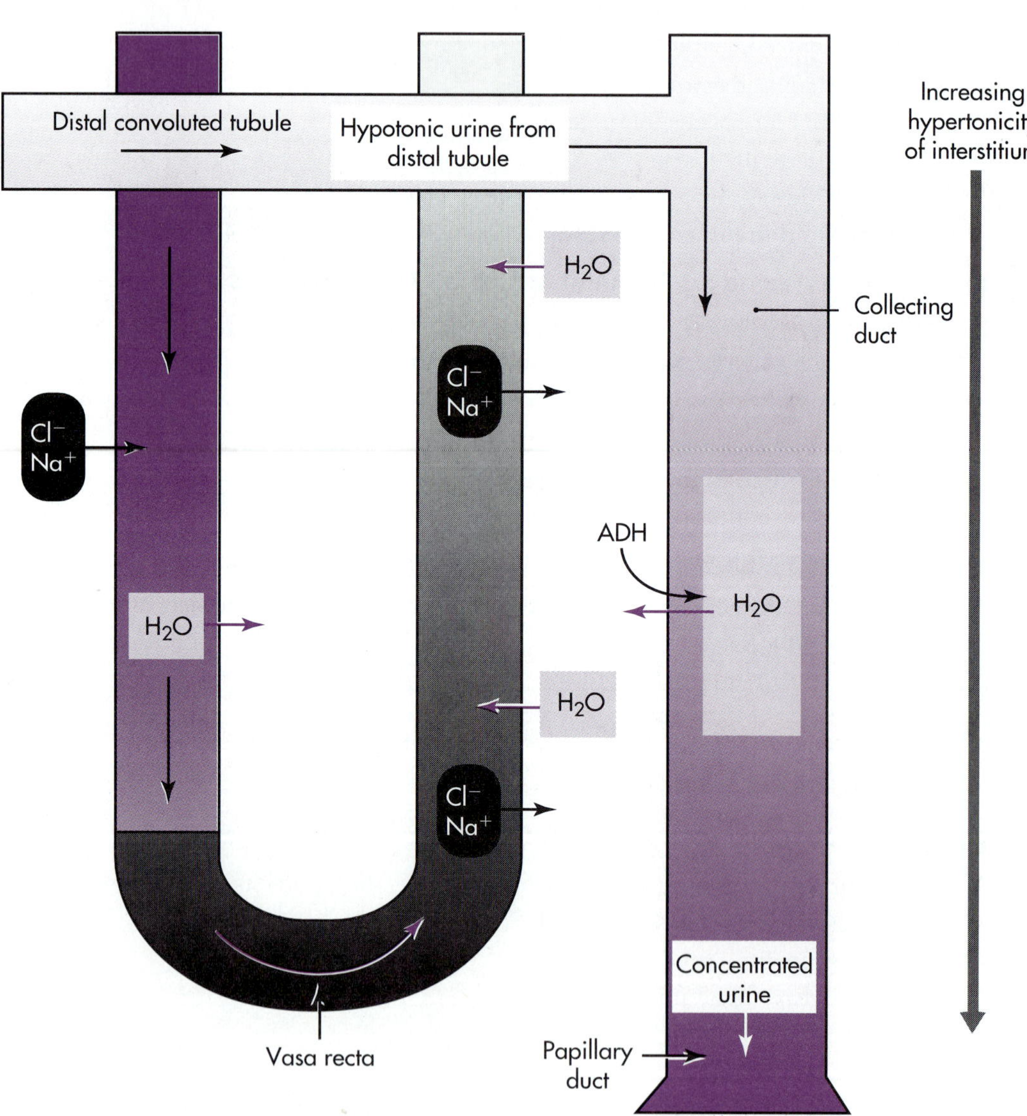

Fig. 16.4 Dilute urine in the collecting duct is concentrated by the osmotic transfer of water from the lumen into the hypertonic medullary tissue from which it is reabsorbed into the hypertonic medullary tissue from which it is reabsorbed into the vasa recta. *(Modified from Stevens A, Lowe JS:* Histology, *Brookfield, Vt., 1992, Gower Medical {London}.)*

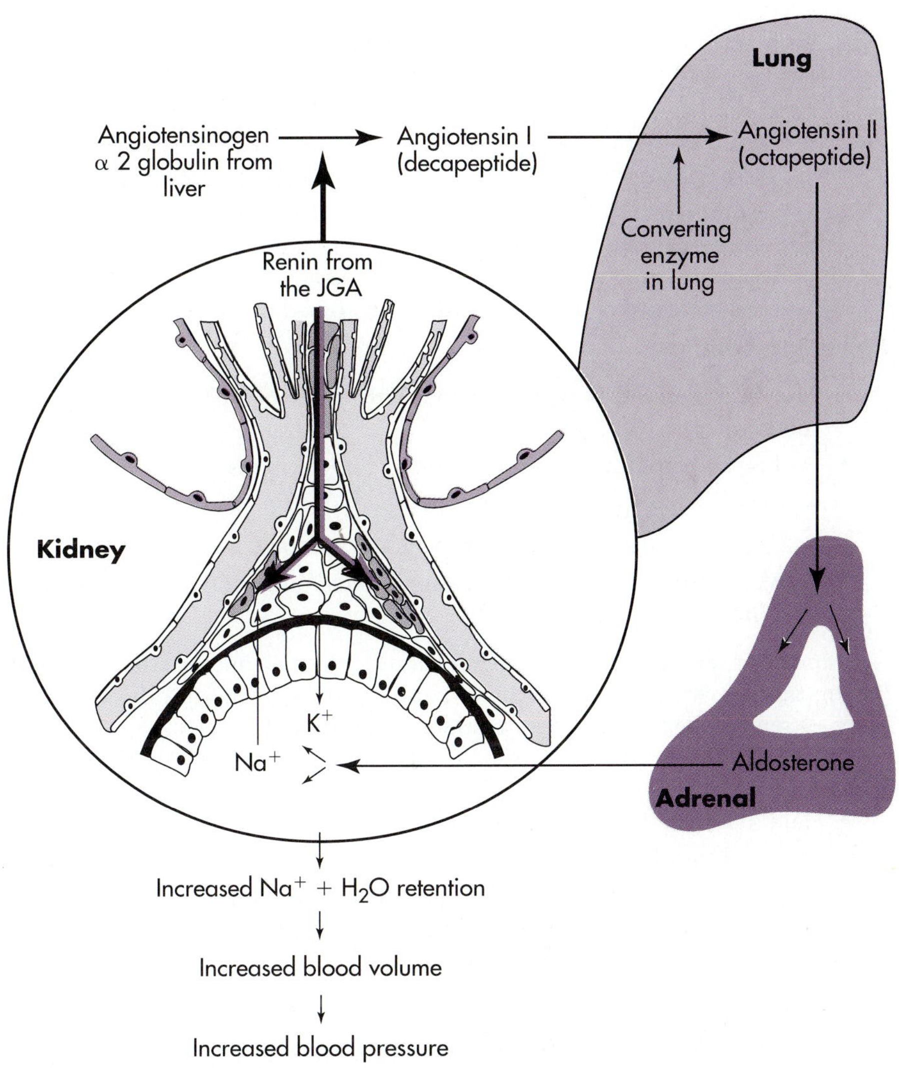

Fig. 16.5 Renin-angiotensin-aldosterone system. Renin secreted by the juxtaglomerular apparatus (JGA) catalyzes the production of angiotensin I from angiotensinogen. Angiotensin I is converted to the active angiotensin II in the lung. Angiotensin II stimulates release of aldosterone from the adrenal cortex. Aldosterone causes the reabsorption of Na^+ ions and water from the distal convoluted tubule. *(Modified from Stevens A, Lowe JS:* Histology, *1992, Gower Medical {London}.)*

- macula densa, specialized cells of DCT
- juxtaglomerular cells, specialized cells in tunica media of afferent arteriole (also in efferent one)
- polkissen cells (lacis cells [pronounced/lah-seé/, French for 'meshwork'])

● **Juxtaglomerular cells**

- Synthesize renin (proteolytic enzyme)
- Angiotensinogen converted by renin to angiotensin II (vasoconstrictor)

The following are steps in Angiotensin II formation. Angiotensinogen is synthesized in liver, is acted on by renin to convert it to Angiotensin, which is converted to angiotensin II in the capillaries of the lung.

Renin   Capillaries of lung

Angiotensinogen ⟶ Angiotensin I ⟶ Angiotensin II

(Synthesized in liver)

- Decrease in blood pressure or oxygenation is detected by afferent arteriole, causes release of renin, increases vacoconstriction, increase blood pressure.
- Angiotensin II appears to act on adrenal cortex to release aldosterone→increases Na^+ resorption in uriniferous tubules→increases blood tonicity→increases osmotic pressure→increase fluid content of blood→increases blood volume→increases blood pressure.

■ Collecting Tubules

- The lumens of DCTs are continuous with those of arched collecting tubules.
- Arched and straight collecting tubules target organs for ADH.
  - ADH makes tubule permeable to water.
  - Urine arriving at collecting tubule is hypotonic.
  - Water leaves tubule to hypertonic interstitium, and urine increases tonicity.

Lumens of several arched collecting tubules are continuous with straight collecting tubules, which fuse to form → papillary duct → minor calyx → major calyx → renal pelvis → ureter → bladder → urethra (Table 16.2).

Epithelium

- Cuboidal in arched collecting tubules
- Increases to columnar in papillary duct
- Transitional epithelium from minor calyx to urethra

BLOOD SUPPLY OF THE KIDNEY

■ Arterial Division

- Renal artery → interlobar arteries (course between pyramids) → arcuate arteries (lie at junction cortex and medulla) → interlobular arteries (run midway between 2 medullary rays) → afferent arteriole → glomerular capillaries → efferent arteriole
- Peritubular plexus (a renal portal system) important in reabsorption. Efferent arterioles→ arteriola recta spuria → capillary network surrounding renal tubules.
- Arteriola recta vera (arises directly from arcuate arteries) forms a capillary network surrounding renal tubules.

■ Venous Division

- Stellate veins (in cortex) → interlobular veins (midway between 2 medullary rays) → arcuate veins (between cortex and medulla) joined by vena recta (from medulla) → interlobar veins (course between pyramids) → renal vein

SUMMARY OF THE EXCRETION OF URINE

- Kidneys carry out functions by
  - filtration of blood plasma
  - selective reabsorption in tubules
  - active secretion in tubules

Table 16.1   *Histologic Features of the Urinary System—Kidney*

ORGAN	EPITHELIUM	SPECIAL FEATURES
Bowman's Capsule	Visceral layer—simple squamous epithelium Parietal layer—simple squamous epithelium	Podocytes
Proximal convoluted tubule	Simple cuboidal epithelium	Microvilli (brush border) Numerous mitochondria
Thin segment of Henle's loop	Simple squamous epithelium	Spaces between cells
Thick ascending limb of Henle's loop	Simple cuboidal epithelium	Numerous mitochondria
Distal convoluted tubule	Simple cuboidal epithelium	Numerous mitochondria
Arched collecting tubule	Simple cuboidal epithelium	
Collecting tubule	Upper portion—cuboidal Lower portion—columnar	
Papillary ducts	Simple columnar epithelium	
Calyces	Transitional	Muscular layers with inner longitudinal and outer circular layer
Renal pelvis	Transitional	Muscular layers with inner longitudinal and outer circular layer

Table 16.2   *Histologic Features of the Urinary System—Postrenal Conducting System*

ORGAN	EPITHELIUM	LAMIA PROPRIA	TUNICA MUSCULARIS	TUNICA ADVENTITIA
Ureter	Transitional	Collagenous and elastic fibers	*Upper portion:* inner, longitudinal; outer, circular *Lower third:* inner, longitudinal; middle, circular; outer, longitudinal	Loose fibroelastic tissue
Bladder	Transitional	Elastic and reticular tissue	Inner, longitudinal or oblique; middle, circular; outer, longitudinal	In nonperitoneal part, fibrosa
Urethra (female)	*Upper portion:* transitional *Lower portion:* stratified squamous with areas of pseudostratified epithelium	Loose connective tissue with elastic fibers; vascular	Inner, longitudinal; outer, circular layers of smooth muscle External sphincter of striated muscle	Fibroelastic tissue
Urethra (male)	*Prostatic portion:* transitional *Membranous portion:* stratified columnar, or pseudostratified *Penile portion:* stratified columnar, or pseudostratified, patches of stratified squamous *External meatus:* stratified squamous	Fibroelastic connective tissue	*Prostatic and membranous portions:* inner, longitudinal; outer circular; sphincter muscle of striated fibers	Fibroelastic tissue

- 1700 liters of whole blood pass through kidneys in a day. About 1.5 liters of urine per day are formed.
- As urine passes through tubules, the concentration of solutes changes.
  - In proximal convoluted tubule, water and solutes are reabsorbed at same rate (isotonicity).
  - Increased tonicity (hypertonicity) as it passes down descending limb of Henle's loop (non–carrier mediated transport of Na^+ into and water out of tubule)
  - Decreased tonicity (hypotonicity) as it passes up ascending limb into DCT (carrier-mediated transport of Na^+ into stroma)
  - Increased tonicity (hypertonicity) as it passes down collecting tubule (non–carrier mediated transport)
  - Diabetes insipidis caused by insufficient ADH

Multiple Choice Review Questions

1. What are the effects of administering ADH to a person with diabetes insipidus?
   a. Increases the tonicity of urine
   b. Decreases the reabsorption of water in collecting tubules of kidney
   c. Increases urine output of kidney
   d. All of the above are correct.

2. Place A beside factors accounted for by non–carrier mediated transport; B beside factors accounted for by carrier-mediated transport.
   _____ Reabsorption of Na^+ from proximal convoluted tubule
   _____ Reabsorption of Na^+ from thick ascending segment of Henle's loop
   _____ Secretion of Na^+ into descending thin segment of Henle's loop
   _____ Reabsorption of water from descending thin segment of Henle's loop

3. Match the cell with its description:
   _____ Microvilli
   _____ Foot processes
   _____ Filled with mitochondria (few microvilli)
   _____ Fenestrated epithelium

   a. Visceral layer of Bowman's capsule
   b. Thick ascending portion of Henle's loop
   c. Endothelium of perivascular plexus
   d. Endothelium of glomerulus
   e. Proximal convoluted tubule

4. Match:
   _____ Causes vascular smooth muscle contraction
   _____ Synthesized in JGA cells
   _____ Synthesized in liver
   _____ Increases Na^+ resorption in DCT

   a. Enzymes that activates angiotensinogen
   b. Substance synthesized by cells of zonula fasciculata
   c. Angiotensinogen
   d. Angiotensin II
   e. Substance synthesized by cells of Z. glomerulosa

5. Arrange the pathway of most of the Na^+ ions in the kidney. (*A* is given.)
   _____ Lumen proximal convoluted tubule
   _____ Arcuate vein
   __a__ Afferent arteriole
   _____ Peritubular plexus
   _____ Glomerular filtrate

Chapter 17

Male Reproductive System

GENERAL

The male genital system (Table 17.1) consists of

- the paired gonads, the testes (singular testis)
- specialized gland-like epithelium that elaborates male gametes (spermatozoa)
- a system of ducts conducting spermatozoa to the surface

    Tubuli recti → rete testis → ductuli efferentes → duct of epididymis → ductus deferens → ampulla of ductus deferens → ejaculatory duct → urethra

- specialized glands that provide nutritive elements and lubricative elements to semen
- seminal vesicles
- prostate
- bulbourethral glands

MICROSCOPIC STRUCTURE AND FUNCTION OF THE TESTIS

■ Structure of the Testis

- The tunica albuginea forms a connective tissue capsule to the testis.
- It is thickened posteriorly to form the mediastinum testis.
- Connective tissue septula extend from mediastinum forming lobules.
    - Each lobule contains 2 to 4 highly convoluted seminiferous tubules.
    - The seminiferous tubule measures 30 to 70 cm long.
    - Seminiferous tubules enter the mediastinum and become continuous with the rete testis.
    - Lining cells of seminiferous tubules—seminiferous epithelium, giving rise to gametes.

■ Functions of the Testis (Fig. 17.1)

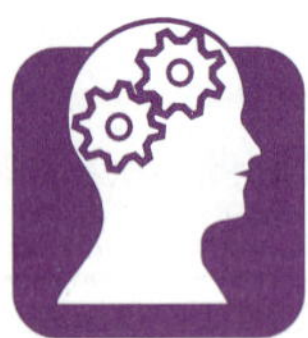

- **Exocrine gland** Seminiferous tubules synthesize a holocrine cytogenic secretion (spermatozoa) forming a compound tubular gland.

- **The testis functions as an endocrine gland.**
    - *Leydig cells (interstitial cells)*
        - Produce androgens (testosterone) and metabolites of other steroids (estrogen and progesterone).

Table 17.1   *Summary of Histologic Characteristics of the Male Reproductive System*

ORGAN	EPITHELIUM	MUSCLE LAYERS	CONNECTIVE TISSUE
Testis			
Seminiferous tubules and spermatogenic cells	Seminiferous epithelium composed of Sertoli cells	None	Basement membrane strengthened by lamellated connective tissue
Tubuli recti (straight tubules)	Simple columnar	None	
Rete testis	Cuboidal or simple squamous	None	Surrounded by dense connective tissue of mediastinum
Ducts			
Ductuli efferentes	Tall columnar ciliated cells alternating with cuboidal secretory cells	Thin circular layer of smooth muscle	Loose connective tissue in spaces between tubules
Ductus epididymidis	Pseudostratified; stereociliated	Circular layer of smooth muscle	Loose connective tissue in spaces between tubules
Ductus deferens (vas deferens)	Pseudostratified Near epididymis; same as ductus epididymidis	Inner longitudinal, middle circular, and outer longitudinal layers of smooth muscle	Loose propria of connective tissue that contains extensive elastic networks Adventitia of connective tissue
Ampulla of ductus deferens	Cuboidal or columnar	Thinner or less regularly arranged than any other parts of ductus deferens	Lamina propria and lamina adventitia
Ejaculatory ducts	Simple columnar or pseudostratified	Muscularis present at beginning	Connective tissue provided with extensive elastic networks
Accessory Glands			
Seminal vesicles	Individual variations Usually pseudostratified but may be columnar	Smooth muscle fibers chiefly circular; external to this Longitudinal fibers may be present	Lamina propria rich in elastic fibers Wall of external connective tissue with elastic nets
Prostate gland	Shows great variation but usually simple columnar or pseudostratified	Smooth muscle fibers in interstitial tissue	Vascular connective tissue with dense elastic networks beneath epithelium Interstitial connective tissue dense with collagenous fibers and elastic networks
Bulbourethral glands (Cowper's glands)	Subject to functional variations In enlarged alveoli, usually flattened In other glandular spaces the cells vary from cuboidal to columnar	Striated and smooth muscle in interstitial tissue	Fibroelastic stroma between tubules
Penis			
Corpora cavernosae	Blood spaces lined with endothelium	Strands of smooth muscle in partitions between cavernous spaces	Collagenous and elastic fibers in tunica albuginea
Corpus cavernosum urethrae (corpus spongiosum)	Blood spaces lined with endothelium	Smooth muscle fibers in inner layer of albuginea Smooth muscle in septa	Abundant elastic networks in albuginea Numerous elastic fibers in septa
Glans penis	Stratified squamous	Circular and longitudinal smooth muscle in walls of veins	Dense connective tissue containing network of anastomosing veins

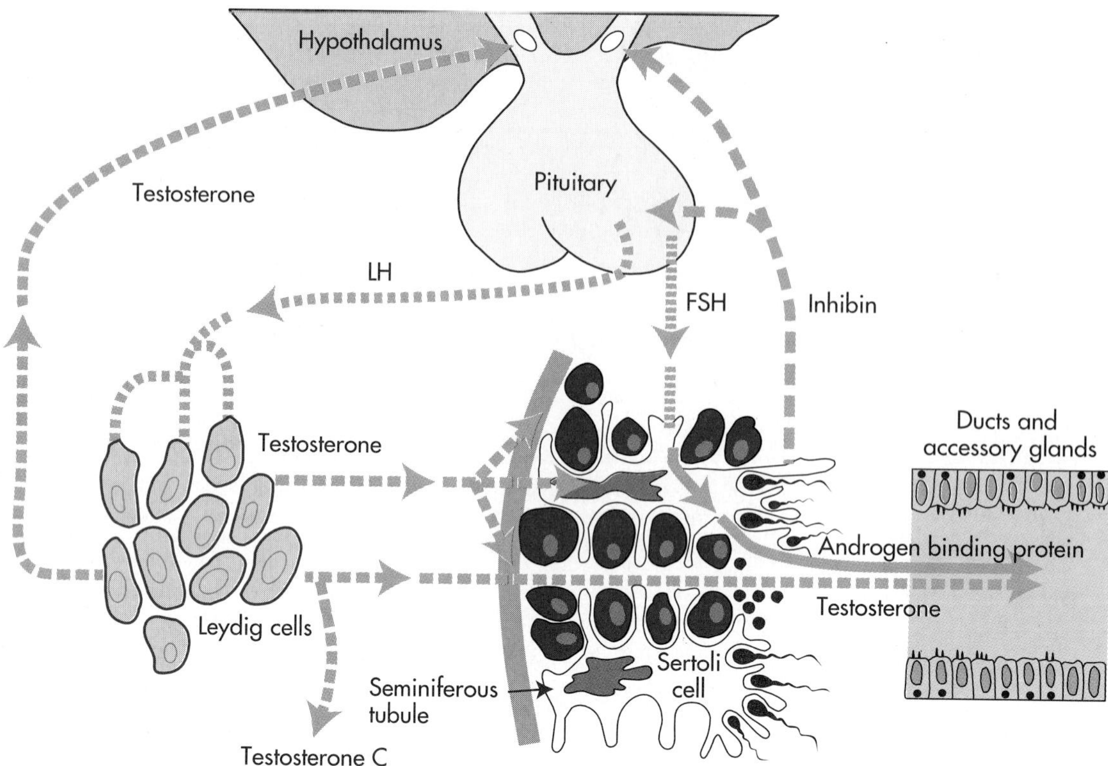

Fig. 17.1 Hormonal control of the male reproductive system. Testosterone, which is produced by the Leydig cells, stimulates spermatogenesis, *A;* maintains the functional activity of the ducts and accessory glands, *B;* maintains secondary sexual characteristics, *C;* and controls the pituitary output of luteinizing hormone (LH), *D;* LH stimulates testosterone secretion by the Leydig cells. Sertoli cells secrete antigen-binding protein (ABP) under the influence of follicle-stimulating hormone (FSH) and inhibin. Inhibin regulates the release of FSH. *(Modified from Stevens A, Lowe JS: Histology, Brookfield, Vt., 1992, Gower Medical {London}.)*

- Leydig cells are under control of luteinizing hormone (LH).

- Testosterone acts on the hypothalamus to control LH-releasing hormone (LH-RH). LH-RH stimulates LH secretion. Testosterone exerts negative feedback on LH secretion.

- Testosterone affects secondary sex characteristics, maintains the integrity of seminiferous tubules and the structure and function of accessory glands and ducts.

- Follicle-stimulating hormone (FSH) also maintains integrity of seminiferous epithelium.

- Testosterone acts on hypothalamus to control FSH-releasing hormone (FSH-RH). FSH-RH stimulates FSH secretion. Testosterone controls FSH through negative feedback.

— *Sertoli cells*

- Sertoli cells synthesize ABP (androgen-binding protein), the production of which is stimulated by FSH.

- They also synthesize inhibin, which acts on the anterior pituitary to decrease FSH release.

Seminiferous Epithelium

■ Spermatogenesis in Seminiferous Epithelium

- Spermatogenesis is the formation of spermatozoa (spermatogenesis = spermatocytogenesis [meiosis] + spermiogenesis).
- Meiosis is the division process by which diploid chromosome number is halved (haploid number).
- Spermocytogenesis is the first stage (spermatogonia → spermatocytes → spermatids). Spermatocytogenesis therefore includes meiosis.
- Spermiogenesis is the second stage in the series of morphologic or physiologic transformations that give rise to mature sperm.

Spermatogenesis does not begin until after puberty. It is under influence of testosterone, which is controlled by LH-ICSH. Before puberty, cells lining seminiferous tubules are supportive cells (Sertoli cells) and spermatogonia (premeiotic cells).

- At the onset of puberty one distinguishes 2 basic types of cells in seminiferous tubules.

  - Sertoli cells
  - Spermatogenic cells (spermatogonia → spermatozoa)

● **Spermatogonia (Fig. 17.2)** Basally located undifferentiated cells that may

- replenish population
- differentiate into the primary spermatocyte

There are basically 2 types of spermatogonia in the seminiferous epithelium.

- Type A spermatogonia (stem cells)

  - Dark cells replenish dark cells or differentiate to form pale cells.
  - Pale cells divide to form type B spermatogonia.

- Type B spermatogonia (derivative cells) give rise to primary spermatocytes, may undergo division to form as many as 16 cells.

Cytoplasmic bridges are synctium-like membranal associations between spermatogonia. These associations are maintained through the spermatid stages. Meiotic synchrony is maintained to spermatid stage through the medium of the cytoplasmic continuities.

● **Spermatocytes**

- Primary spermatocytes undergo last duplication of DNA and enter prophase I → metaphase I (reductional division) → 2 secondary spermatocytes (haploid cells).
- Secondary spermatocytes → metaphase II (equational division) → 2 spermatids.
- Thus 1 primary spermatocyte forms 4 spermatids.

Spermatid undergoes spermiogenesis → spermatozoa (singular, spermatozoon).

Stages of spermatogenesis occur in lumenward gradient (Fig. 17.3).

- Basal cells—spermatogonia (earliest stages)
- Surface cells—spermatozoa (later stage)

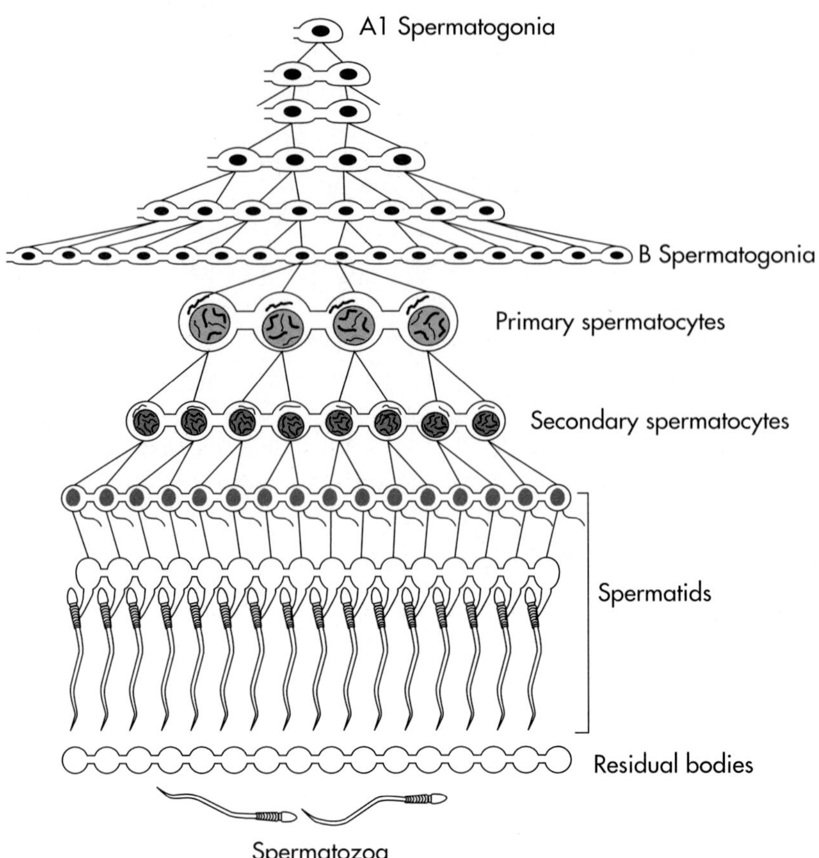

Fig. 17.2 The clonal nature of spermatazoa. The earliest spermatogonia divide to produce separate daughter cells. Once committed to differentiation the cells of all subsequent generations are connected by intercellular bridges. During the spermatid stage the cells shed their residual bodies to become separate cells. *(Modified from Junqueira LC, Carneiro J:* Basic histology, *East Norwalk, Conn., 1992, Appleton & Lange.)*

• Approximately 22 days are spent as a primary spermatocyte. It takes 64 days to go from the most mature spermatogonia to the developed spermatozoon.

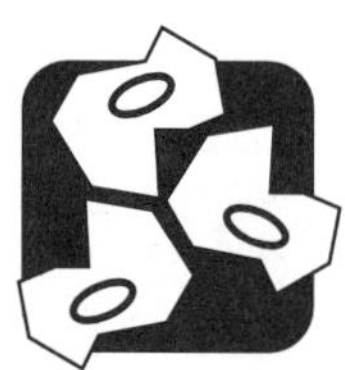

■ **Cell Cycle of Seminiferous Epithelium** Only cells in DNA synthesis in seminiferous epithelium are spermatogonia and interphase primary spermatocytes. Before entering meiosis, primary spermatocytes synthesize DNA. DNA synthesis then ceases (Fig. 17.4).

Measure amounts of DNA in various cells (C = gamete amount of DNA)

- Spermatogonia (2C to 4C)
- Primary spermatocyte in prophase of meiosis I (4C)
- Secondary spermatocyte (2C)
- Spermatid (C)
- Fertilization restores 2C DNA synthesis to 4C DNA.

● Important consequences of meiosis

- Gamete contains the haploid chromosome number.

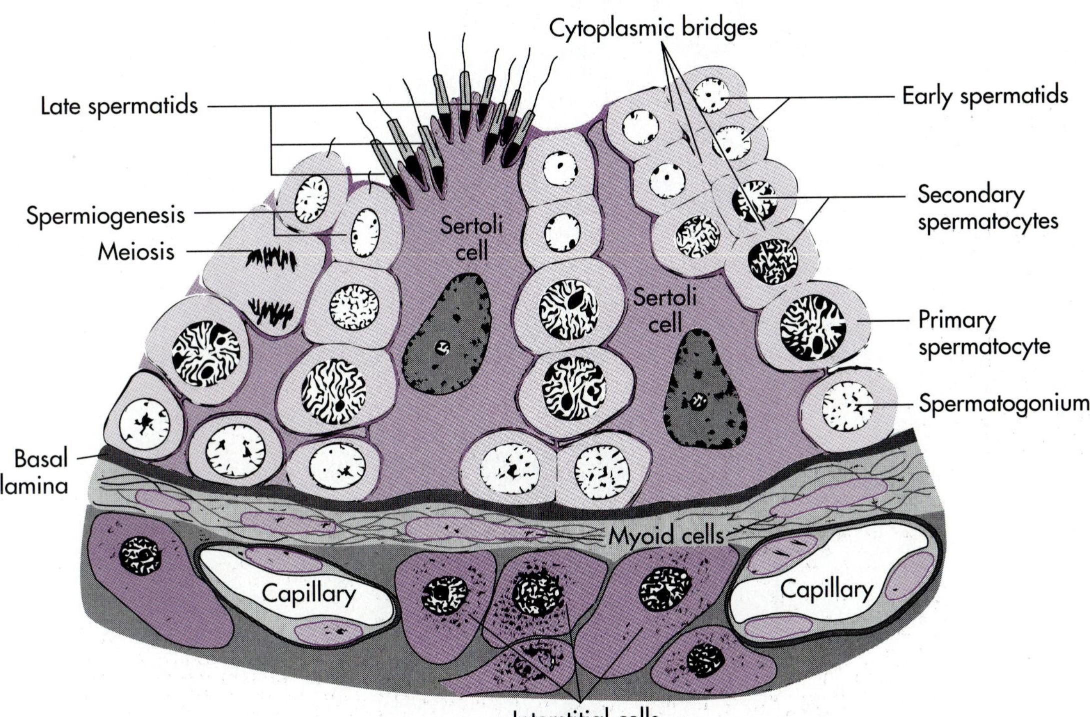

Fig. 17.3 Seminiferous tubule and interstitial tissue. The section shows the lumenward gradient of spermatogenic cells and their relationship to Sertoli cells. *(Modified from Junqueira LC, Carneiro J:* Basic histology, *East Norwalk, Conn., 1992, Appleton & Lange.)*

- Gamete contains either an X or a Y chromosome (sex determination).

Spermiogenesis—transformation of spermatid to mature sperm
Organelles of spermatid undergo specialization (Fig. 17.5)

- Small carbohydrate-containing granules appear in association with the Golgi apparatus. Several such granules fuse to form acrosomal granule in acrosomal vesicle. Granule localizes at one end of nucleus.
- Membrane of acrosome vesicle adheres to nuclear envelope and spreads over nucleus forming
    - acrosomal granules
    - acrosomal cap (nuclear cap)
- Spermatid elongates and acrosome substance spreads in acrosome cap. Golgi detaches to form residual Golgi zone.
- Nucleus becomes increasingly condensed, and the chromatin is heterochromatinized.
- Centrioles migrate to posterior pole of nucleus and situate at right angles to one another.
- One of centrioles (distal centriole) gives rise to flagellum.
- Both centriole and base of flagellum migrate to nuclear envelope. Proximal centriole forms the basal body.
- A small ring of cytoplasm forms around the flagellum close to the distal centriole. It slides along the flagellum becoming the annulus of the midportion of the spermatozoa. Mitochondrial sheath forms.

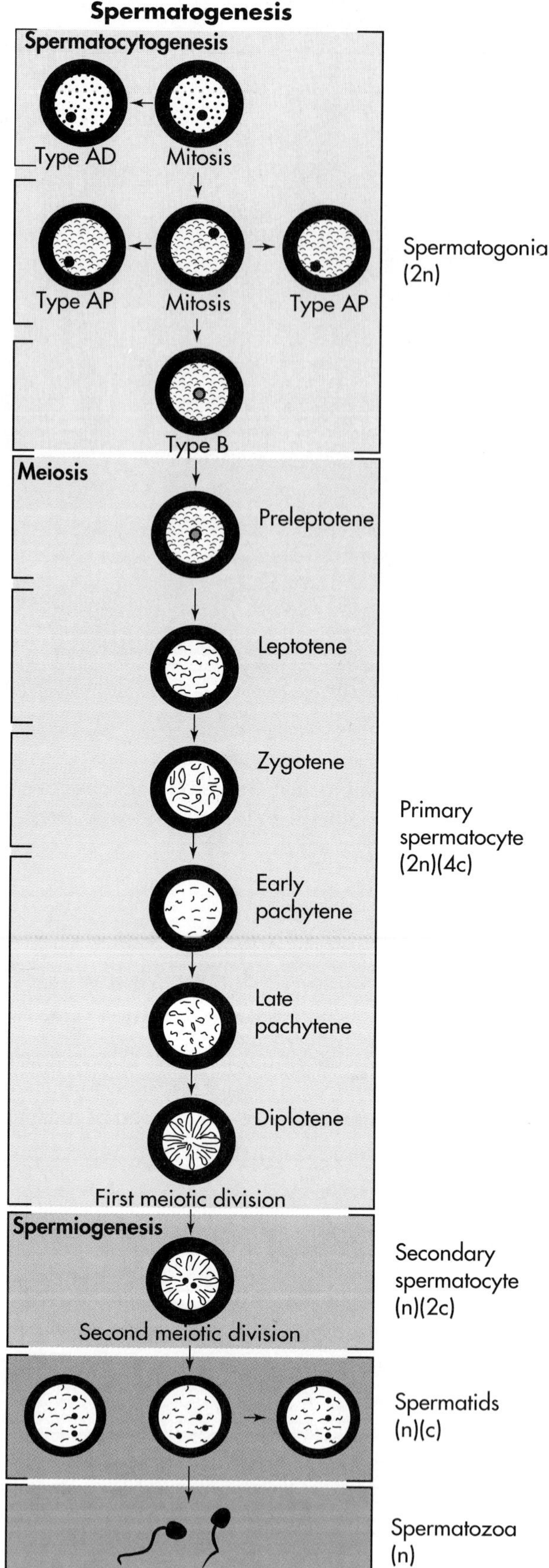

Fig. 17.4 Spermatogenesis and meiosis. Spermatogenesis begins with division of spermatogonia to give rise to the Ad, the Ap, and the type B spermatogonia. The type B spermatogonium, having completed DNA replication, enters into prophase of the first meiotic division as a primary spermatocyte. The cell completes the reductional division of meiosis to give rise to the secondary spermatocyte. Without an intervening interphase the cell undergoes the second meiotic division to give rise to haploid spermatids. The spermatids undergo spermiogenesis to give rise to the spermatozoa. *(Modified from Stevens A, Lowe JS:* Histology, *Brookfield, Vt., 1992, Gower Medical {London}.)*

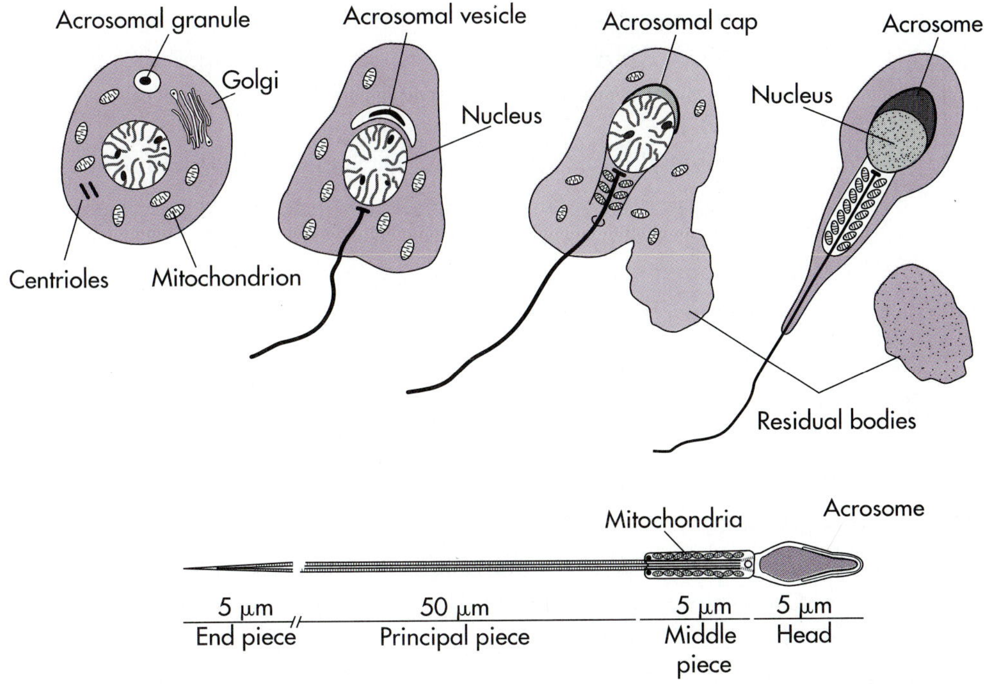

Fig. 17.5 *Above,* Principal changes that a spermatid undergoes during spermiogenesis. *Below,* Structure of a mature spermatozoon. *(Modified from Junqueira LC, Carneiro J:* Basic histology, *East Norwalk, Conn., 1992, Appleton & Lange.)*

- A large piece of cytoplasm is cleaved off the sperm head, forming an anucleate mass.

■ **Cell Associations in the Seminiferous Epithelium and Duration of Spermatogenesis in Man-Humanity** A single section through the seminiferous tubule doesn't show all the stages. A given area may reveal groups in 4 or 5 well-defined stages. Individual stages have a tendency to be present in association with other specific stages.

Clear-cut association groups can be recognized. The clear-cut association groups are accounted for by long duration of entire process.

When cells of all groups are placed in a series, they show a continuity of events characteristic of a cycle.

● Duration of spermatogenesis

- Only spermatogonia and interphase primary spermatocytes become labeled with [^{3}H] thymidine after 1-hour exposure to isotope.
- Takes approximately 50 to 60 days before fully developed sperm are labeled.

■ **Mature Spermatazoon (Fig. 17.5)**

● Head

- The nucleus occupies most of the sperm head.
- As spermiogenesis begins, chromatin begins to clump (heterochromatinization).
- Clumping continues until the entire nucleus is filled with heterochromatin.
- DNA in the nucleus is highly organized crystalline nucleoprotein.

- There is a switch from histone to protamine.
- Virtually all RNA synthesis ceases during spermatogenesis.
- Changes during spermiogenesis must involve preformed messenger RNA.
- The acrosomal cap is a membrane covering two thirds of the nucleus.
  - Carbohydrate-containing material is spread throughout cap.
  - It is believed to contain hyaluronidase.
  - It contains some proteolytic enzyme (zonalysin) associated with the inner acrosomal membrane.
  - Plasma membrane

● **Neck**

  - Dense funnel of coarse longitudinal fibers continuous with midpiece

● **Tail**

  - Midpiece
  - Axial fiber bundle (2 central singlets + 9 doublets in microtubule)
  - Coarse circumferential fibers continuous with those in neck
  - Mitochondrial helix

● **Principal piece (55 µm length)**

  - Axial fiber bundle continuous with midpiece
  - Coarse circumferential fibers continuous with midpiece

● **End piece**

  - Axial fibers continuous with principal piece
  - Coarse fibers end

Spermatozoa are not motile when they are formed. They move from the seminiferous tubule through the rete testis by formation of fluid in the seminiferous tubule and resorption of fluid in the ductus epididymidis. Spermatozoa in the ductus epididymidis and ductus deferens are moved by peristalsis. The movement of spermatozoa is activated by the secretion of genital glands.

SERTOLI CELLS AND THE BLOOD-TESTIS BARRIER (FIG. 17.6)

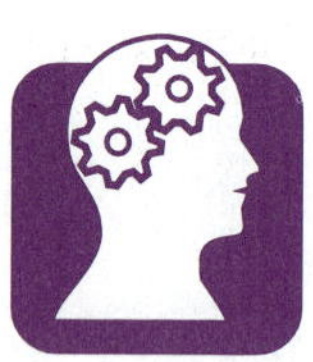

■ Sertoli Cells

- Sertoli cells are tall, columnar cells extending from the basement membrane to the lumen. They support, protect, and help nurture germ cells.
  - FPM
  - They remain after degeneration of the germ cells.

■ Blood-Testis Barrier

- Sertoli cells are connected to one another by zonulae occludentes to separate spermatogonia from other stages of spermatogenesis.
- Tissue fluid must pass through Sertoli cell to reach spermatocytes, spermatids, and spermatozoa.

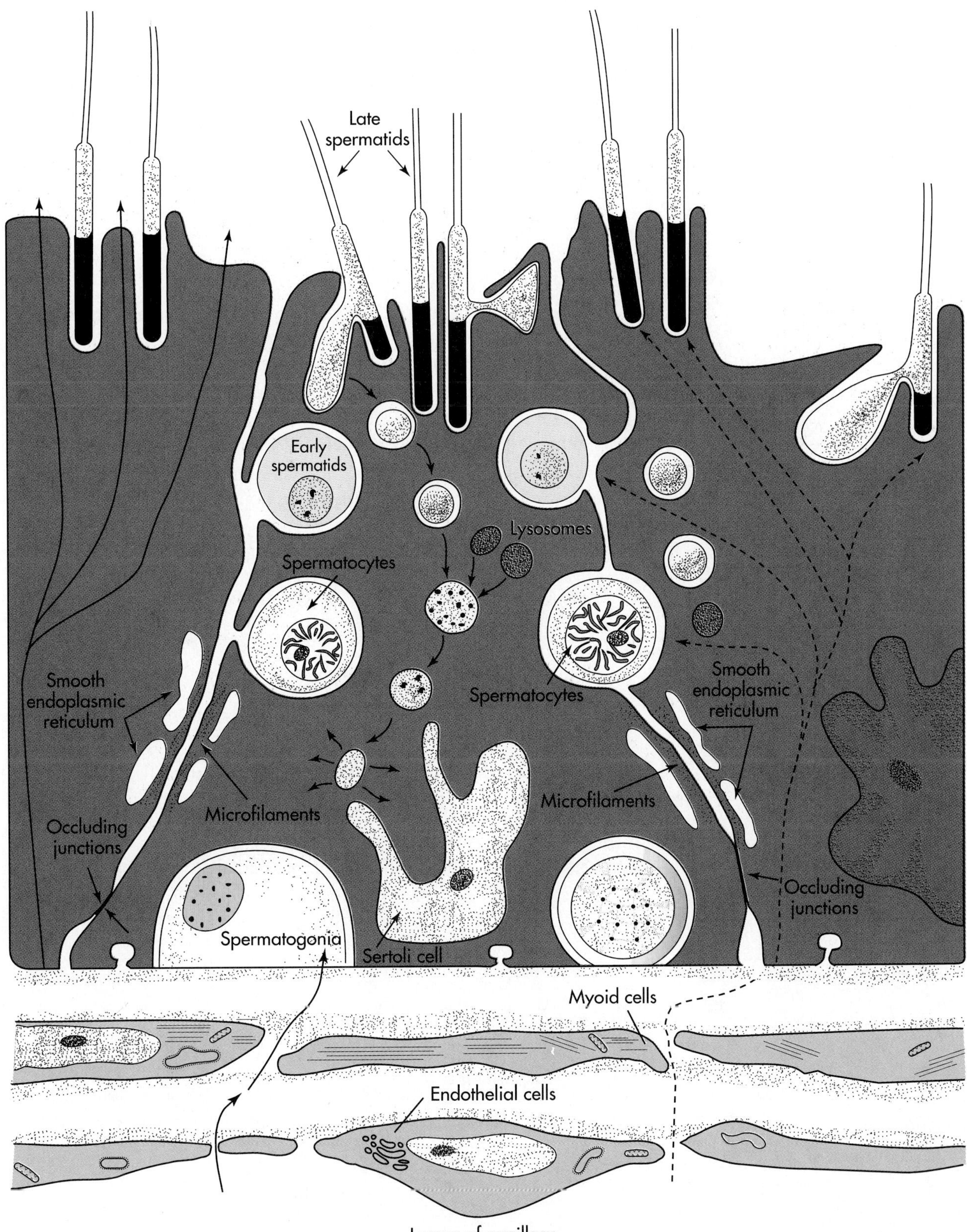

Fig. 17-6 The blood-testis barrier. The Sertoli cells divide the seminiferous tubules into two compartments. The basal compartment is occupied by the spermatogonia. The adluminal compartment is separated from the basal compartment by the zonula occludens. Cells in the process of spermatogenesis are enveloped by Sertoli cells in this compartment. *(Modified from Junqueira LC, Carneiro J:* Basic histology, *East Norwalk, Conn., 1992, Appleton & Lange.)*

- Foreign protein from postmeiotic germ cells is kept out of the bloodstream by the zonula occludens, preventing possible antibody induction.

■ Control of Testosterone Secretion

- Sertoli cells produce ABP, which favors local storage of testosterone to maintain spermatogenesis.
- They also secrete inhibin $\rightarrow$ decrease FSH.
- Sertoli cells envelope the spermatogenic cells and phagocytose residual bodies of spermatozoa.
- They also secrete fluid.

■ Semen Production

- Spermatozoa are swept from the seminiferous tubule and lumen of the ductus epididymidis by current formed by the fluid secreted in seminiferous tubules by Sertoli cells and absorbed in the ductus epididymidis.
- The efferent ductules and ductus epididymidis are storage regions.
- At the time of ejaculation, muscular contractions of ductus epididymidis, ductus deferens, and urethra force the release of spermatozoa.
- Sequence at ejaculation—secretion of Cowper's and Littre's glands, the prostate, release of spermatozoa, and then secretion of seminal vesicles

● Seminal vesicle

- Mucoid secretion, rich in fructose
- Secretion contains factors for coagulation of semen and antiagglutination of spermatozoa.

● Prostate

- Thin secretion is rich in acid phosphatase.
- Secretion contains prostaglandins (uterine contraction).
- Corpora amylacea increase in aging.

● Bulbourethral (Cowper's) glands lubricate urethra.

● Littre's glands lubricate urethra.

- Semen—seminal plasma + spermatozoa
- Spermatozoa, about 300 million per ejaculate
- Seminal plasma, about 3 ml (secretions of accessory glands)

MULTIPLE CHOICE
REVIEW QUESTIONS

1. In terms of their genetic constitution, the two spermatids formed from a single cell during the second meiotic division

    a. have either an X or a Y chromosome, but not both.
    b. are nearly identical.
    c. are very different.
    d. A and B are correct.
    e. A, B, and C are correct.

2. In a secondary spermatocyte in metaphase of meiosis II, one finds

    a. 23 chromosomes.
    b. 46 chromatids.
    c. an amount of DNA equivalent to that found in a somatic G_1 diploid cell.
    d. A and B are correct.
    e. A, B, and C are correct.

3. A person drinks water that is accidentally contaminated with [^{3}H] thymidine. He drinks only this water for 2 months. What would be the most advanced stage of spermatogenesis that has incorporated the label into DNA 2 months after he began to drink the water?

    a. Spermatogonia
    b. Primary spermatocytes
    c. Secondary spermatocytes
    d. Early spermatids
    e. Fully developed spermatozoa

4. Tritiated thymidine is administered to an adult for 1 week. A biopsy is taken at the end of that week and fixed for autoradiography. Place A beside cells that would be labeled; B beside cells that would not be labeled.

    _____ Spermatogonia
    _____ Oocyte in primordial follicle
    _____ Primary spermatocyte
    _____ Spermatid

5. Match the organelle with its function:

    _____ Elaboration of acrosome
    _____ Synthesis of testosterone
    _____ Synthesis of androgen-binding protein
    _____ Formation of blood-testis barrier

    a. Primary spermatocyte
    b. Golgi of spermatid
    c. RER of Sertoli cell
    d. SER of Leydig cell
    e. Zonula occludens of Sertoli cell

Chapter 18

Female Reproductive System

GENERAL

The organs discussed in this chapter include the ovary, oviduct, uterus, vagina, external genitalia, breast, and placenta. The histophysiologic characteristics of these organs is complicated by the changes that occur during the menstrual cycle and during pregnancy. The time when menses first occurs is **menarche. Menopause** is a variable period of time during which cyclic changes become intermittent and eventually cease. During the **postmenopausal period** there is a slow, progressive involution of this system.

OVARY

■ General

- External covering of simple squamous or cuboidal epithelium, erroneously still referred to as "germinal epithelium"
- Tunica albuginea under epithelial surface
- **Cortex** of **ovarian follicles** containing **oocytes**
- **Medulla** of vascular, highly cellular connective tissue

■ Ovarian Follicles

- Primordial germ cells (**oogonia**) migrate from yolk sac endoderm into ovary early in embryonic period.
- Oogonia increase in number by mitosis until fifth to seventh fetal month resulting in 3 million oogonia per ovary.
  - Many die by **apoptosis, or programmed cell death (atresia),** resulting in only 200,000 per ovary at the time of menarche.
  - Many enter **prophase I** of **meiosis** and stay there until stimulated to continue meiosis by **follicle-stimulating hormone (FSH).**
  - Those in prophase I of meiosis are **primary oocytes** (Fig. 18.1).
- Peripheral to the primary oocyte in an ovarian follicle there is:

Epithelium resting on a basement membrane outside of which is ovarian stroma: both the epithelium and its adjacent stromal covering are endocrine tissues.
  1. **Primordial follicle**—single layer of squamous epithelium.
  2. **Primary follicle**
     - With single layer of cuboidal epithelium—**unilaminar primary follicle**
     - With stratification of epithelium—**multilaminar primary follicle;** during the growth of the epithelium an amorphous zone appears between the primary oocyte and the follicular epithelium—**zona pellu-**

184

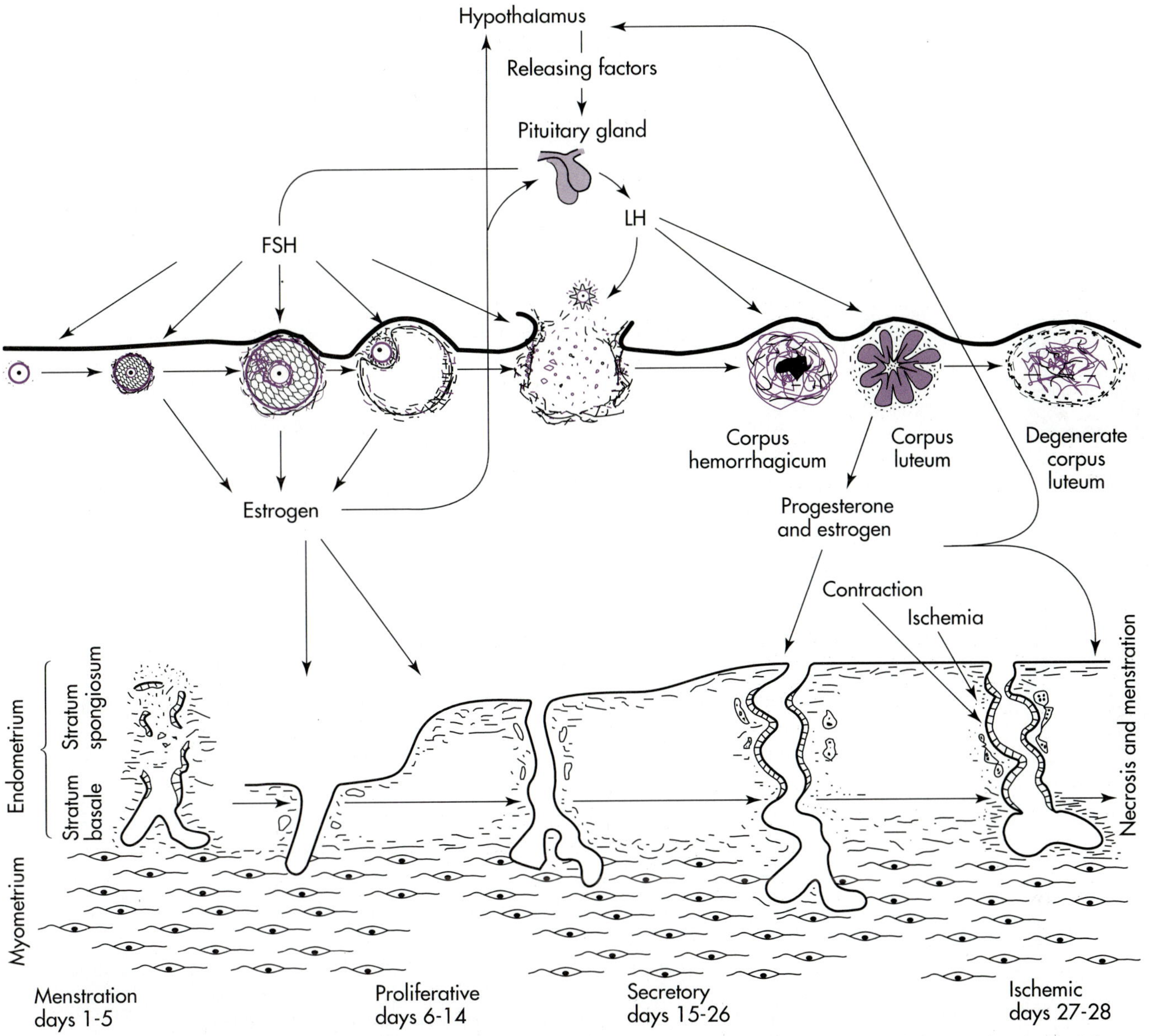

Fig. 18.1 Overview of the interrelationships between the hypothalamus and pituitary gland and the ovarian and endometrial cycles. *FSH,* Follicle stimulating hormone; *LH,* leutinizing hormone.

cida (ZP), which is formed by contributions from both the oocyte and the follicular epithelium, and each has surface projections into the ZP. As these growth changes occur, the oocyte differentiates by increasing the number of mitochondria, Golgi complexes, RER, and free polysomes.

3. **Secondary follicle**—fluid (liquor folliculi)–filled spaces appear in stratified follicular epithelium; spaces coalesce to form **antrum** (antral follicle). Oocyte is still in prophase I of meiosis—primary oocyte. Establishment of antrum causes oocyte to reside in a mound of follicular cells (**granulosa cells**)—**cumulus oophorus.**

4. Mature, or **graafian, follicle** exists for 1 or 2 days before ovulation.

Granulosa cells attached to zona pellucida elongate forming **corona radiata,** which will accompany the oocyte during and after ovulation.

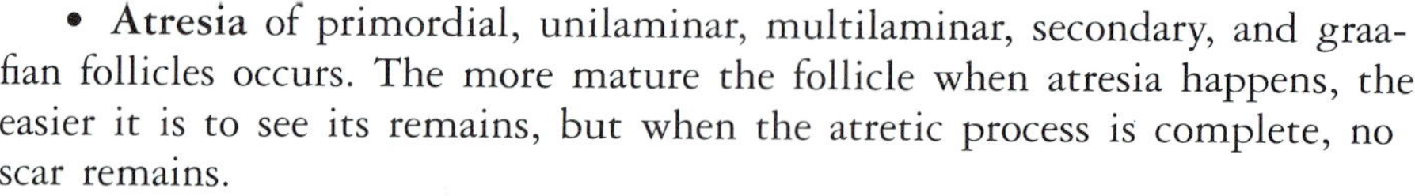

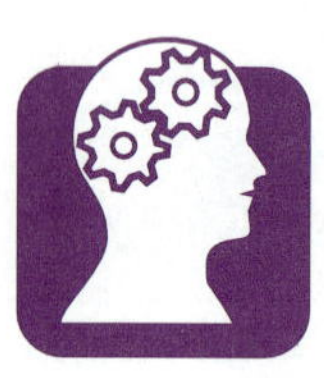

- **Atresia** of primordial, unilaminar, multilaminar, secondary, and graafian follicles occurs. The more mature the follicle when atresia happens, the easier it is to see its remains, but when the atretic process is complete, no scar remains.

5. Stroma

Closest to the follicle is the highly vascularized **theca interna,** an endocrine hormone–secreting zone; cells contain SER and make **androstenedione,** which is converted (requiring FSH) to **estrogen** by nearby granulosa cells.

Peripheral to theca interna is the nonendocrine stroma **theca externa.**

- After menarche, monthly and alternating between the ovaries, groups of 5 to 15 follicles start to grow and differentiate under the influence of **FSH.**

Normally only one follicle completely matures and ovulates; the others undergo atresia. In the normal reproductive life of a woman only about 450 ova are ovulated; the rest undergo atresia.

As a group of follicles begins to grow (unilaminar $\rightarrow$ multilaminar $\rightarrow$ secondary $\rightarrow$ graafian), the number of granulosa cells increases, thus the level of estrogen increases.

■ Ovulation

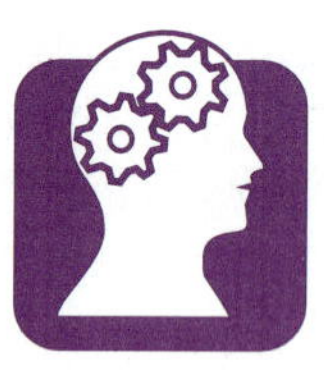

- Meiosis I is completed by the primary oocyte just before ovulation: **ovulated ovum** is a **secondary oocyte** arrested in **metaphase II.**
- Unequal cell division during meiosis I results in one large secondary oocyte (2C DNA, 23 chromosomes each with 2 chromatids = 46 chromatids) + one tiny secondary oocyte, the first polar body; both surrounded by the ZP. Since both the secondary oocyte and the first polar body contain 23 chromosomes, they are haploid.
- Ovulation occurs through a weak area, or stigma, on ovarian surface, probably caused by reduced blood flow because of pressure from the Graafian follicle.
- Ovulated secondary oocyte in peritoneal cavity briefly; must be "caught" by **fimbria of oviduct;** if missed by fimbria and fertilized, there can be an abdominal pregnancy.
- Requires a surge of **luetinizing hormone (LH);** induced by rising level of estrogen acting on hypothalamo-hypophyseal system. Rising level of estrogen also causes an increase in LH receptors on the granulosa cells.
- If ovulated secondary oocyte is not fertilized, it dies; fertilizable life of ovum is about 24 hours.

■ Fertilization

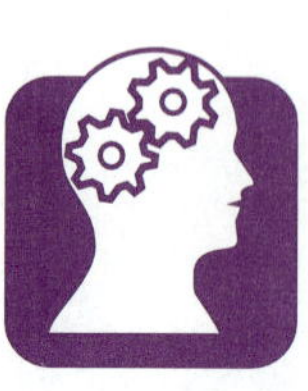

- If ovulated secondary oocyte is fertilized:
  - Sperm penetrates corona radiata; **hyaluronidase** digestion and movements of sperm tail; **acrosomal reaction**—sperm plasma membrane over acrosome becomes fused at points forming fenestrations through which acrosomal contents (hyaluronidase and proteolytic enzymes released); **zonalysin** attached to inner acrosomal membrane liquefies small slit in ZP; plasma membranes of ovum and sperm head fuse producing, in effect, a single cell.
  - Ovum completes **meiosis II,** forming a second polar body and a large mature gamete, the nucleus of which is the **female pronucleus** (1C DNA, 23 chromosomes, haploid, 23 chromatids; only one sex chromosome, an X).
- The ovum completes meiosis II and forms the female pronucleus, the

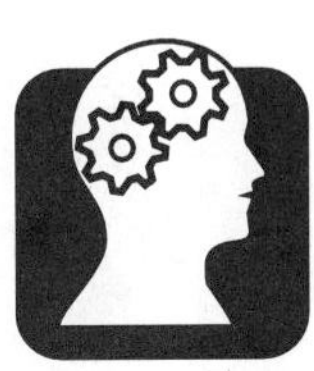

sperm head forms the **male pronucleus** (1C DNA, 23 chromosomes, haploid, 23 chromatids; only one sex chromosome, and it can be either X *or* Y).

- Then each pronucleus undergoes one round of **DNA synthesis;** so 1C DNA becomes 2C DNA; 23 chromosomes containing one chromatid each become 23 chromosomes, each with 2 chromatids; the **zygote** now contains a total of 4C DNA, 46 chromosomes, and 92 chromatids housed in the 2 pronuclei.

- The two pronuclei meet (**syngamy**) but do not fuse; nuclear membranes dissolve, and chromosomes line up on equatorial plate ready for first mitotic or cleavage division; zygote stage ends and embryogenesis begins.

- Fertilization causes the ovum to become **metabolically activated.**

  - Lysosomes released
  - Some enzyme systems activated
  - Protein synthesis enhanced
  - Multiple nucleoli formed in female pronucleus

- **Block to polyspermy**

  ZP and vitelline membrane become impermeable

- Errors of fertilization

  - **Polyspermy:** two sperm enter; zygote has 2 male and 1 female pronuclei; embryo is triploid; incompatible with life; spontaneous abortion

  - **Polygyny:** failure to emit second polar body; 2 female and 1 male pronuclei; triploidy

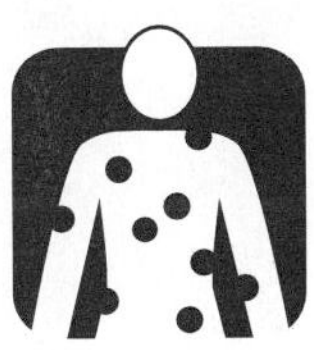

■ Corpus Luteum

- An endocrine gland formed from collapsed remains of ovulated graafian follicle.

- Its formation requires presence of **LH.**

- Granulosa cells become luteinized—**granulosa lutein cells;** lots of SER; produce increasing amounts of **progesterone;** with time rising progesterone level progressively inhibits LH production; LH necessary for life of corpus luteum (CL); CL commits suicide; i.e., it has been a **corpus luteum of menstruation;** this "suicide" is prevented by presence of **HCG** (human chorionic gonadotropin) produced by trophoblast cells of embryo; HCG maintains CL as **corpus luteum of pregnancy.**

- Theca interna cells become luteinized—**theca lutein cells;** lots of SER; produce estrogen.

- Progesterone and estrogen from CL of menstruation of CL or pregnancy maintain endometrium in secretory phase until menses or parturition respectively; progesterone "quiets" myometrium.

- CL of pregnancy also produces **relaxin,** which softens pubic symphysis, promotes dilatation of cervix, and "quiets" myometrium.

- After life of CL of menstruation or CL of pregnancy they scar—**corpus albicans.**

Uterus

■ Wall

- **Perimetrium:** serosa or adventitia depending on peritoneal reflections.

- **Myometrium:** smooth muscle that can undergo **hypertrophy** and hy-

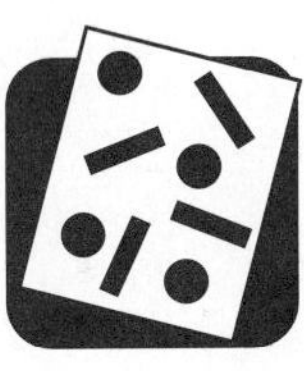

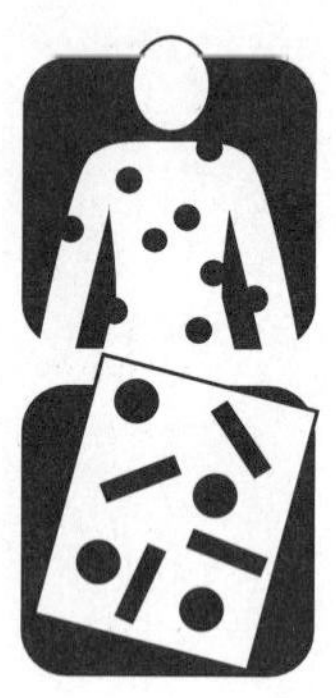

perplasia, especially during pregnancy; activity of myometrial smooth muscle enhanced by estrogen, depressed by progesterone and relaxin; supportive connective tissue stroma; benign tumor composed of smooth muscle cells and fibroblasts—**fibromyoma**—**fibroid.**

- **Endometrium:** inner lining or mucosa composed of surface epithelium of simple columnar cells; endometrial glands, and highly vascular stroma (lamina propria).
  - **Functionalis** layer is superficial four fifths, which sloughs and repairs with each menstrual cycle.
  - **Basalis** layer is deep fifth, which does not slough during menses; functionalis layer is repaired or rebuilt from basalis layer.
  - **Endometriosis:** presence of endometrial tissue ectopically, usually in myometrium by direct extension but also in extrauterine sites.

■ Endometrium During Menstrual Cycle

- Cycle begins on first day of menses or bleeding—day 1.
- **Menses—days 1 to 4;** functionalis layer sloughs off and is removed—menstrual phase of menstrual cycle.
- **Proliferative phase—days 5 to 14;** functionalis layer rebuilt from basalis layer; repair stimulated by estrogen; end signaled by ovulation.
- **Secretory phase—days 15 to 27;** dependent on formation of corpus luteum release of progesterone; progesterone acts on estrogen-primed endometrium causing endometrial glands and arteries to coil and the columnar cells of the glands to accumulate **glycogen** first in the basal region of each cell (early secretory phase); later glycogen moves to apical portion of cell (late secretory phase); in late secretory phase stroma becomes edematous.
- **Premenstrual phase—days 27 and 28;** if no fertilization, no implantation, no HCG; corpus luteum "commits suicide" by inhibition of LH due to rising level of progesterone; death of CL causes abrupt drop in estrogen and progesterone production, which in turn causes contraction of coiled arteries and **ischemia** of tissue distal to contracted segment; ischemic tissue undergoes **necrosis** (not apoptosis); endometrial arterial walls leak RBCs into stroma, eventually break open—**hemorrhage** and menstrual flow.

ENDOCRINOLOGY

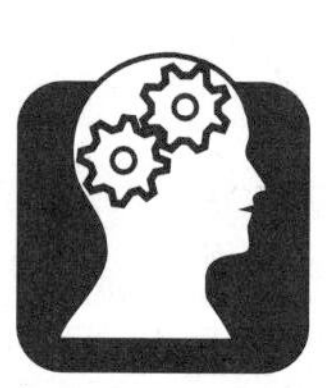

- **FSH** and **LH** from pituitary gonadotrophs stimulate group of primordial ovarian follicles (5 to 15) to grow and mature.
- Increased numbers of cells in enlarging follicles causes rising level of **estrogen.**
- Rising level of estrogen (estradiol and estrone)
  - Initiate proliferative repair of sloughed functionalis layer from the remaining basilis layer.
  - Negative feedback on **FSH-RH** production
  - Positive feedback on **LH-RH** production
    - **LH surge**
    - Results in proper **FSH:LH ratio**
    - **Induces ovulation**
    - Postovulatory LH levels necessary for establishment of corpus luteum
- Rising level of **progesterone** from corpus luteum causes:
  - Estrogen-primed proliferative endometrium to change to **secretory endometrium**

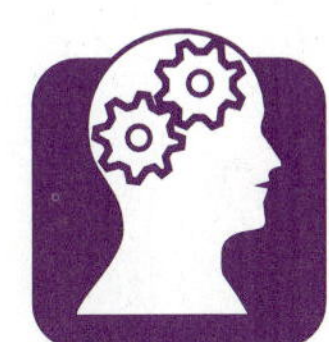

- Negative feedback on **LH-RH,** resulting in less and less LH and death of corpus luteum if **HCG** not present.
- Death of CL causes level of progesterone and estrogen to drop, causing:
  - contraction of coiled arteries and entry into premenstrual and then menstrual phases
  - loss of negative feedback on LH-RH and FSH-RH. FSH and LH levels begin to rise; repeat from top.

Oviduct

- **Four Regions**
  - **Infundibulum,** or funnel-shaped end with finger-like **fimbria**
  - **Ampulla,** or dilated region, proximal to infundibulum; fertilization occurs here.
  - **Isthmus,** or nondilated region, proximal to ampulla
  - **Pars intramuralis** or that part coursing through the uterine wall
- **Three Layers**

  - **Mucosa (with longitudinal folds)**
    - Simple columnar epithelium
      - **Ciliated cells** (cilia) beat toward uterus.
      - **Secretory cells** produce viscous liquid film; nourishment for ovum, zygote, early embryo.
      - Epithelial cells are tallest during proliferative phase; shortest in late secretory-premenstrual phase.
    - Underlying lamina propria (stroma)

      Becomes edematous during premenstrual phase
  - **Muscularis**
    - Inner circular smooth muscle
    - Outer longitudinal smooth muscle
    - Contractions of both layers of smooth muscle
      - Stimulated by presence of estrogen
      - Inhibited by presence of progesterone
  - **Serosa**

Cervix

- Lower cylindrical part of uterus
- Epithelial lining of simple columnar cells secretes **mucus.**
- **Cervical glands** secrete mucus; more viscous during pregnancy; more watery at midcycle, which helps movement of sperm in cervical canal, uterus, oviduct.
- Portio vaginalis—distal lowermost end protruding into vagina, surrounded by fornices; covered by stratified squamous parakeratinized epithelium
- Cervical epithelium
  - **Cell desquamation** is basis for Pap smear **exfoliative cytology.**
  - Five cell types found in Pap smear:
    Basal, parabasal, intermediate, precornified, cornified surface

- Estrogen stimulates cell differentiation; cells that desquamate during proliferative phase are more mature; have pyknotic nuclei and cytoplasmic keratin.
- During secretory phase desquamating cells are less mature; Pap smear contains more parabasal, intermediate, and fewer cornified cells.

VAGINA

- **Three-layered Wall**
  - **Mucosa**

    Stratified squamous parakeratinized epithelium

    - Cells synthesize and accumulate **glycogen.**
    - Glycogen is deposited in vaginal lumen as cells slough.
    - "Benign" bacteria utilize glycogen, release **lactic acid** causing normal **low pH,** which inhibits growth of pathogenic bacteria.
    - Glycogen content
      Highest at midcycle; pH at midcycle lowest
      Lowest at late secretory, pH rises, and susceptibility to infection increases

    — *Epithelium thickest during proliferative phase (estrogen)*
    — *Lamina propria*
      - Rich in elastic fibers
      - No glands
      - Highly vascularized. These vessels are source of fluid **exudate** during sexual excitement.

    — *No submucosa*
  - **Muscularis**
    - Mostly longitudinal smooth muscle
    - Some circular smooth muscle closest to lamina propria
  - **Adventitia**
    - Rich in elastic fibers

EXTERNAL GENITALIA

- **Clitoris**
  - Homologous in development and structure to penis
  - Erectile tissue in two bodies, end in rudimentary glans clitoris

- **Labia Minora**
  - Folds of skin with core of dense irregular connective tissue

- **Labia Majora**
  - Folds of skin also but with large amount of adipose connective tissue and thin layer of smooth muscle—developmentally homologous to scrotum

- **Glands of Bartholin**
  - Open into each side of vestibule
  - Homologous to bulbourethral glands in male
  - Secrete mucus

MAMMARY GLAND (FIG. 18.2)

■ **Before Puberty**

- **Lactiferous sinuses** and **ducts**

■ **At Puberty**

- Sprouting/branching of deep ends of lactiferous ducts forms large numbers of **alveolar glandular units.**
- Significant accumulation of **adipose** tissue
- Above driven by **estrogen**
  - Male breast responds to estrogen also.
    - Placental estrogen crosses into fetal blood ("witch's" milk in newborn male).
    - **Gynecomastia,** or development of adult male breast, e.g.: Alcoholic cirrhosis: liver cannot chemically "detoxify" estrogen from zona reticularis of adrenal gland; estrogen circulates; increased cirrhosis, increased level of estrogen, increased development of breast

■ **Adult**

- 15 to 25 lobes of compound tubuloalveolar glands, each with its own

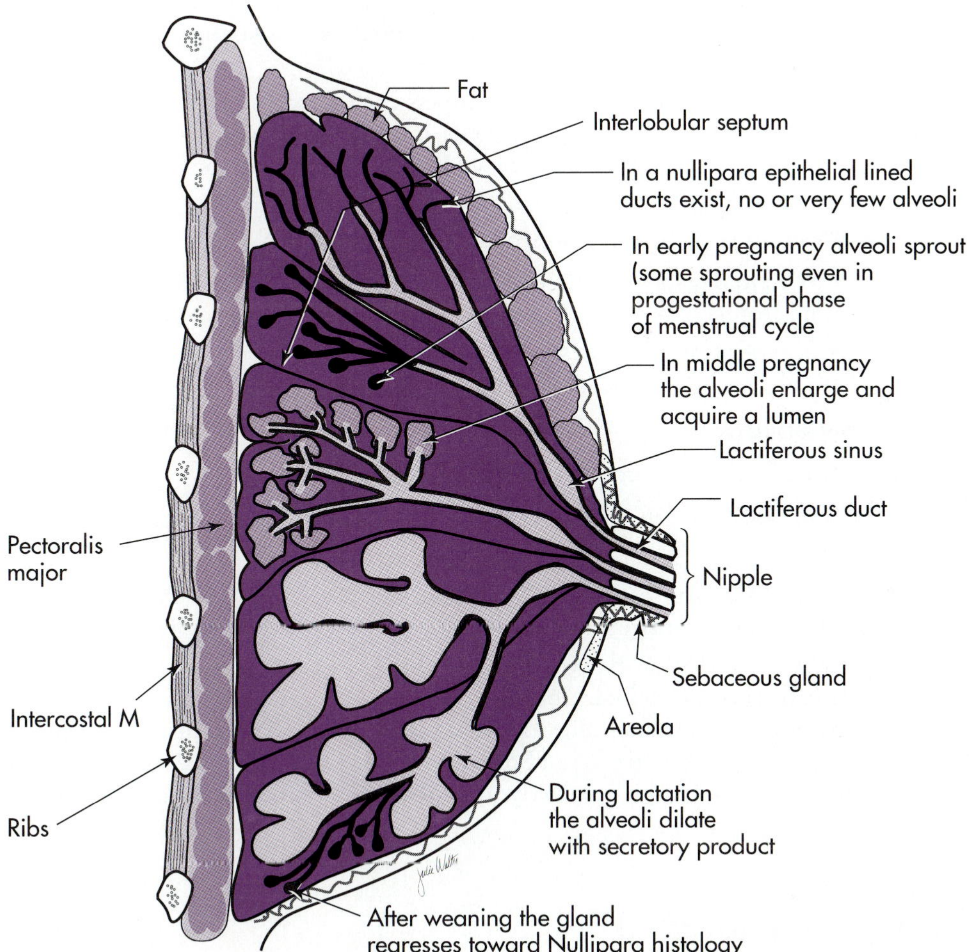

Fig. 18.2 Gross and microscopic anatomy of the breast at different stages in development.

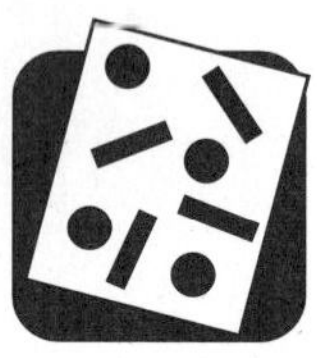

lactiferous duct and lactiferous sinus; lobes separated by dense connective tissue septa; lobes contain adipose connective tissue.

- Secretory alveoli immediately surrounded by loose areolar connective tissue

- **Intralobular ducts** → **interlobular ducts** → **lactiferous ducts** → **lactiferous sinuses** in nipple

- Alveolar glandular epithelium dormant until pregnancy; during secretory phase of menstrual cycle adipose tissue increases, some growth of ducts and alveoli, and the breast enlarges and becomes more nodular.

■ **Pregnancy**

Intense growth and development of alveoli caused by presence of **estrogen, progesterone, prolactin,** and **human placental lactogen**

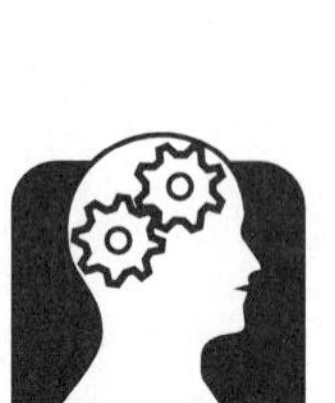

- Glandular epithelial cells

  - Cytoplasmic fat droplets
  - Secretory vacuoles containing **milk proteins**
  - Both greatly increased during **lactation**
  - Secretion of **apocrine** type (apex of cell included in secretory product)
  - Milk proteins and lipids exocytosed into lumen of alveolus with **lactose, lactalbumin,** and **immunoglobulins (passive immunity** for suckling infant); first secretion after birth is **colostrum,** which has less fat and more protein than later milk.

- Stellate **myoepithelial** cells encompass each alveolus between alveolar epithelium and its basal lamina; will contract in response to **oxytocin** release from **pars nervosa** in response to newborn suckling at nipple (mother "lets down").

  - Breast feeding keeps prolactin levels high.
  - Weaning leads to a loss of **prolactin** and involution

    - Alveoli degenerate; entire cells slough, removed by connective tissue macrophages.
    - Size of breast decreases.
    - Myoepithelial cells do not degenerate.

■ **Postmenopausal**

- Parenchyma and stroma decrease.

■ **Breast Cancer**

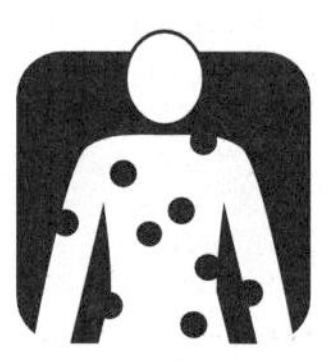

- 90% arise in ductal, not glandular, epithelium.
- **Noninfiltrating intraductal carcinoma**

Confined within basement membrane; begins as atypical proliferation of ductal epithelium, which eventually fills lumen of duct.

- **Infiltrating ductal carcinoma**

Malignant ductal epithelial cells locally invade through basement membrane; usually accompanied by reactive fibrosis, even some calcification; malignant cells can break into area lymph vessels (lymphatic spread), venules (hematogenous spread).

PLACENTA (FIG. 18.3)

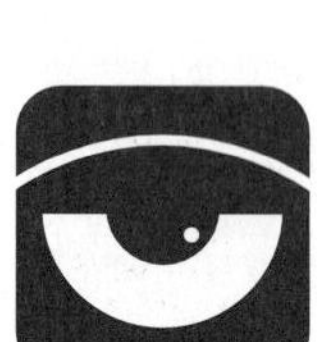

■ **General**

- Metabolic exchange between mother and fetus

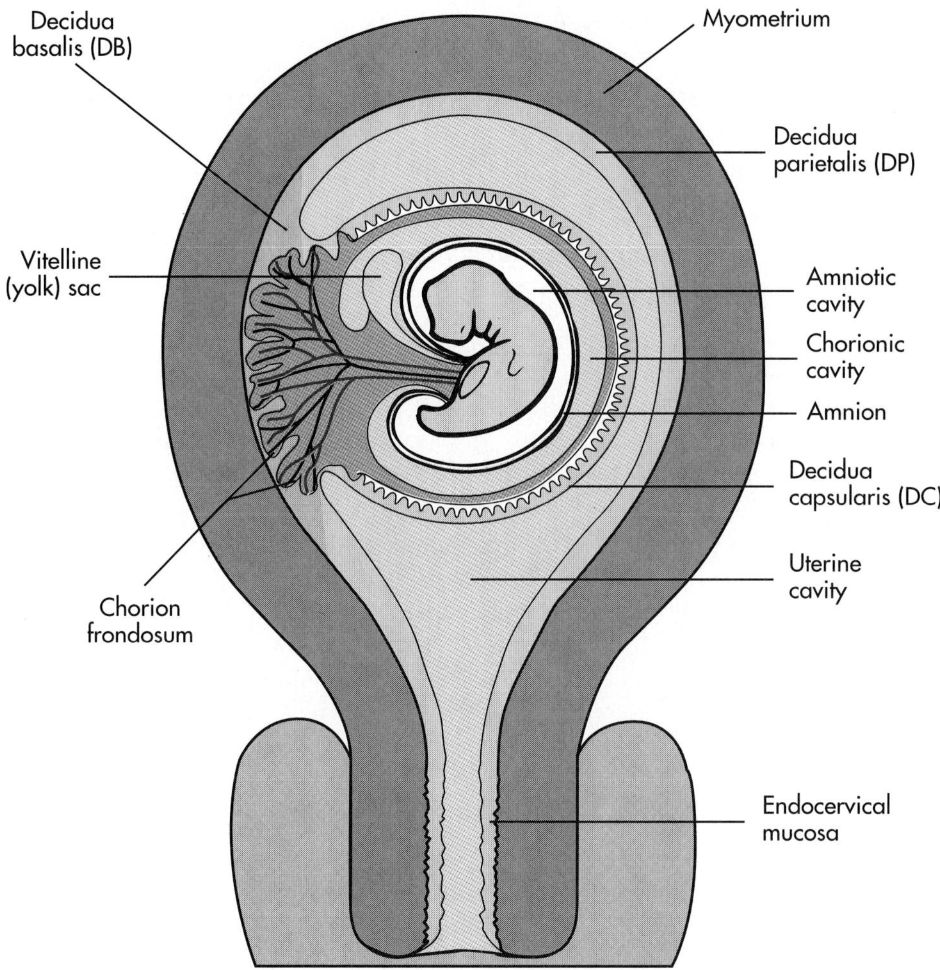

Fig. 18.3 Overview of the pregnant uterus and the membranes and cavities associated with pregnancy.

- More of a **sieve** than a barrier
- Endocrine organ
- **Estrogen, progesterone, human chorionic gonadotropin, human placental lactogen,** and others
  - Fetal component: **chorion frondosum** (bearing villi)

    - **Syncytiotrophoblast:** outer syncytial layer
    - **Cytotrophoblast:** inner cellular layer
    - Basement membrane
    - Fetal connective tissue, blood vessels

  - Maternal component: **decidua basalis** of endometrium subjacent to chorion frondosum

Other decidua

- **Decidua capsularis:** overlies conceptus
- **Decidua parietalis:** remainder of decidualized endometrium not found in decidua basalis or decidua capsularis. DP + DC fuse at midpregnancy, obliterating the uterine cavity.

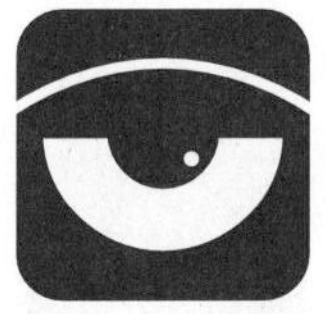
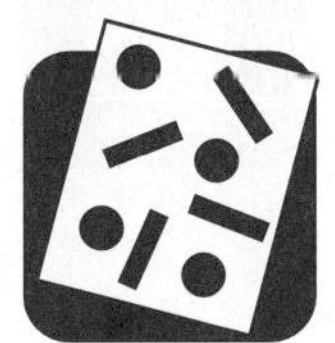
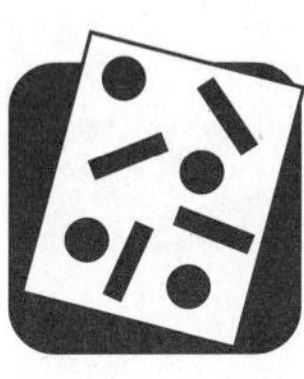

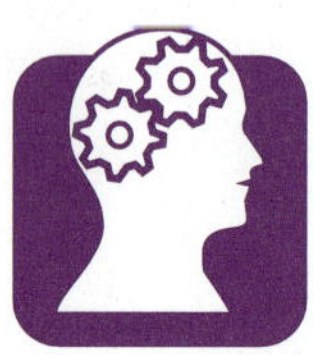

- **Decidual reaction**
  - Stromal response of endometrium to implantation
  - Stromal cells increase in size, become polyhedral, fill up with glycogen and lipid—**decidual cells**
  - Prevents excessive invasion of trophoblast

■ **Villi**

- **Fingerlike projections of fetal component**
- **Developmental stages**

  - **Previllous stage:** outer syncytiotrophoblast with **lacunae** containing **maternal blood** and secretions from endometrial glands; inner layer of cytotrophoblast

  - **Primary villus:** projections with solid core of cytotrophoblast surfaced by syncytiotrophoblast; no mesodermal core; stick into lakes of maternal blood in lacunae of syncytiotrophoblast

  - **Secondary villus:** core of fetal mesoderm, but no blood vessels have differentiated from this yet; covered by layer of cytotrophoblast, which in turn is surfaced by syncytiotrophoblast.

  - **Tertiary villus:** same as secondary, but vessels present in mesodermal core; as they age syncytiotrophoblast thins in some regions, forms knots in others; cytotrophoblast layer becomes intermittent; branches of umbilical arteries in villi carry deoxygenated fetal blood, branches of umbilical vein carry oxygenated (80% oxygen saturation) fetal blood.

- **Types and distribution of villi (Fig. 18.4)**

  - **Anchoring** or **stem:** large, extend from chorionic plate and attach to decidua basalis, forming outer cytotrophoblastic shell, which interfaces with maternal decidua basalis; **fibrinoid** deposits separate fetal zone from maternal zone (Nitabuch's **membrane**).

  - **Floating** or **free:** smaller divisions or branches off stem; float in intervillous space (previously lacunae of syncytiotrophoblast) filled with maternal blood. Early, villi found in entire chorionic vesicle; remain and develop at embryonic pole forming chorion frondosum; decrease and disappear at abembryonic pole forming chorion laeve.

■ **Cotyledons**

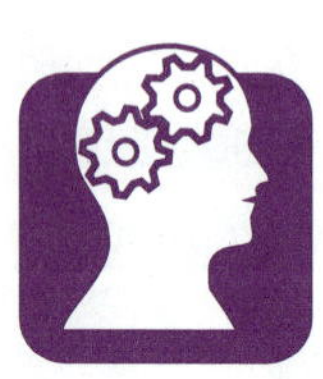

- During fourth and fifth months septa from **decidua basalis** grow toward but never reach chorionic plate.
- Decidual septa divide placenta into 10 to 35 chambers (cotyledons).
- Maternal arteries and veins open into **intervillous space** within each cotyledon; arterial blood under high hydrostatic pressure spurts toward chorionic plate, loses pressure, falls over villi, showering fetal villi with highly oxygenated blood and returning deoxygenated blood to maternal lungs.

■ **Placental Membrane (Sieve): Structure**
Maternal blood in intervillous space of cotyledon

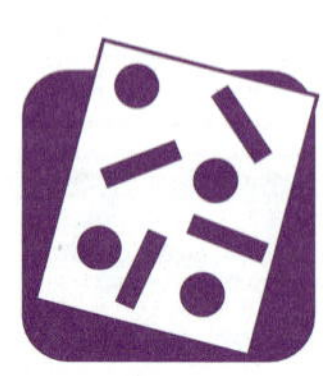

- Syncytiotrophoblast
  - **True syncytium**—multinucleated mass of cytoplasm
  - Arises from daughter cells produced by cytotrophoblast
  - **Microvilli** on **surface bathed in maternal blood**
  - **Pinocytotic vesicles:** tremendous transport activity—absorptive zone

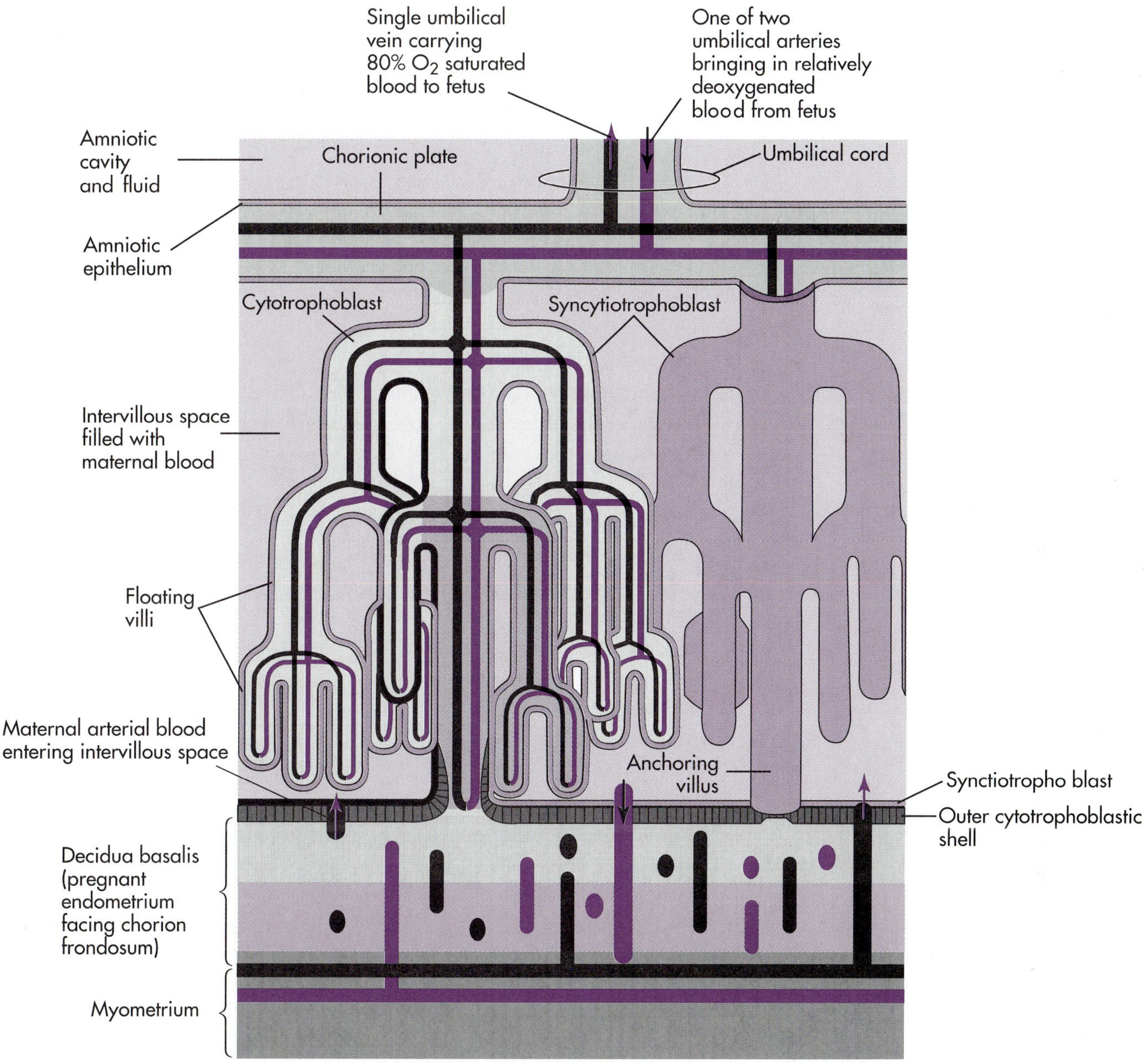

Fig. 18.4 Detailed look at the vascular tree of fetal blood vessels within free or anchored villi and their relationships to maternal blood in the intervillous space and the decidua basalis of the endometrium.

- **SER, RER, Golgi bodies, mitochondria**—secretory zone **HCG, HPL, estrogen, progesterone**
- Thins in late pregnancy

● **Cytotrophoblast**

- **Individual cells,** held together by desmosomes
- No ultrastructural indication of synthetic activity
- **Mitotically active**—some daughter cells added to syncytiotrophoblast
- Discontinuous as pregnancy proceeds, allowing syncytiotrophoblast to sit on basement membrane

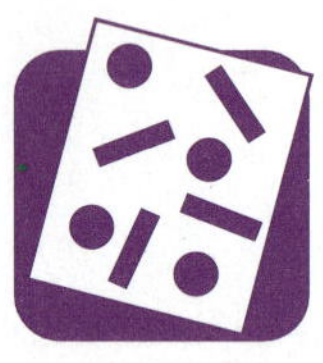

- Basement membrane of cytotrophoblast
- Perhaps fetal stromal cells (connective tissue core of villus)
  - Fibroblasts and connective tissue fibers
  - **Hofbauer** cells: fetal macrophages or histiocytes
- Basement membrane of fetal capillary
- Fetal endothelium
- Fetal blood

■ Placental Membrane: Transport

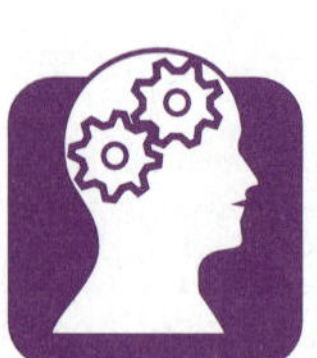

- Simple diffusion, facilitated diffusion, active transport, pinocytosis
- Substances transferred
  - **Gases:** oxygen, carbon dioxide
  - **Nutrients:** water, free fatty acids, amino acids, vitamins, glucose
  - **Waste products:** urea, uric acid, bilirubin, etc.
  - **Hormones**
  - **Electrolytes**
  - **Antibodies**
    - **Passive immunization** of fetus by means of maternal antibody
    - (IgG) against diphtheria, smallpox, measles but not whooping cough or chickenpox
  - **Drugs**
    Thalidomide, nicotine, sedatives, analgesics, cocaine, and heroin (fetal drug addiction)
  - **Infectious agents**
    Rubella, measles, encephalitis, poliomyelitis, syphilis, etc.
  - **Blood**
    - Some small amount of exchange between fetus and mother
    - Rh factor and **erythroblastosis fetalis**

■ Abnormalities

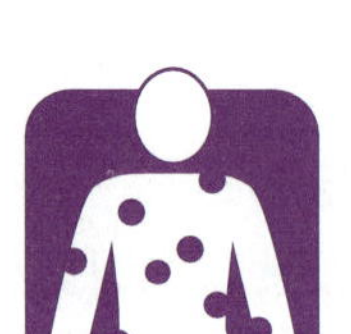

- Placenta succenturiata: accessory lobule of placenta connected by vessels to main placenta
- Battledore placenta: marginal attachment of cord
- Velamentous insertion of cord: umbilical cord inserts beyond placental margin
- Placenta accreta: trophoblastic invasion beyond normal depths
- Choriocarcinoma: malignancy of trophoblast
- Placenta previa: implantation in lower segment of uterus
  - Lateral PP: no obstruction of internal cervical os
  - Marginal PP: partial obstruction of os
  - Central PP: complete covering of os

■ Placenta and Fetal Membranes in Twins

- Fraternal, or dizygotic
  - Two amnions
  - Two chorions

- • Two placentas
- • But could be fused
- **Identical, or monozygotic**
  - — *96%—division of embryonic disk or inner cell mass*
    - • Two amnions
    - • One chorion
    - • One placenta
  - — *4%—earlier division of embryo at 2-cell stage up to morula*
    - • Two amnions
    - • Two chorions
    - • Two placentas
    - • (Same as for fraternal twins)
  - — *Rare (0.2%)—late but incomplete division of embryo*
    - • Conjoined twins
      - • One amnion, one chorion, one placenta

Fetal Cells in Maternal Blood

• Some trophoblast cells break free during invasive implantation, gain access to maternal bloodstream, can lodge in lung, disappear after birth (allograft rejection).

• Other fetal cells in maternal blood—lymphocytes and nucleated RBCs

• If harvestable, as by flow cytometry after being marked with fluorescent tags against fetal antigens, grow in vitro and **karyotype** fetus

MULTIPLE CHOICE REVIEW QUESTIONS

1. All the following describe the ovarian cycle *except*

    a. changes in shape and number of follicular cells.
    b. production of more oocytes.
    c. antrum formation within region of follicular cells.
    d. increase in diameter of oocyte nucleus.
    e. formation of zona pellucida.

2. All the following are events in female reproductive cycles *except*

    a. increased muscular activity of uterine tube in estrogenic phase.
    b. thinning of vaginal epithelium in menses.
    c. LH affects estrogen and progesterone levels, whereas FSH affects only estrogen level.
    d. atresia in ovary with corpus luteum.
    e. decreasing estrogen level just before ovulation increases FSH-RF release.

3. The large cell resulting from the division event occurring immediately after fertilization contains (do not include the sperm in your calculation):

    a. 4C DNA, 46 chromosomes, 92 chromatids.
    b. 2C DNA, 46 chromosomes, 46 chromatids.
    c. 2C DNA, 23 chromosomes, 46 chromatids.
    d. 2C DNA, 23 chromosomes, 23 chromatids.
    e. 1C DNA, 23 chromosomes, 23 chromatids.

4. As you study a Pap smear, you observe the presence of many cells with pyknotic nuclei and keratin in the cytoplasm. From which phase of the menstrual cycle did this smear come?

    a. Menses
    b. Proliferative
    c. Secretory
    d. Premenstrual

5. Which of the following structures produces HCG?

    a. Hofbauer cell
    b. Outer cytotrophoblastic shell
    c. Nitabuch's membrane
    d. Syncytiotrophoblast
    e. Cytotrophoblast

Chapter 19

Endocrine System

GENERAL

Cells need to communicate with each other and even themselves. Cells communicate directly with each other through gap junctions and cell surface molecules. Neurons communicate by direct structural pointing or targeting of a messenger to the target cell. Cells can communicate with each other over short or long distances by means of **chemical messengers,** which have specific receptors on the target cell.

- **Autocrine:** from self to self

- **Paracrine:** chemical messenger moves through tissue fluid or over a surface. **Epidermal growth factor (EGF)** uses the paracrine mode because EGF is a component of saliva. As saliva coats epithelial surfaces in the GI tract the EGF is delivered to its target, the surface epithelium. Licking applies EGF directly to a wound on the skin (e.g., dogs and cats licking surface wounds on themselves or others).

- **Endocrine:** chemical messenger carried in blood to target; messenger: a hormone. Hormones can have a general target (e.g., **insulin**) or a specific target, e.g., **TSH (thyroid-stimulating hormone).**

- **Control of Endocrine Function**

- **Nervous**

    - Oxytocin release in response to infant suckling at nipple

- **Nonneural**

    - Direct

        - Hormone level regulated by product of action of the hormone

            - Blood level of **parathyroid hormone (PTH)** determined by blood level of calcium; low calcium directly stimulates PTH release → osteoclasts liberate stored calcium → blood level of calcium increases.

            - Blood level of glucose increasing; **insulin** production increases → more glucose enters cell, lowering blood level of glucose.

    - Indirect

        Third party involved and interposed between hormone and its action on its target and the feedback of that effect on hormone production; third party: **releasing hormones** of hypothalamus, e.g.:

        — *Hypothalamohypophyseothyroid axis* Starting point: decrease in blood level of thyroid hormone; detected by neurons in hypothalamus to trigger release of **TRH (thyroid–releasing hormone),** i.e., the "third party"; TRH is transported over a short axon system to be released in capillaries, which form one part of a **portal system;** TRH in capillary blood is collected into a portal vein, which then branches

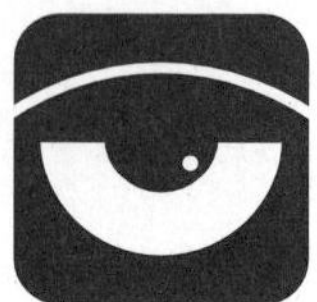

into a second capillary network in the **pars distalis,** where the TRH leaves the blood and finds its target cell, a type of **basophil,** which releases **TSH; TSH**'s target is the follicular epithelium in the thyroid gland; under TSH "bombardment" this epithelium releases T_3 and T_4; blood level of thyroid hormone increases; this **negatively feeds back** on the TRH neurons, lowering the production of TRH.

■ Ductless System

- Exocrine: uses an epithelial duct system to transport secretory product.
- **Endocrine:** does not use a duct system—ductless, but uses capillaries and other blood vessels as functional ducts, i.e., secretion directly into the bloodstream.

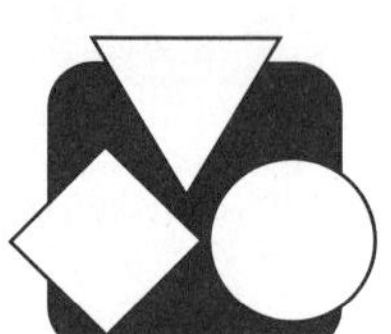

ENDOCRINE ORGANS AND TISSUES

- **Pituitary** or **hypophysis, thyroid, parathyroid, adrenal, islets of Langerhans, testis, ovary, placenta,** and **pineal gland**
- If the hormone produced is a **steroid,** the cell makes it on **SER.**
- If the hormone is a **peptide** or **polypeptide,** the cell makes it on **RER.**
- If the hormone is a **glycoprotein** both SER and RER are used.
- Some hormones are synthesized and released immediately—no storage phase.
- Other hormones are synthesized and stored before release:
  - **Intracellularly** as secretory granules before release
  - **Extracellularly** in follicles
    - Thyroid
    - Pars intermedia

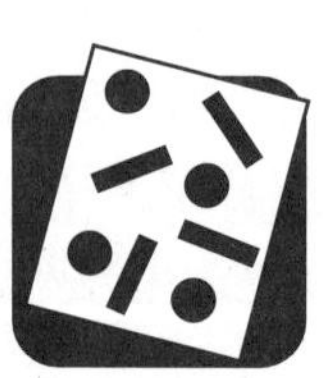

PITUITARY GLAND, OR HYPOPHYSIS (FIG. 19.1)

- Attached to base of brain (**hypothalamus**) by a stalk, the **infundibulum**
- Develops from two different sources
  - **Oral ectoderm** (Rathke's pouch), roof of oral cavity
  - **Neural ectoderm** from the floor of the developing brain
- Two major regions
  - **Adenohypophysis** is derived from oral ectoderm; divided into 3 regions—**pars distalis, pars tuberalis,** and **pars intermedia.**
  - **Neurohypophysis** is derived from neural ectoderm; two regions—**pars nervosa** and **infundibulum.**
- Blood supply to and from the hypothalamus and hypophysis is unique and plays an important role in histophysiologic characteristics of the gland.
  - Superior hypophyseal arteries arise from circle of Willis.
  - Inferior hypophyseal arteries arise from internal carotid arteries.
  - These vessels form 2 capillary beds that are connected to each other by one or more portal veins, i.e., the **hypothalamo-hypophyseal portal system.**
- Hormones produced by the adenohypophysis and the neurohypophysis are

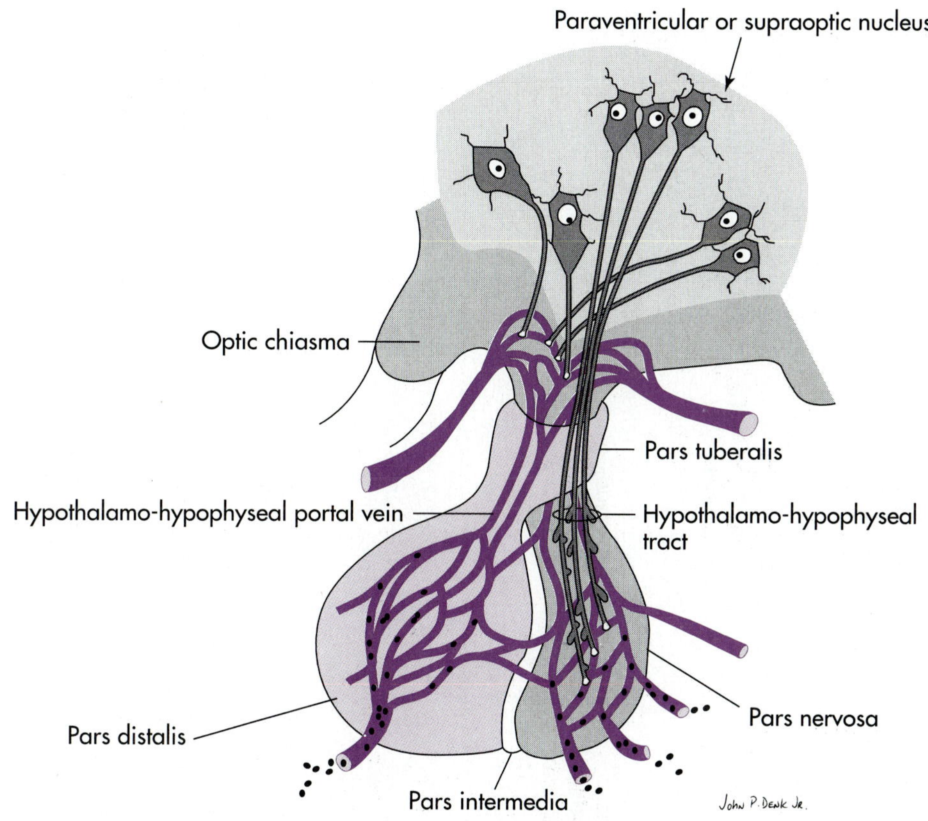

Fig. 19.1 Structure-function relationships between the hypothalamus and the hypophysis for both vascular and neural routes of intercellular communication.

known by their acronyms (see Table 19.1 for the functional importance of each of these hormones):

- **TSH** : Thyroid-stimulating hormone
- **FSH** : Follicle-stimulating hormone
- **ACTH** : Adrenocorticotropic hormone, or corticotropin
- **LH**   : Luteinizing hormone
- **STH** : Somatotropic hormone
- **ICSH** : Interstitial cell–stimulating hormone
- **LTH** : Lactogenic hormone, or prolactin
- **MSH** : Melanocyte-stimulating hormone
- **ADH** : Antidiuretic hormone

PARS DISTALIS AND PARS TUBERALIS

Two major types of cells situated in cords or clumps adjacent to capillaries or sinusoids:

- ■ **Chromophobes (Hate Color):** probably exhausted chromophils
- ■ **Chromophils (Love Color)**
  - ● Acidophils
    - • **Somatotrophs:** 350 to 400 nm granules; growth hormone, or **somatotrophin (STH)**

202

Table 19.1 *Effects of Endocrine Hormones*

Hormone	Type of Hormone	Produced By	Target Organ	Major Effect	Endocrine Disorders— Hyper- (+) or Hypofunction (−)
Anterior Pituitary—Pars Distalis					
TSH	Glycoprotein	Basophil	Thyroid	Synthesis and release of thyroid hormone	(+) = Hyperthyroidism (−) = Hypothyroidism
FSH	Glycoprotein	Basophil	Ovarian follicle	Growth of ovarian follicle	
LH (ICSH)	Glycoprotein	Basophil	Testis Ovarian follicle	Spermatogenesis Growth of follicle, corpora lutea formation	
			Interstitial cells of testis	Stimulate testosterone secretion	
ACTH	Polypeptide	Basophil	Adrenal cortex	Secretion of corticosteroid hormones	(−) Hypoadrenalism (Addison's Disease) (+) Hyperadrenalism (Cushing's Syndrome)
LTH (lactogenic) Prolactin	Protein	Acidophil	C. lutea Mammary gland	Progesterone secretion Milk secretion	
Growth hormone or somatotrophic hormone	Protein	Acidophil	Liver to cause release of IGF-1 (insulin-like growth factor-1, formerly known as somatomedin), which stimulates growth in epiphyseal plates	Growth	(+) Gigantism, acromegaly (−) Dwarfism
Anterior Pituitary—Pars Intermedia					
MSH (in lower animals)	Polypeptide	Basophilic cells	Skin	Dispersion and synthesis of melanin	
Posterior Pituitary—Pars Nervosa					
ADH	Peptide	Cells in SO and PV nuclei of hypothalamus	Smooth muscle of blood vessels	Increase hypertension (pressor effect)	
			Collecting ducts of kidney	Increase water resorption (antidiuretic effect)	(−) Diabetes insipidis (no water conservation from urine) unconcentrated urine, thirsty
Oxytocin	Peptide	Same	Smooth muscle of uterus Smooth muscle of mammary gland	Contraction Expel milk (suckling puppies, mother "lets down")	

Hypothalamus Releasing factors	Peptides	Neurosecretory cells	Anterior pituitary	Release tropic hormones	
Thyroid Gland T$_3$, T$_4$	Modified amino acid	Epithelial cells	Most cells	Increase basal metabolic rate	(+) Increase BMR, weight loss, exophthalmos, leads to parenchymous goiter (−) Myxdema, cretinism, colloid goiter
Thyrocalcitonin	Peptide	C cells	Bone	Decreased bone resorption, decrease blood Ca^{++}	
Parathyroid Gland PTH	Polypeptide	Chief cells	Bone and others	Increase bone resorption, increase blood Ca^{++}	(+) Osteitis fibrosa (−) Hypocalcemia, muscle tetany
Adrenal Cortex Mineralocorticoids (aldosterone)	Steroid	Zonula glomerulosa	Kidney	Control Na$^+$ and K$^+$ balance	(−) Addison's disease (loss of Na$^+$) Cushing's syndrome
Glucocorticoids	Steroid	Zonula fasciculata	Liver	Convert protein to glycogen	(−) Addison's disease (low blood glucose)
Gonadocorticoids	Steroid	Zonula reticularis	Male accessory sex glands and ducts	Development of secondary sex characteristics	(+) In female, pseudohermaphroditism
Adrenal Medulla Epinephrine and norepinephrine	Aliphatic amine	Chromaffin cells	Nerve endings and other tissues	Fight or flight	(+) Pheochromocytoma; histologically benign but clinically malignant, inappropriate release of catecholamines

ACTH, Adrenocorticotropic hormone; *ADH,* antidiuretic hormone; *FSH,* follicle-stimulating hormone; *ICSH,* interstitial cell–stimulating hormone; *LH,* luteinizing hormone; *LTH,* lactogenic hormone; *MSH,* melanocyte-stimulating hormone; *PTH,* parathyroid hormone; *PV,* paraventricular nucleus; *SO,* supraoptic nucleus; *STH,* somatotropic hormone; *T$_3$,* triiodothyronine; *T$_4$,* thyroxine; *TSH,* thyroid-stimulating hormone.

Continued.

Table 19.1 *Effects of Endocrine Hormones—cont'd.*

Hormone	Type of Hormone	Produced By	Target Organ	Major Effect	Endocrine Disorders— Hyper-(+) or Hypofunction (−)
Pancreatic Islets of Langerhans					
Insulin	Polypeptide	B cell	Most cells	Permeability to glucose	(−) Diabetes mellitus (+) Insulin shock
Glucagon	Polypeptide	A cells	Liver	Breakdown glycogen to glucose; hyperglycemic effect	
Somatostatin	Polypeptide	D cells	Islet A and B cells: STH acidophils of pars distalis	Suppress insulin/glucagon and growth hormone release	
Pineal Body					
Melatonin	Modified amino acid	Chief cells	Gonads	Inhibits development of gonads	(−) Precocious sexual development (+) Delayed sexual development Gonads

- **Mammotrophs:** 200 nm granules in nonlactating condition; 600 nm granules during lactation **prolactin, or lactogenic hormone (LTH)**
- Basophils
  - **Thyrotrophs:** 110 to 160 nm granules (**TSH**)
  - **Gonadotrophs:** 150 to 250 nm granules (**FSH** and **LH**, same cell can do both)
  - **Corticotrophs:** 250 to 350 nm granules (**ACTH**)

Pars Intermedia

Small zone of tissue with follicles that contain a pale staining colloid; no known function in the human. This is not true for lower animals, in whom this region produces melanocyte-stimulating hormone (MSH).

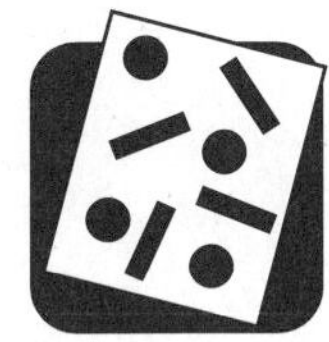

Pars Nervosa

- Composed of **pituicytes,** which are similar to the glial cells of the CNS, i.e., stromal elements
- Parenchymal cells are neurons with cell bodies in the **paraventricular** and **supraoptic** nuclei of the hypothalamus.
- Axons of these neurons form the **hypothalamo-hypophyseal tract.**

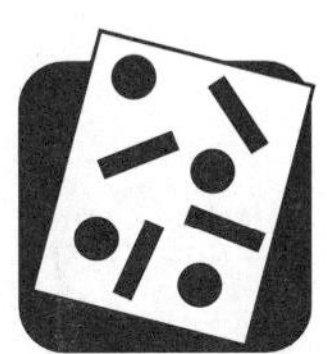

Two hormones are synthesized by different neurons in both of these nuclei: **oxytocin** and **ADH.**

- Transported down this long axon system to terminals near capillaries in the pars nervosa
- Transported with the help of carrier proteins called **neurophysins**
- Hormones accumulate; stored in axon terminals; swollen axon terminals: **Herring** bodies

Hypothalamus receives input from the peripheral nervous system (PNS), e.g., infant suckling at the nipple. At first no milk to swallow, infant aggressively sucks, nervous stimulation of the nipple affects PNS → CNS → supraoptic and paraventricular nuclei of hypothalamus → oxytocin synthesis and release → bloodstream → myoepithelial cells of breast → contract → squeeze milk from alveoli → duct system → removed by negative pressure → infant quiets down (mother has "let down").

Pituitary gland is "**master gland**"; i.e., it controls many other endocrine organs by secretion of stimulating hormones such as TSH, FSH, and ACTH. Master itself, however, is under control of the hypothalamus, which receives neural input from other regions of the nervous system.

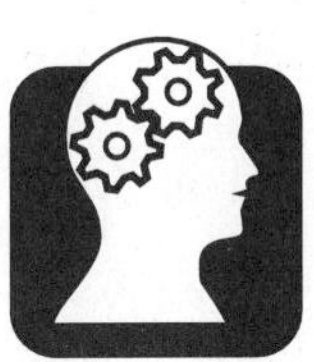

■ **Hypothalamo-hypophyseal Tract**
  - A **long axon** system transporting oxytocin and ADH from site of synthesis to site of release

■ **Hypothalamo-hypophyseal Portal System** A **short axon** system transporting **releasing hormones** (TRH, FSH-RH, etc.) from hypothalamic neuron cell bodies → short axons → capillaries → portal vein → second capillary bed in pars distalis → exit to target acidophil or basophil. In this way the hypothalamus controls the pars distalis and pars tuberalis. Most of the hormones traveling from the hypothalamus to the pars distalis and pars tuberalis are releasing hormones, but one of these hypothalamic hormones is inhibitory for the release

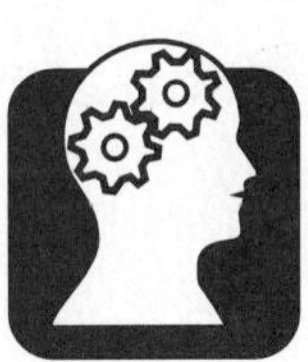

of prolactin and is called **prolactin-inhibiting hormone (PIH).** For release of prolactin, PIH must be inhibited (inhibition of an inhibitor is release).

THYROID GLAND

- Composed of follicles lined by **follicular epithelial cells.** Each follicle contains a pinkish **colloid** material that is the extracellular storage site for thyroid horomone, i.e., **thyroglobulin.**

- Interposed between follicular cells are **C cells,** or **parafollicular** cells, which make **calcitonin.**

- **Tetraiodothyronine (T_4)** and **triiodothyronine (T_3)**

- Blood **iodide** is taken up by follicular epithelial cells, oxidized to **iodine,** transported to colloid at cell surface where **tyrosine** residues are **iodinated extracellularly** forming first mono-, then di-, tri- and tetra-iodothronines. Glycoprotein moiety manufactured in follicular epithelial cells, secreted into follicle lumen where it complexes with iodinated thyronines to form **thyroglobulin.**

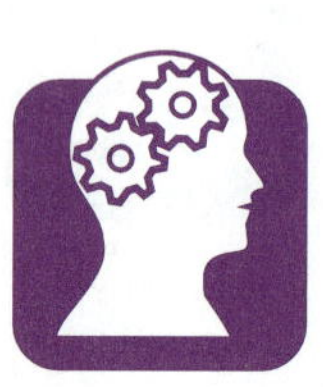

- When more T_3 and T_4 are needed, thyroglobulin is taken up into vesicles by the follicular cells; lysosomal proteolytic enzymes break it down into T_4, T_3, T_2, and T_1, with T_4 and T_3 being the functional thyroid hormones.
- The follicular epithelium is stimulated to perform these functions (synthesis + storage + release) by **TSH.**
- Tall columnar follicular epithelium indicates cells actively breaking down thyroglobulin and releasing thyroid hormone. Presence of squamous-appearing follicular cells indicates the opposite state of activity, i.e., a storage state or production of thyroglobulin instead of its breakdown. TSH acts on the thyroid to increase

  - iodine uptake
  - rate of synthesis of thyroglobulin
  - rate of iodination
  - secretion of T_4 and T_3
  - height of the follicular epithelium

Calcitonin is synthesized by the C cells in response to a decrease in the blood level of calcium and therefore is antagonistic to parathyroid hormone and suppresses bone resorption.

PARATHYROID GLAND

- The parathyroid gland has a characteristic fibrofatty stroma and two versions of its parenchymal cells, the **chief,** or **principal,** cells:

  - Dark cytoplasm is full of granules
  - Light cytoplasm has few granules, hormone was released
  - Normal ratio of L:D is 3:1

- Principal cells release parathyroid hormone (parathormone, PTH) in direct response to a decreasing blood calcium level. PTH acts to raise blood level of calcium by increasing the activity of osteoclasts and increasing the intestinal absorption of calcium. Vitamin D is required for proper intestinal absorption of calcium.

- **Oxyphil** cells occur singly or in clusters and have very acidophilic cytoplasm containing numerous mitochondria. The number of oxyphils increases with age. The function of oxyphils is not fully understood.

Adrenal Gland

• Develops from a dual origin, reflected in the histophysiologic features of its two major regions, the **cortex** and the **medulla.**

   • Cortex develops from mesoderm near the root of the dorsal mesentery.

   • Medulla develops from **neural crest** cells, parenchyma of medulla equivalent to **postganglionic neurons** of the **sympathetic** division of the autonomic nervous system.

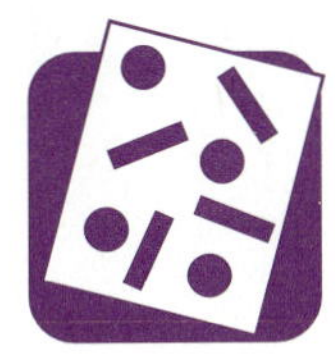

■ **Cortex (3 Distinct Regions from Capsule Toward Medulla)**

   ● **Zona glomerulosa,** or a zone of parenchyma arranged in clumps or like glomerular masses

   ● **Zona fasciculata** in which cords of cells run radially inward from the zona glomerulosa

   ● **Zona reticularis** is a region of anastomosing cords between the zona fasciculata and the medulla.

      • All these regions have abundant sinusoids, which serve as the functional ducts for the parenchymal cells.

      • Over 40 steroid compounds can be isolated from the adrenal cortex.

      • Zona glomerulosa produces **mineralocorticoids.**

      • Zona fasciculata produces **glucocorticoids.**

      • Zona reticularis produces **androgens** and **estrogens.**

      • **Zona glomerulosa: aldosterone** (a mineralocorticoid)

         • Target is the renal tubule.

         • Decreases the reabsorption of potassium

         • Increases the reabsorption of sodium. If sodium is being reabsorbed into the bloodstream, chloride will eventually follow it, and this process will increase the sodium chloride concentration in the blood. Water will be drawn to this to dilute it to normal tonicity. If water is added to blood the blood volume will increase. The enlarged blood volume will increase blood pressure.

   Atrial natriuretic peptide (ANP), or **atriopeptin,** is antagonistic to aldosterone. ANP is synthesized and released by atrial cardiomyocytes in response to their degree of stretching, which is reflective of the volume of blood in the atrial chambers. ANP promotes **natriuresis,** or the loss of sodium into the urine, which water will follow (duiresis).

      • **Zona fasciculata: hydrocortisone** (a glucocorticoid)

         • Increases the level of amino acids in blood and tissue fluid

         • Increases glycogen synthesis in the liver

         • Mobilizes fat depots

         • Suppresses growth

         • Causes a reduction in lymphatic tissue and antibody production

         • Stabilizes cell membranes I

         • Is a steroid hormone, and so the cells of the zona fasciculata have well-developed SER, intracellular fat stores

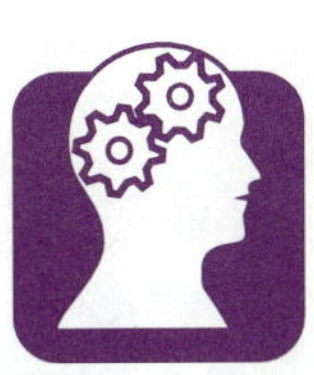

      • **Zona reticularis: androgens** and **estrogens** (there is a little bit of male in every female and a little bit of female in every male). In the male alcoholic with severe cirrhosis, hepatocytes have decreased in number. One

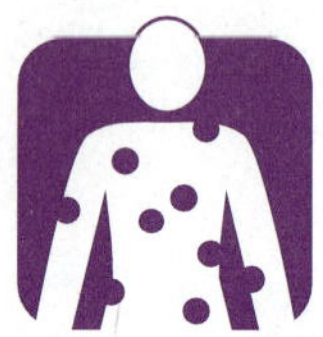

function of the hepatocyte is to "detoxify" certain natural compounds such as estrogen. If the function of the liver is compromised because of the loss of hepatocytes from alcoholic poisoning and replacement of that lost tissue with scar tissue (**cirrhosis**), then abnormal amounts of estrogen will be allowed to circulate. The male breast can respond to this elevated level of estrogen with development and enlargement, i.e., **gynecomastia.**

■ Medulla

- Parenchymal cells of the medulla stain brown when potassium dichromate is used—**chromaffin** cells.
- Synthesize and release the **catecholamines epinephrine** and **norepinephrine.**
- Equivalent to **postganglionic** cells of the **sympathetic** nervous system the hormones released—**sympatheticomimetic**
  - 75% of the catecholamines released after stimulation of the adrenal medulla is epinephrine.
  - 25% is norepinephrine.

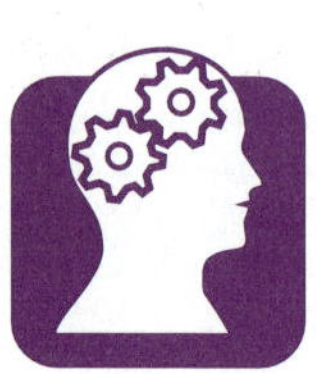

- Together epinephrine and norepinephrine cause
  - Increased heart rate
  - Increased blood pressure
  - Conversion of liver glycogen to glucose

PANCREATIC ISLETS OF LANGERHANS

- Small islands of endocrine tissue in the exocrine pancreas
- Three types of cells

  1. **Alpha cells** contain water-soluble granules of **glucagon.** Glucagon causes the breakdown of glycogen to glucose in the liver and therefore is a **hyperglycemic** factor antagonistic to insulin, which is a **hypoglycemic** factor.
  2. **Beta cells** produce alcohol-soluble granules of **proinsulin. Insulin** acts on the cell membrane of most cells moving glucose from blood into cells. A deficiency in insulin results in the disease **diabetes mellitus,** or **type I diabetes.** It may be an autoimmune disease in which the defense system destroys islet tissue.
  3. **Delta cells** produce **somatostatin.**
     - Suppresses the release of insulin and glucagon by a paracrine mode
     - Suppresses the release of growth hormone from the pars distalis by an endocrine mode

PINEAL BODY, OR EPIPHYSIS CEREBRI

- Develops as an outgrowth of the third ventricle of the brain
- Parenchymal cells called **pinealocytes,** or **chief cells**
- Interstitial cells equivalent to glial cells
- Mixed in with these two cell types are many nerve fibers originating from areas of the CNS and also postganglionic sympathetic nerve fibers

Produces **melatonin** from **serotonin**

- Melatonin has an **antigonadotropic** effect; destruction of the pineal body in a child (as by a neoplasm) can result in precocious sexual development. Administration of melatonin delays the onset of puberty and gonadal development.

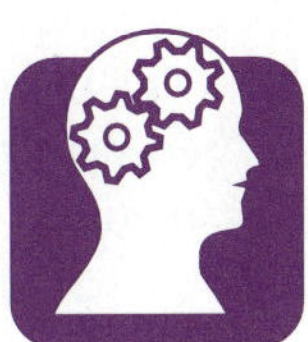

- Light-dark cycle and melatonin

  - Rats raised in continuous darkness (DD)—high melatonin level—no estrus cycle

  - LL (continuous light)—low level of melatonin—low antigonadotropic effect—early estrus

  - Normal circadian (LD) cycle
    Melatonin levels high during nocturnal phase; low during diurnal phase; threefold fluctuation

  - Light information from eye to pineal body
    Retina → optic nerves → median forebrain bundle → brainstem → thoracic spinal cord → intermediolateral gray → preganglionic sympathetic fibers → sympathetic chain → superior cervical ganglion → carotid arterial plenus → cerebral vessels → pineal gland

- **Corpora arenacea** (brain sand, sand bodies) has distinguishing characteristic

  - Increase with age
  - Useful internal landmark for neuroradiologists

Multiple Choice Review Questions

1. The principal stimulus for the secretion of epinephrine and norepinephrine from the adrenal medulla is derived from
   a. ACTH.
   b. corticotropin-releasing factor.
   c. sympathetic preganglionic nerves.
   d. aldosterone.
   e. hypo-osmolarity of the blood.

2. One constant feature of all endocrine glands is
   a. their great vascularity.
   b. the ability to regenerate their specialized cells.
   c. their dependence on the hypothalamus and pituitary for stimulation.
   d. the storage of large amounts of their respective hormones.
   e. their dependence on the autonomic nervous system to control their secretion.

3. Match the cell type with its hormone:
   a. Hypophyseal acidophil
   b. Hypophyseal basophil
   c. Hypophyseal chromophobe
   d. Hypothalamic neuron
   e. None of the above
   _____ TSH
   _____ TSH-RG
   _____ ACTH
   _____ Somatotrophin
   _____ FSH
   _____ Glucagon

Chapter 20

Sense Organs

EYE

■ **General** With respect to the eye, "inner" refers to or toward the centermost part of the eye, and "outer" refers to points away from the centermost point. From inside to outside the eye has three major layers or tunics (Fig. 20.1):

● **Photosensitive retina**

- **Receptors** (the **rods** and **cones**) and other neurons that are transmitters of visual information through the optic nerve to the brain

Optic nerve leaves eye at optic papilla or disk.

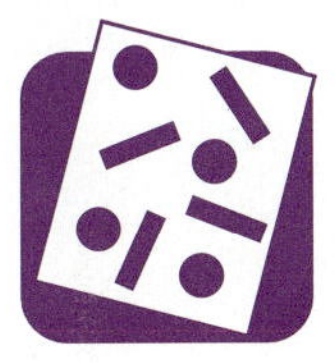

- No receptors here; this is the blind spot.
- Nonphotosensitive parts of the retina are found on the ciliary body and on the iris.

The transition region between the photosensitive retina, composed of 10 different layers of cells and their connections, and the nonphotosensitive retina form the **ora serrata.**

● **Vascular middle coat, the uvea, which has three subdivisions**

- **Choroid:** highly vascular (nutrition to outer half of retina)
- **Ciliary body** (special part of uvea peripheral to lens): ciliary processes project toward lens.
- **Iris** (special part of uvea anterior to lens)
  - Opening in center is **pupil**
  - **Constrictor muscle** of pupil
  - **Dilator muscle** of pupil

● **Tough, fibrous corneoscleral coat for protection and shape.** In addition to the three major layers of the eye there are some cavities or chambers.

- **Anterior chamber**
  Posterior to cornea and anterior to iris
  Contains aqueous humor

- **Posterior chamber**
  Bounded by iris, lens, and ciliary body
  Contains aqueous humor

- **Vitreal cavity**
  Posterior to lens and ciliary body, anterior to optic disk
  Contains vitreous humor

Path that light takes from the environment to the receptors in the retina (with some side trips to pick up some histophysiologic concepts that strongly influence the light path)

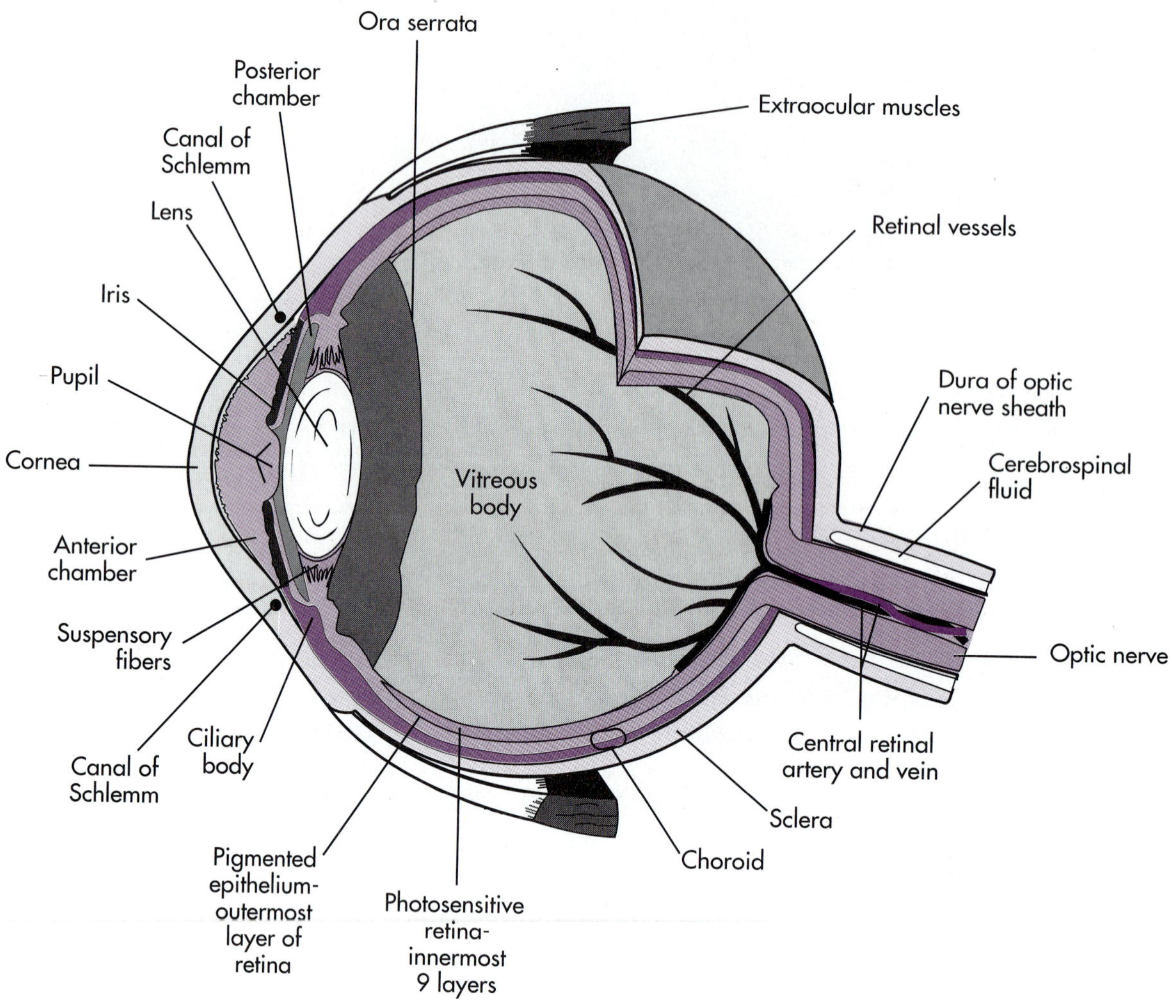

Fig. 20.1 General anatomy of the eyeball including its tunics and chambers.

- ■ **Cornea (Avascular, Nourished by Diffusion from Tears and Aqueous Humor)**
  - ● Stratified squamous wet epithelium
    - • Repairs quickly
    - • Many free nerve endings (very sensitive)
    - • Well-studied circadian rhythm in mitotic index
      - • Circadian rhythm: 1 cycle every 24 ±4 hours
      - • At peak there are 20 to 25 mitotic figures per 1000 cells
      - • At trough time there are 1 or 2 mitotic figures per 1000 cells
  - ● Basement membrane (of Bowman)
  - ● Substantia propria
    - • Thin lamellae of collagen fibers, each layer having a different direction of fibers
    - • Fibroblasts
  - ● Basement membrane (of Descemet)
    - • Endothelium

- Amazingly all 5 major layers are transparent.
- The cornea is the main site for refraction of light entering the eye.

■ Aqueous Humor in Anterior Chamber

■ Pupil of Iris

■ Aqueous Humor of Posterior Chamber

Now we will take a side trip and discuss some of the histophysiologic aspects of the iris and how the diameter of the pupil is controlled.

- Anterior surface of iris is a discontinuous layer of fibroblasts and melanocytes.
- Loose, pigmented, vascular connective tissue core
- Posterior surface covered by double layer of heavily pigmented epithelium, which some authors refer to as the iridic (variants: iridal, iridial, iridian) portion of the retina. The outermost layer of cells is the adult derivative of the outer layer of the optic cup. The innermost layer of cells is the adult derivative of the inner layer of the optic cup.

- **Sphincter of pupil** is flat ring of smooth muscle around margin of pupil. Innervated by parasympathetic postganglionic neurons from the ciliary ganglion by the short ciliary nerves. Short ciliary nerves also innervate the ciliary muscle so that it and the sphincter of the pupil work in concert; i.e., during **accommodation for near vision** there is contraction of the ciliary muscle, which releases tension on suspensory ligaments of lens (see below) and a contraction of the sphincter of the pupil, limiting the amount of light passing through the pupil. This is very similar to selecting a smaller aperture on your camera to prevent overexposure of the film.
- **Dilator of pupil** is smooth muscle radially arranged around pupil.

  - Innervated by the sympathetic division of the autonomic nervous system
  - When these sympathetic fibers fire, the dilator contracts and pulls the margins of the pupil, thereby increasing the diameter of the pupil. The eye drops that are used to dilate eyes contain epinephrine, which is a sympathicomimetic drug.

■ Lens

Biconvex, covered with a capsule

- Thick carbohydrate-rich layer on its entire outer surface
- Cuboidal epithelium on the anterior one half of the lens
- At the equator of the lens the epithelial cells are columnar and migrate into the substance of the lens becoming lens fibers (6-sided prisms), which are elongated cells that have lost their nuclei and have filled their cytoplasm with a special class of proteins called *crystallins*.

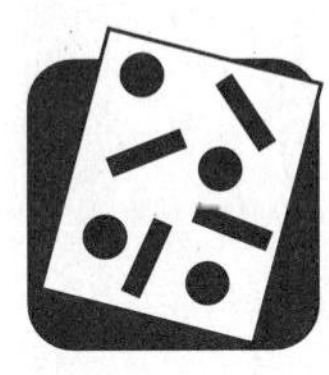

- The lens is avascular and receives its nourishment from the aqueous humor in the posterior chamber and from the vitreous body.
- The lens is responsible for taking the light initially refracted by the cornea and focusing it on a special region of the retina where the sharpest vision is perceived, i.e., the **fovea centralis.**

The natural elasticity of the lens allows it to change shape. Thus it will fatten or thicken when it is "left alone" or when the tension on the ciliary zonules is released by contraction of ciliary muscle when the short ciliary nerves fire and the eye is accommodating for near vision. As one ages, this elasticity decreases, thus the need for "Ben Franklin" reading glasses beginning at 40 to 50 years of age to compensate for the inability of the lens to get as thick as it used to in its younger days.

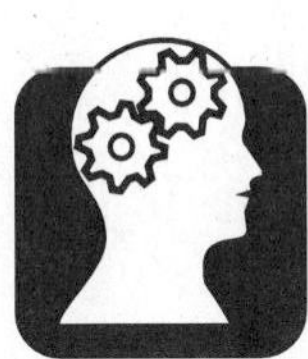

The lens is held in place or suspended from the **ciliary processes** of the circular ciliary body by a system of fibers that constitutes the **ciliary zonule** or zonule of Zinn.

The ciliary processes are about 70 radially arranged ridges on the surface of the ciliary body. The processes give rise to the zonule fibers of the ciliary zonule.

The **ciliary body** is composed mostly of smooth muscle fibers arranged in several planes. In **accommodation for near vision** the short ciliary nerves fire causing contraction of the ciliary muscle. This releases tension on the ciliary zonule and the lens assumes its natural, thick, fat, or unstretched-out shape, So in accommodation for near vision, as in reading these words, especially for prolonged periods of time (studying for the USMLE Part I) your eyes get or feel "tired" (prolonged and constant contraction of the ciliary smooth muscle). To rest your eyes, which really is a resting or noncontraction of the ciliary muscle, you look up and away from the book and accommodate for far vision. At first this seems backwards: that is, how can contraction of a muscle result in a release of tension on something? Remember that the lens is suspended in the center of a circle. Contraction of the circle decreases its diameter and takes tension off the ciliary zonules, allowing the lens to return to its normal, thick shape i.e., accommodation for near vision. Relaxation of the circle will return tension to the ciliary zonules, and this pulls the lens thin, i.e., accommodation for far vision.

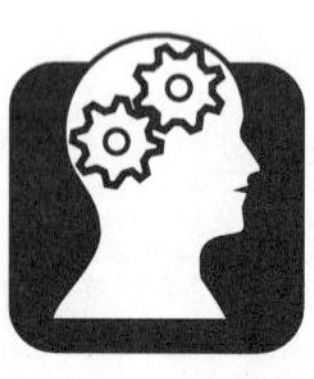

Ciliary portion of retina (nonphotosensitive) covers ciliary body and processes. This epithelium is two cells thick with the outer layer pigmented and the inner layer unpigmented. This epithelium produces the aqueous humor.

- **Aqueous humor**

  - Formed on surface of ciliary body
  - Fills and passes through posterior chamber to **anterior chamber**
  - Leaves anterior chamber through the **trabecular meshwork,** a labyrinthine system of minute passages among endothelial lined trabeculae on the inside of the limbus of the eye (area where the cornea merges with the sclera)
  - **Canal of Schlemm:** a flat, endothelial lined vessel full of aqueous humor leaving the anterior chamber
  - Aqueous veins arise from canal of Schlemm and empty into episcleral veins
  - If the exit of aqueous humor through the canal of Schlemm to the aqueous veins to the episcleral veins is compromised, for example, by an inflammatory or aging process, the result will be an increased **intraocular pressure** (normal production of aqueous humor but less than normal drainage of this fluid), which is **glaucoma.** An increased intraocular pressure is dangerous because it can be transmitted to the retinal vessels and compromise the blood flow in these vessels, which can result in ischemia to the cells of the retina, and blindness results.

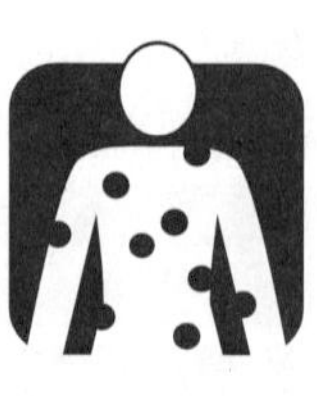

- **Vitreous Body**

  - Gelatinous mass
  - Structureless
  - 99% water

- **Retina, a 10-layered Structure with the Layers Named from Inside to Outside (Fig. 20.2)**
    1. Inner limiting membrane

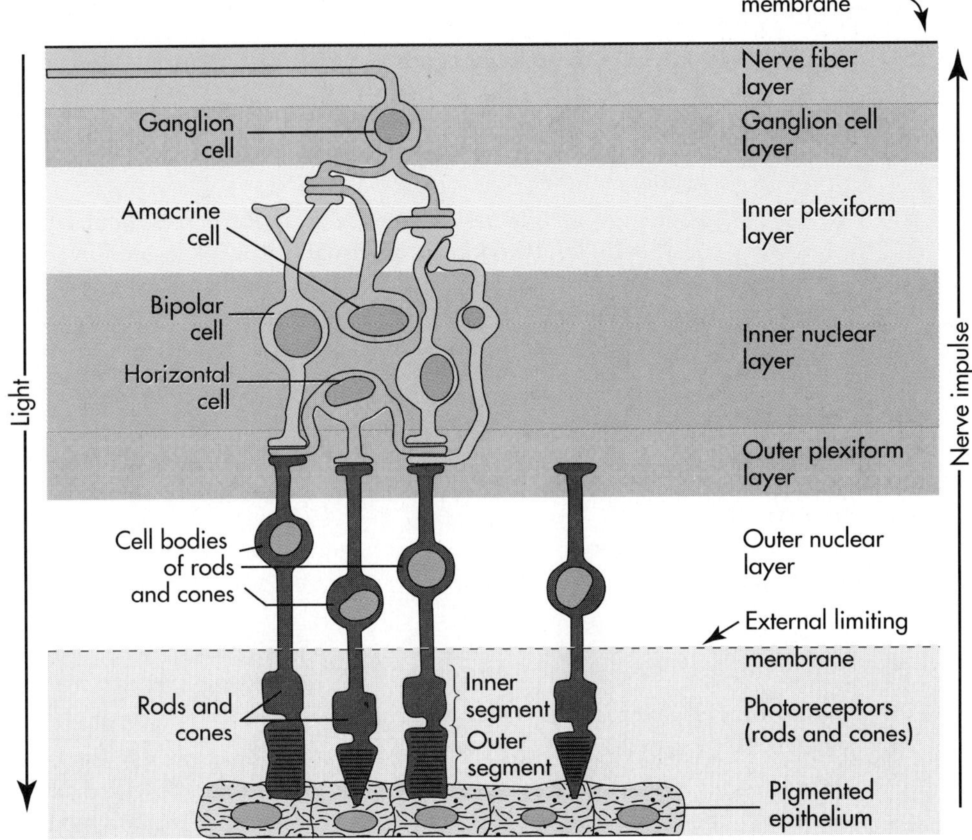

Fig. 20.2 Diagram of the 10 layers of the retina and the paths that light takes into the retina and nerve impulses take exiting the retina.

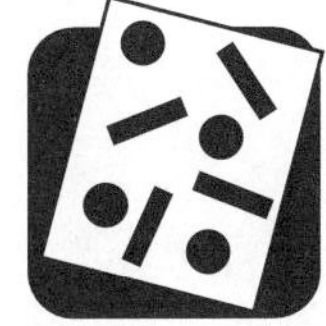

    2. **Layer of optic nerve fibers:** unmyelinated axons of ganglion cells converging toward optic papilla

    3. **Layer of ganglion cells:** third-order, multipolar, neurons, i.e., the terminal neuron of the retina

    4. **Inner plexiform layer:** area of many synapses between axons of the second-order, or bipolar, neurons and dendrites of the ganglion cells

    5. **Inner nuclear layer:** nuclei of the second-order neurons (bipolar)

    6. **Outer plexiform layer:** area of many synapses between the axons of the rods and cones (first-order neurons) and the dendrites of the second-order, or bipolar, neurons

    7. **Outer nuclear layer:** nuclei of rods and cones

    8. **Outer limiting membrane:** actually a row of junctional complexes between photosensitive cells, which appears as a line, the limiting membrane

    9. Layer of **rod and cone inner and outer segments**

  10. **Pigmented epithelium:** absorbs light

- Prevents reflection from uvea and sclera
- Protects sensitive ends of rods and cones
- Phagocytosis of apical, discarded lamellae from rods and cones

Remember that for light to get to the sensitive ends of the rods or cones it passes through at least nine layers of retinal tissue (except in the fovea centralis).

Neuron Path that Visual Information Takes from Rods and Cones to Optic Nerve

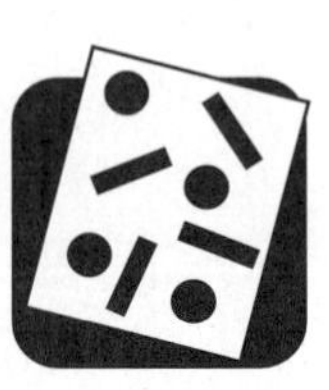

- **Rod,** a first-order neuron that responds to low light situations and perceives visual information in shades of gray

  — *Outer segment*

    - Slender cylinder
    - Large number of parallel lamellae arranged perpendicularly to long axis of cylinder. Rhodopsin, or visual purple, is located in these lamellae. These lamellae are "born" at the inner segment region of the outer segment and migrate to the tip of the cell where they are shed and then phagocytosed by the pigment cells of the retina (layer 10).

  — *Inner segment: usual complement of cytoplasmic organelles*

- **Cone,** also a first-order neuron that is morphologically similar to the rod but has a larger inner segment. Cones detect higher intensities of light and greater visual detail and come in three basic types.

    - Red absorbing
    - Blue absorbing
    - Green absorbing

- **Inner nuclear layer (second-order neuron)**
- **Ganglion cell layer (third-order neuron)**
- **Other:** In addition to the **rods** and **cones (first-order neurons),** the **bipolar neurons (second-order neurons)** and the **ganglion cells (third-order neurons),** there are two other types of cells involved in passing and modifying the visual information being gathered and transmitted by the retina.

    - **Horizontal cells** can be found in the outer plexiform layer of the retina. They connect photoreceptor cells with each other laterally.
    - **Amacrine cells** are found in the inner plexiform layer of the retina where they connect bipolar neurons with other bipolar neurons as well as connecting a single bipolar cell with several ganglion cells.

Fovea Centralis

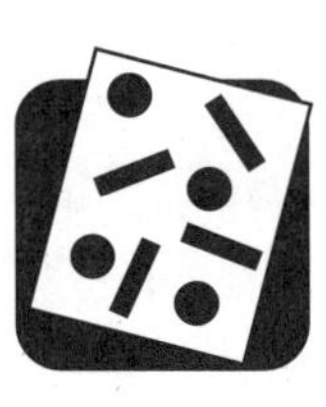

- A specialized region of acute vision located in the center of a yellowish-pigmented region of the retina just lateral to the **optic papilla (blind spot),** i.e., the **macula lutea**
- Region of most distinct vision
- All layers of the retina are missing out to the outer nuclear layer; this allows free passage of rays of light to cones.
- The fovea centralis is rod-free: pure cones.

Accessory Organs of Eye

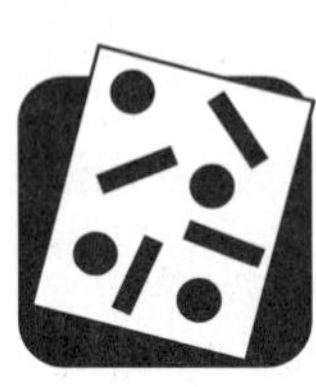

- Eyelid (from anterior to posterior)

  — *Integument*

    - Hairs
      - Small all over
      - Large hairs at edge of lid are the *eyelashes.*
    - Sebaceous glands associated with eyelashes are called the *glands of Zeis.*

- Sweat glands, or the glands of Moll, have ducts opening into eyelash follicles.
- A sty is an infected gland of Moll or Zeis (zeisian sty).

— *Orbicularis oculi (skeletal muscle)*

— *Palpebral fascia (tarsal plate)*

- Superiorly attached to strands of smooth muscle (Müller's muscle)
- **Glands of Meibom** (sebaceous glands): openings form a single row in front of free edge of lid. The secretory product of the meibomian glands keeps the normal tear film in the eye.

— *Palpebral conjunctiva,* a stratified squamous wet epithelium that is continuous with the same covering the white of the eye, i.e., the bulbar conjunctiva. The bulbar and palpebral conjunctivae meet in the superior and inferior fornices of the conjunctival sac.

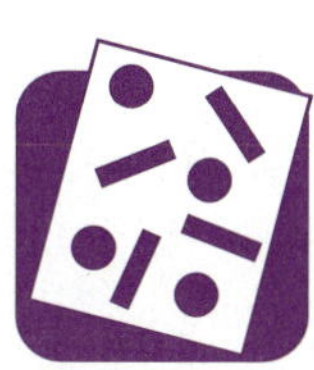

- Lacrimal gland

  - Serous acini secreting a watery product, the tears, which contain a bactericidal substance

Some Interesting Clinicopathologic Conditions Associated with the Eye

- Horner's **ptosis,** or a drooping of the upper eyelid due to destruction of cervical sympathetic ganglia by, e.g., a carcinoma of the apex of lung. This in effect is a denervation of Müller's muscle, which is the smooth muscle that is responsible for holding the superior eyelid up when the eye is open. The action of Müller's muscle is overridden by voluntary contraction of the orbicularis oculi when you blink your eye.

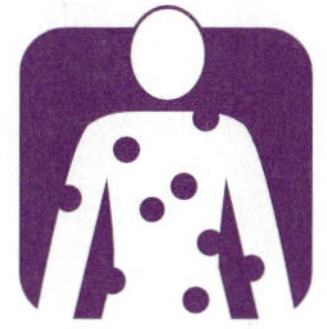

- Aniridia

  Deletion of chromosome number 11
  90% of the children with aniridia have Wilms's tumor, a cancer of the kidney arising from embryonic nephrogenic tissue.

- Squamous cell carcinoma of the epithelium of the cornea or bulbar or palpebral conjunctivae

EAR

Three Major Divisions

- Outer ear

  - Auricle
    - Elastic cartilage
    - Integument
  - External auditory meatus
  - Elastic cartilage (externally); bony canal (internally)
  - Integument
    - Sebaceous glands
    - Modified sweat glands called *ceruminous glands*
    - The combined secretion of the two above is ear wax.

- **Middle ear**
  - Auditory (eustachian) tube
  - Tympanic cavity
    - Auditory ossicles
      - **Malleus**
      - **Incus**
      - **Stapes** (M-I-S; from lateral to medial)
    - Chorda tympani
    - Tendons of tensor tympani (cranial nerve V) and stapedius (cranial nerve VII)

  These muscles contract in a reflex fashion in response to loud sounds (not fast enough for sudden loud sounds like a gun shot) and thereby can lessen the vibration of the ossicles.

  - **Tympanic membrane**
    - Connective tissue core (mesoderm)
    - Covered laterally by thin skin (ectoderm)
    - Covered medially by simple cuboidal epithelium (endoderm)
- **Inner ear**
  - *Membranous labyrinth;* complicated system of ducts: **semicircular ducts, sacculus, utriculus,** and **cochlear duct**
    - Filled by **endolymph**
    - Constructed of ectodermally derived, simple squamous epithelium with patches of special sensory epithelium, i.e.:
      - **Maculae** of **utricle** and **saccule**
      - **Cristae** of each ampulla of each of the 3 semicircular ducts
    - Surrounded by **perilymph**
    - Suspended in a system of bony canals called the **bony labyrinth;** e.g., semicircular canals

Macula (of Utricle; of Saccule)

- Columnar sustentacular cells
- Hair cells: microvilli embedded in a gelatinous mass that contains **otoliths** (crystals of calcium carbonate)
- When the head is inclined, the weight of the otoliths causes a change in position of the jelly of the maculae, thus position in space is perceived.

Crista Ampullaris (One for Each Semicircular Duct)

- Hair cells with microvilli embedded in a gelatinous mass which is the **cupula.**
- When head rotates, the cupula is moved, the hairs of the hair cells are distorted, and rotation is perceived.

The Bony Cochlea is Filled with Perilymph (High in Na$^+$)

- Divided by the **basilar membrane** into 2 subdivisions (Fig. 20.3)
  - Scala vestibuli
  - Scala tympani

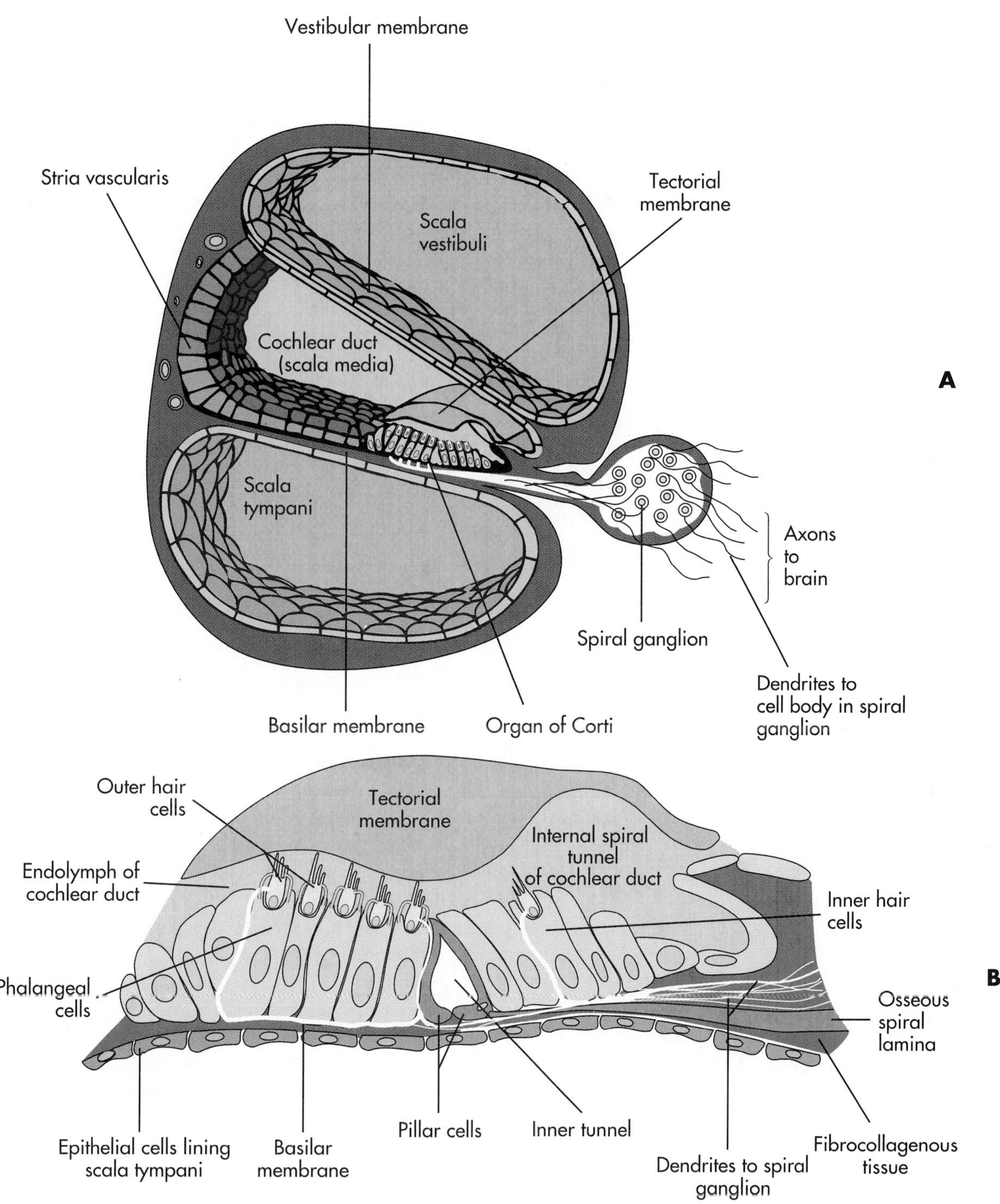

Fig. 20.3 **A,** The inner ear featuring the organ of Corti and its neural projection to the spiral ganglion and beyond. **B,** Details of the organ of Corti.

- The scala vestibuli is separated from the cochlear duct by the **vestibular membrane.**
- Attached to the basilar membrane is the **organ of Corti.**
- The cochlear duct is filled with endolymph (high in K^+).
- Sources of endolymph and perilymph
  - Endolymph
  - In general, most cells of the membranous labyrinth are geared up ultra-structurally for synthesis and secretion and are believed to be directly involved in the metabolism of endolymph.
  - Thus the **stria vascularis,** the **spiral prominence** (both being components of one wall of the cochlear duct), and the extrasensory cells of the cristae and maculae, as well as the other cells of the membranous labyrinth, are involved in the production of endolymph.
  - Perilymph
    - Source in debate
    - Possibly an ultrafiltrate of blood or possibly derived from CSF
    - Perilymphatic spaces are functionally connected to the subarachnoid space.

- **Organ of Corti**
  - **Supporting cells**
  - **Hair cells**
    - Inner
    - Outer
    - Inner and outer hair cells separated by a tunnel (inner tunnel)
  - **Tectorial membrane:** a cuticle type of arrangement into which the tips of the hair cells are embedded.

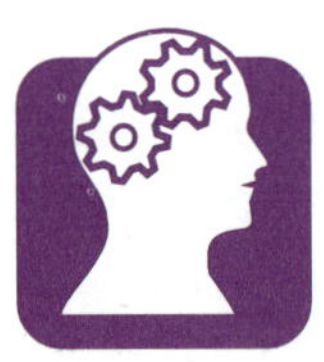

- **Histophysiology of Hearing**
  - Vibrations in air→tympanic membrane→auditory ossicles (amplitude of vibrations increased about $10 \times$ by M-I-S)→foot of stapes→**oval window**→perilymph of scala vestibuli→vestibular membrane→endolymph of cochlear duct, basilar membrane, and scala tympani→**round window** (rapidly bulges and retracts in rhythm with pressure changes in perilymph)
  - Pressure changes cause oscillations of basilar membrane. A specific pitch (frequency) results in greater movement in one specific area of basilar membrane. For example, high tones cause maximal vibration of basilar membrane nearest round window; low tones cause maximal vibration near **helicotrema** (at apex of cochlea where the scala vestibuli and the scala tympani communicate with each other).
  - When the basilar membrane moves, the hair cells of the organ of Corti move and the hairs of the hair cells are distorted.
  - Stimulus conducted over nerve fibers to the spiral ganglion; from spiral ganglion to brain where the original vibrations are interpreted as sound

OLFACTORY MUCOSA

A special region in the superior aspect of each nasal cavity consisting of an **olfactory epithelium,** which like regular respiratory epithelium is pseudostratified but without goblet cells, and the supportive lamina propria, which contains the olfactory glands.

- ■ **Olfactory Epithelium**
    - ● **Bipolar neurons, or olfactory cell:** Has an **apical dendrite,** which has a swollen area called the **olfactory vesicle** from which several nonmotile cilia spread out over the surface. These long processes contain the olfactory receptors. The basal part of the olfactory bipolar neuron is an axon that enters the lamina propria to join other axons from adjacent bipolar neurons, together eventually forming the olfactory nerve, or cranial nerve I.
    - ● **Sustentacular or support cells:** columnar cells giving nutritional and physical support to the olfactory bipolar neurons.
    - ● **Basal cells:** undifferentiated reserve cells, the daughters of which can differentiate into support cells.

- ■ **Olfactory Lamina Propria**
    - • Loose areolar connective tissue containing bundles of axons of the olfactory bipolar neurons and the **olfactory glands of Bowman**
    - • These glands are composed of serous acini, which deliver the secretory product to the surface through a duct system. Odoriferous substances are trapped or dissolved in this watery secretion.

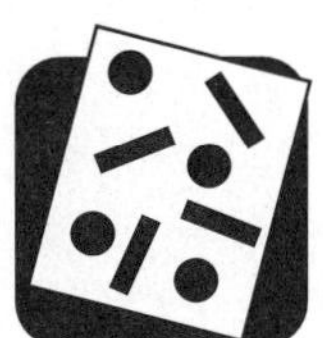

Taste Buds

- • Taste buds are pale, oval structures found in the epithelium covering the fungiform, foliate, and circumvallate papillae. Each taste bud contains three cell types:
    - • Neuroepithelial cells, which have apical microvilli passing through the taste pore, or the small opening in the taste bud on its epithelial surface
    - • Support cells
    - • Basal cells

MULTIPLE CHOICE REVIEW QUESTIONS

1. Which of the following descriptions best describes the "blind spot":
   a. Optic disk or papilla
   b. Macula lutea
   c. Fovea centralis
   d. Ora serrata
   e. Canal of Schlemm

2. Choose the correct pathway for the circulation of aqueous humor: 1, anterior chamber; 2, pupil; 3, formation by ciliary process; 4, canal of Schlemm; 5, episcleral veins.
   a. 1-2-3-4-5
   b. 3-2-1-4-5
   c. 1-5-3-4-2
   d. 1-5-4-2-3
   e. 3-4-5-1-2

3. Arrange the following items in proper sequence for normal hearing: (1) Sound vibrations in air, (2) tympanic membrane, (3) oval window, (4) perilymph of scala vestibuli, (5) endolymph of cochlear duct.
   a. 1-2-3-4-5
   b. 1-2-4-5-3
   c. 1-2-5-4-3
   d. 1-2-4-3-5
   e. 1-2-5-3-4

4. Where do the anterior and posterior chambers of the eye communicate with each other?
   a. Optic disk
   b. Canal of Schlemm
   c. Pupil
   d. Ora serrata
   e. Through ciliary zonules

5. This region secretes a substance that functions as a barrier to the movement of water:
   a. Stria vascularis of cochlear duct
   b. Olfactory mucosa
   c. Macula of the utricle
   d. Glands of Meibom
   e. Ciliary processes

Answers and Explanations to Multiple Choice Review Questions

CHAPTER 1: INTRODUCTION: LEVELS AND BIOLOGICAL ORGANIZATION AND TECHNIQUES

1. Answers a, a, a, d, e:
Convert each to its corresponding value for the match.

2. Answer d:
The smallest structure is an intracellular organelle (mitochondrion).

a: The digestive system is an entire system.
b: Red blood cell is an entire cell.
c: Connective tissue represents a collection of tissues.
e: The stomach is an entire organ.

3. Answer b:
Autoradiography specifically labels macromolecules when they are synthesized in a cell or tissue and then enables the following of these molecules through the cells. Autoradiography can be used to study the synthesis and processing of a cell component.

a: Immunocytochemistry enables staining of a specific molecule, but newly synthesized and previously labeled molecules are not distinguished.
c: Staining with H and E enables visualization but cannot distinguish newly synthesized from other molecules.
d: Staining with osmium tetroxide enables visualization but cannot distinguish newly synthesized from other molecules.
e: Freeze fracture reveals nothing about synthesis of a molecule.

4. Answers a, c, c, b, b:

a: Mitochondrion is an organelle.
c: The heart is an organ.
c: The stomach is an organ.
b: Epithelium is a tissue.
b: Muscle is a tissue, although the term *muscle* is also used to describe an organ.

5. Answer c:
Immunocytochemistry can specifically identify polypeptides as antigens.

a: Autoradiography labels newly synthesized molecules but is nonspecific.
b: Staining with H & E is nonspecific.
d: Uranyl acetate staining is nonspecific.
e: Freeze-fracture is nonspecific.

CHAPTER 2: CELL BIOLOGY: CYTOPLASMIC ORGANELLES

1. Answer b:
A zonula occludens completely surrounds the cells forming a permeability seal.

a: A nexus provides channels from one cell to an adjacent one.
c: A macula adherens is simply a spot weld on the surface holding two cells together.
d: A zonula adherens is a zone that holds two cells together.
e: A macula occludens is a spot weld and does not surround the cell. Material can pass between the two cells avoiding the region of the occludens.

2. **Answer c:**
   The P face would show tails of phospho-lipid molecules and granules formed by intrinsic membrane proteins.

   a: Extrinsic membrane proteins are found on the membrane surface.
   b: Polar heads of phospholipid molecules are found on membrane surface.
   d: Carbohydrate-containing oligosac-charides are found on the external surface.
   e: All of the statements describe the cell coat.

3. **Answer e:**
   The cell coat of the intestinal epithelial cell may act as a filter. The cell coat is rich in carbohydrate groups. It may be covalently linked to amino acids and intrinsic membrane proteins. The poly-saccharides of the cell coat may be re-sponsible for recognition sites on the membrane.

4. **Answers c, b, d, e, a:**

   c: Exocytosis is movement in bulk out of the cell.
   b: Pinocytosis is cellular drinking (droplets of H_2O); H_2O molecules enter the cell by noncarrier mediated transport.
   d: Fatty acids enter the cell by non-carrier mediated transport.
   e: Charged molecules enter by active transport.
   a: Phagocytosis (cellular eating) describes the uptake of a solid material (like a bacterium).

5. **Answers b, e, a, d, c:**
   From the outside, you first encounter a, the oligosaccharides of the cell coat, b, the polar heads of phospholipid mole-cules in the external bilayer, c, the non-polar tails of phospholipid molecules in the external bilayer, d, the E face, and then e, the P face.

6. **Answer c:**
   The only autophagic activity listed is the digestion of mitochondria because these are intrinsic to the cell.

   a: Bacteria originate outside of the cell.

b: Invading virus particles originate outside of the cell.
d: Contents of a phagocytic vesicle originate outside of the cell.
e: A collagen fiber from the surrounding connective tissue originates outside of the cell.

7. **Answer e:**
   None of these proteins are coded for the mitochondrial genome and synthesized on mitochondrial ribosomes; therefore, their synthesis would not be affected by chloramphenicol.

   a: Proteins of the mitochondrial membrane are coded for by nuclear genes synthe-sized on free cytoplasmic polysomes.
   b: Kreb cycle enzymes are synthesized on free cytoplasmic polysomes.
   c: Cytoplasmic ribosomal proteins are synthesized on free cytoplasmic poly-somes.
   d: Lysosomal enzymes are coded for by nuclear genes and synthesized on RER.

8. **Answer d:**
   The number of polysomes decreases since the ribosomes continue to move off the mRNA, protein synthesis decreases, and since no more messages are available, the 40S and 60S subunits do not form the 80S ribosomes but remain as subunits in the cytoplasm.

   a: Since ribosomes translocate on mRNA, but no more attach, the number of polysomes decreases. However, other options are also correct.
   b: Protein synthesis decreases because there are no more polysomes. However, other options are also correct.
   c: The number of free 40S and 60S subunits increases because ribosomes attach from polysomes releasing 40S and 60S sub-units. However, other options are also correct.
   e: At least one option is correct.

9. **Answers d, a, a, c, c:**

   d: Mitochondrial ribosomal RNA is synthesized on mitochondrial DNA.

a: Proteins synthesized for secretion
(intestinal enzymes) are synthesized
on the RER.
a: Lysosomal enzymes are synthesized
on RER.
c: Hemoglobin is an intracellular protein
and is synthesized on free polysomes.
c: Mitochondrial proteins of the TCA cycle
are intracellular proteins and are synthesized on free polysomes.

10. **Answers b, d, a, c, e:**
Synthesis on RER, to SER, to transfer
vacuole, to Golgi, and exocytosis.

b: Transfer vacuole carries from SER.
d: Protein is packaged in secretory vacuole
in Golgi.
a: Proteins are synthesized on RER to SER.
c: Transfer vacuole fuses with Golgi.
e: Secretory vacuole releases to the outside
by exocytosis.

CHAPTER 3: CELL BIOLOGY: NUCLEUS AND CELL DIVISION

1. **Answer d:**
The cells would accumulate at metaphase
and have 6.0 picograms of DNA.

a: Is the amount of DNA in a gamete.
b: Is the amount of DNA in a G1 phase
cell.
c: Some S phase cells would contain 4.5
picograms.
e: Is the amount of DNA found in a polyploid cell.

2. **Answers a, a, a, c, b:**
The number of sex chromatin bodies
equals the number of X chromosomes
minus one.

a: No sex chromatin bodies.
a: No sex chromatin bodies.
a: No sex chromatin bodies.
c: 2 sex chromatin bodies.
b: 1 sex chromatin body.

3. **Answer b:**
Since there are cells with different chromosome constitutions, it would have to
have been a mitotic event, and since some

of the cells have an additional chromosome, it must have arisen by nondisjunction.

a: In meiotic nondisjunction, all cells would
have the same chromosome constitution.
c: Anaphase lagging can only give rise to
cells with less chromosomes, not cells
with extra chromosomes.
d: Anaphase lagging can only give rise to
cells with less chromosomes, not cells
with extra chromosomes.
e: Deletion does not change chromosome
number.

4. **Answer a:**
The first meiotic division, which has already occurred, is a separation of paired
chromosomes; in this case, the X and the
Y chromosome. The meiotic second division represents an equational giving rise
to two X or two Y chromosomes.

b: The cell gives rise to only 2 cells.
c: As a result of the first meiotic division
the cell has either an X or a Y chromosome.
d: The cell gives rise to only 2 cells.

5. **Answer e:**
Since you are blocking conversion of
the precursor to 18S and 28S RNA, the
amount of fibrillar region would increase
because it contains the 45S precursor, but
the amount of granular region and cytoplasmic ribosomes would decrease since
the precursor is not processed. The number of ribosomal genes would remain
constant.

a: 45S RNA synthesis continues, but there
is no conversion to 18S and 28S and fibrillar components that represent 45S
precursor increase. However, other options are also correct.
b: No conversion of 45S RNA to 18S and
28S RNA, which appears in the granular
area. However, other options are also correct.
c: Since there is no more 18S and 28S RNA
processed and no more ribosome biosynthesis, the number of ribosomes decreases. However, other options are also
correct.

d: The number of ribosomal genes is not affected. However, other options are also correct.

6. **Answer d:**

Heterochromatin is converted to euchromatin, decreasing the amount of heterochromatin. Since heterochromatin was inactive in RNA synthesis, this increases RNA synthesis in the nucleus and genes previously not expressed because they lay in heterochromatin are now expressed.

a: The polyanions would cause a decrease in the amount of heterochromatin in the nucleus. This would lead to other effects.
b: Although the total RNA synthesis would increase, this would then lead to the expression of genes previously not expressed. The heterochromatin would be converted to euchromatin, thus decreasing the total heterochromatin.
c: An increase in total RNA synthesis would lead to the expression of genes, which were previously repressed in the heterochromatin.
e: At least one option is correct.

7. **Answer d:**

Unlike euchromatin, heterochromatin is inert genetically and shows little if any RNA synthesis, but like euchromatin, it contains DNA and histone.

a: Although heterochromatin is genetically inert, other correct properties are also listed.
b: Although heterochromatin is inactive in RNA synthesis, it is also relatively genetically inert and contains DNA and histone protein.
c: Heterochromatin does contain DNA and histone protein. However, it is also genetically inert and inactive in RNA synthesis.
e: At least one option is correct.

8. **Answers b, b, d, e, a:**

b: The nucleolus organizer and the chromosomal secondary constriction are the same thing and are the site on the chromosome that contains genes coding for rRNA.

b: The nucleolus organizer and the chromosomal secondary constriction are the same thing and are the site on the chromosome that contains genes coding for rRNA.
d: The fibrillar area of the nucleolus contains 45S RNA precursor.
e: The granular area contains 18S and 28S RNA in 40S and 60S subunits.
a: There is no nucleolar membrane.

Chapter 4: Epithelial Tissue

1. **Answer c:**

The basal body contains 9 triplet microtubules.

a: 7 doublet microtubule arrangements are unknown.
b: 9 doublet and 2 central singlet microtubules found in body of cilium.
d: 9 doublet microtubules not known without singlet.
e: 9 doublets and singlet microtubule unknown.

2. **Answer b:**

The SER, which has many of the enzymes involved in steroid biosynthesis, is the site.

a: RER is the site of protein synthesis.
c: The nucleus is the site of DNA and RNA synthesis.
d: The Golgi is the site of protein processing.

3. **Answer b:**

The continuous replicating VIM cells are located in the basal layer, and they provide the stem cell population to replace cells lost at the surface.

a: The cells on the surface are nonreplicating FPM cells.
c: The intermediate layer has some DIM cells but no stem cells.
d: The underlying connective tissue does not contribute to the epithelial cell population.

4. **Answers c, d, e, b, a:**

c: Keratin is a protective protein.

d: The SER of the liver parenchymal cell contains enzymes involved in drug detoxification.

e: The Golgi is the site of protein packaging for secretion.

b: The nexus contains channels for direct intercellular communication.

a: Microvilli of the intestinal epithelial cell increase the surface area for absorption.

5. Answers a, d, c, a, d:

a: This contains the stem cell population of SSE.

d: These are highly differentiated surface cells.

c: Capillary endothelial cells replicate themselves very rarely and are RPM cells.

a: This cell provides for replacement of ciliated surface cell.

d: These are highly specialized FPM cells.

CHAPTER 5: CONNECTIVE TISSUE

1. Answers e, c, d, b, a:

e: Plasma cells synthesize humoral antibodies.

c: Mast cells synthesize heparin.

d: Fibroblasts synthesize tropocollagen.

b: Adipose cells store triglyceride.

a: Macrophages demonstrate phagocytosis.

2. Answers b, c, a, e, d:

b: Proline is immediately hydroxylated on synthesis of alpha chain.

c: Procollagen is formed from proalpha chains immediately after synthesis.

a: The proalpha chain is synthesized.

e: Tropocollagen polymerizes extracellularly for form collagen fibers.

d: Procollagen is secreted from cell; there peptidases on the cell surface convert it to tropocollagen.

3. Answer c:
The drug would interfere with cross linking. Tropoelastin would continue to be synthesized, but the elasticity is dependent on extensive cross linking of the random coiled molecule.

a: Elasticity decreases due to decreased cross linking.

b: Tropoelastin continues to be synthesized but not converted to elastin.

d: Tropoelastin continues to be synthesized.

e: The periodicity of collagen is 64 nm.

4. Answers a, b, a, a, a:

a: The number of monocytes in the connective tissue increases during chronic infection.

b: Vitamin C is necessary for hydroxylation of proline and procollagen synthesis.

a: Cross links in collagen increase as the molecule ages.

a: Hyaluronic acid restricts movement of large molecules in ground substance.

a: Acute infections demonstrate an increase in neutrophils.

5. Answer a:
Tropocollagen measures 280 nm in length.

b: The periodicity of collagen is 64 nm.

c: The periodicity of collagen is 64 nm.

d: Tropocollagen is rich in proline and hydroxyproline.

e: The microfibrillar component of elastic fibers is not tropocollagen.

CHAPTER 6: NERVOUS TISSUE

1. Answers c, d, a, b, d:

c: Oligodendrocytes are found in white and gray matter.

d: Collagen fibers are not found in white or gray matter.

a: Cell bodies of neurons are only found in gray matter.

b: Myelin is found mainly in white matter.

d: Endoneurium is not found in gray matter.

2. Answers b, d, c, a, c:

b: Neurons synthesize neurotransmitters.

d: Astrocytes mediate nutrition to neurons.
c: Oligodendrocytes and Schwann cells elaborate myelin.
a: Microglia demonstrate phagocytosis.
c: Schwann cells synthesize myelin.

3. Answers b, c, c:

b: Nissl substance decreases during chromatolysis.
c: There is no increase in the number of neurons after birth.
c: There is no connective tissue in the gray and white matter.

4. Answer c:

There is no stem compartment of neurons, which are FPMs and cannot be replaced if destroyed.

a: Microglia are RPMs and can replace damaged cells.
b: Oligodendrocytes are RPMs and can replace damaged cells.
d: Astrocytes are RPMs and can replace damaged cells.

5. Answers e, a, d, c, b:

A, From the axon out, one would encounter, B, the myelin sheath of the Schwann cell, C, the endoneurium, D, perineurium and, E, the epineurium.

CHAPTER 7: MUSCULAR TISSUE

1. Answers a, e, d, c, b:

a: The carbon atoms atomic weight is 12.
e: G actin's molecular weight is 40 kd.
d: Myosin's is 500 kd.
c: Many actin and myosin molecules make up a myofilament.
b: Thick and thin myofilaments comprise the myofibril.

2. Answer a:

Thick filaments are only found in A band.

b: Thick filaments are made up of hundreds of myosin molecules.
c: Thin filaments are attached to the Z line.
d: Thin filaments are localized in the A and I bands.

e: At least one option is correct.

3. Answers c, a, b, b, a:

c: A band length is constant.
a: The length of H band changes with relaxation and contraction.
b: The length of I band changes with relaxation and contraction.
b: Release of calcium from sarcoplasmic reticulum initiates contraction.
a: Thickness of fiber increases during contraction.

4. Answers d, e, a, c, b:

d: T tubules are located at the A-I intercept in skeletal muscle.
e: Myosin is located in thick filaments.
a: The A band's length remains constant during contraction and relaxation.
c: T tubules are located at Z line in cardiac muscle.
b: Actin is located in thin filaments, and the I bands contain only thin filaments.

5. Answer b:

There are no T tubules in smooth muscle.

a: Smooth muscle contains actin and myosin.
c: Smooth muscle contains abundant gap junctions.
d: Smooth muscle contains abundant mitochondria.

CHAPTER 8: INTEGUMENTARY SYSTEM

1. Answers d, b, c, a, d:

d: FPMs are found in the s. granulosum and s. corneum.
b: DIMs in s. spinosum.
c: RPMs are found in the ducts of glands.
a: VIMs are found in the s. basale.
d: Chromatophores are FPM cells.

2. Answer d:

All are correct.

Cytosine arabinoside would inhibit DNA synthesis in s. basale and s. spinosum. Therefore cells could not divide and replace cells sloughed from the surface (causing thinning of the skin and stopping DNA synthesis in the base of the hair follicle, which would stop growth).

3. **Answer b:**
   Melanocytes synthesize melanin.

   a: Melanophores accumulate melanin but do not synthesize it.
   c: Chromatophores accumulate melanin but do not synthesize it.
   d: At least one option is correct.

4. **Answers a, d, b, e, c:**
   From the basal layer to the surface a, s. basale; b, s. spinosum; c, s. granulosum; d, s. lucidum; e, s. corneum.

5. **Answer d:**
   Chromatophores are found in the dermis, melanophores in the s. spinosum and s. basale, and melanocytes in the s. basale.

CHAPTER 9: CARTILAGE, BONE, AND JOINTS

1. **Answer c:**
   Volkmann's canals interconnect Haversian systems.

   a: Volkmann's canals contain blood and lymph vessels, not processes of osteocytes.
   b: Canaliculi interconnect lacunae.
   d: Volkmann's canals interconnect Haversian systems; they are not components of a Haversian system.
   e: Volkmann's canals are not components of interstitial lamellae.

2. **Answer b:**
   Growth hormone stimulates proliferation of the chondrocytes in the zone of proliferation in the epiphyseal plate. This is interstitial growth.

   a: The process of calcification due to the hypertrophy of the chondrocytes is not influenced by growth hormone.
   c: Osteoblasts and fibroblasts located in the osteogenic and fibrous layers of the periosteum respectively are probably influenced by growth hormone in relation to the growth in width of the diaphysis of

the long bone, but the question asked for which of the choices was "most" sensitive to growth hormone.
   d: Osteoblasts of the metaphysis also probably respond to the presence of growth hormone, but not to the degree or strength that proliferating chondrocytes do.
   e: Osteoblasts respond to serum calcium levels. If low, osteoblastic activity increases. If high, osteoblastic activity decreases.

3. **Answer c:**
   Skeletal muscle—fibrous layer of periosteum—osteogenic layer of periosteum—outer circumferential lamellae—Haversian system and its canal—inner circumferential lamellae—endosteum—bone marrow.

   a, b: Endosteum is the layer on the innermost aspect of the bone, right next to the bone marrow and therefore would be far away from a skeletal muscle located on the outside of the periosteum.
   d: Inner circumferential lamellae would not be next in the sequence after osteogenic layer of the periosteum with Haversian systems also being a part of the sequence. The Haversian systems are in the compact bone between the inner and the outer circumferential lamellae.
   e: Haversian canal would not be in the correct sequence given that the osteogenic layer of the periosteum is also a part of the sequence.

4. **Answer a:**
   Bone marrow - osteoblast - fresh osteoid - mineralized osteoid - calcified cartilage.

   b, c: With osteoblast in the sequence, it has to come before unmineralized osteoid.
   d: Mineralized osteoid cannot be second in the sequence with unmineralized osteoid and osteoblast choices in the sequence.
   e: Calcified cartilage cannot come before osteoblast in this anatomical arrangement.

5. **Answer d:**
   The osteoclast releases the contents of its lysosomal vesicles onto the surface of

the bone matrix, which is being broken down. The pH of this microenvironment is below 7.0.

    a: Hypertrophied chondrocytes release alkaline phosphatase, which will be involved in the precipitation of calcium phosphate in the cartilage matrix.

    b: Osteocytic osteolysis recaptures the most recent calcium added to the bone matrix and does not involve the release of lysosomal hydrolyases.

    c: Osteoprogenitor cells are relatively undifferentiated and serve as a source for osteoblasts and osteoclasts. They are not differentiated enough to be involved in the release of lysosomal hydrolyases.

CHAPTER 10: THE RESPIRATORY SYSTEM

1. Answer d:

By the time the respiratory tree reaches the alveoli, no ciliated cells are present.

    a: Type II pneumocytes are found in the alveolar septa.

    b: Endothelial cells lining the alveolar capillaries are a very important component of the alveolar septum.

    c: Type I pneumocytes are a very important component of the alveolar septum.

    e: Alveolar macrophages, since they wander over the alveolar surface, can transiently be a component of the alveolar septum.

2. Answer a:

The true vocal fold is covered by stratified squamous wet epithelium.

    b: The true fold does not contain any glands at all.

    c: The true fold does not contain any cartilage of any kind.

    d: The false fold is superior to the true fold.

    e: The true fold does not contain any cartilage of any kind.

3. Answer d:

The great alveolar cell or the type II pneumocyte is the cell source for surfactant.

    a: Goblet cells make mucus, not surfactant.

    b: Type I pneumocytes are the very thin surface lining of the alveolus, and they are covered by the surfactant coat, but they do not manufacture it.

    c: Dust cells or alveolar macrophages are not involved in the production of surfactant.

    e: Bronchiolar glands produce some mucus, not surfactant.

4. Answer c:

The dust cell wanders over the alveolar surface and is thick enough to be a hindrance to gas exchange. It is not a component of the air-blood barrier.

    a , b, d, e: All other choices are characteristic components of the blood-air "barrier" or interface with the pneumocyte type I being closest to the air and the endothelial cell closest to the blood. Since both of these cells have their own basal laminae there can be two basal laminae or one thicker, shared basal lamina.

5. Answer c:

Of the choices listed, the Clara cell count would be highest in the terminal bronchioles.

    a: These immediate branches of the trachea do not contain Clara cells.

    b: Bronchi containing hyaline cartilage in plates or little pieces also do not contain more than a few Clara cells relative to the terminal branches of the bronchial tree.

    d: Interalveolar septa are too far down the respiratory tree to have more than an occasional Clara cell.

    e: The pores of Kohn are interalveolar pores, which are holes between adjacent alveoli.

CHAPTER 11: THE CARDIOVASCULAR SYSTEM

1. Answer b:

Arterioles have thick walls relative to the size of the lumen. This is reflective of the high hydrostatic pressure they carry and help maintain.

a: A thick adventitia and a large lumen better describes a vein.

c: A thin media plus a large lumen better describes a vein.

d: A large blood-filled lumen better describes a venous structure.

e: Large amounts of elastic fibers in the tunica media would describe an elastic artery such as the aorta or pulmonary trunk or their immediate branches. Arterioles are down at the other end of the tree.

2. **Answer d:**

This is the correct sequence of layers or sublayers of the wall of an artery from inside to outside.

a: Next to blood in the lumen one would not encounter adipose tissue as the next structure encountered on the way out through the vessel wall.

b: Although smooth muscle cells are in the wall, they would come after the subendothelial CT and the internal elastic membrane.

c: The subendothelial CT has to come between the blood and the internal elastic membrane.

3. **Answer d:**

The zonula occludens (ZO) is a part of the junctional complex between epithelial cells lining the GI tract (enterocytes) and some other epithelial cells. It is a fusion of the outer leaflets of the two opposing membranes. ZO is not a component of the intercalated disc found in cardiac muscle.

a, b: Both of these are found in the transverse part of an intercalated disc. Also in the transverse part of an intercalated disc one can find macula occludens.

c: Gap junctions or nexi are found in the lateral parts of the intercalated disc or that part of the intercalated disc that runs parallel to the long axis of the muscle fiber.

4. **Answer d:**

Conducting and distributing arteries do not have valves.

a - c: All of these structures do have valves preventing the backflow of fluid.

5. **Answer c:**

Lymph capillaries have the thinnest wall of all and therefore are the easiest for cancer cells to invade.

a, b: Capillaries, whether of the fenestrated or continuous type, would be the next easiest to break into because both of these have very thin walls but not as thin as lymph capillaries.

d: A venule would be thicker than any of the capillaries and would resist invasion longer because of its thicker wall.

e: The vessel with the thickest wall in all of the choices is the arteriole, and because of this relatively thicker wall, the arteriole would be the last of the vessels listed to be completely invaded.

CHAPTER 12: BLOOD

1. **Answer c:**

In this disease bacteria are not killed inside the PMN. When the PMN dies viable bacteria are released. A genetic defect has resulted in the absence of hydrogen peroxide.

a: Chediak-Higashi is characterized by a lag in the initiation of the fusion of the lysosomes with the ingested bacteria.

b: Chronic inflammation in this question assumes that there is no genetic defect and that a long standing infection in a CT area will eventually resolve.

d: Any anemia would indicate something wrong with the RBC pool whether it is numbers of RBCs or the concentration of the hemoglobin in them.

e: CML is a type of leukemia in which undifferentiated stages of hematopoiesis end up circulating in the peripheral blood.

2. **Answer e:**

In the PMN the granules are lysosomes or membrane bound bags of enzymes.

a: There are no true pigments in a PMN.

b: The lysosomes in the cytoplasm of the PMN were made in the RER-Golgi.

c: Mitochondria have nothing to do with the specific granules or lysosomes.

d: Plasma cells synthesize and release immunoglobulins; this has nothing to do with PMNs.

3. **Answer d:**

Eosinophils make up about 3% of a normal differential count.

a: This percent is associated with PMNs.

b: This percent is associated with lymphocytes.

c: This percent is associated with monocytes.

e: This percent is associated with basophils.

4. **Answer d:**

Spectrin is a major cytoskeletal molecule.

a: Lysosomes have nothing to do with the cell cytoskeleton.

b, c: Adult or fetal hemoglobin are not cytoskeletal components.

e: The glycocalyx is the cell coat on the cell surface (E surface of the plasmalemma).

5. **Answer b:**

Both the basophil and the mast cell contain IgE on their cell surface. When this antibody reacts with the appropriate antigen, the cell degranulates and releases heparin, histamine, SRS, etc.

a; c-e: These cells are not involved in the immediate hypersensitivity reaction and do not contain IgE antibody receptors on their cell surface.

CHAPTER 13: BONE MARROW

1. **Answer b:**

Of all the stages listed the pronormoblast is the youngest or the least differentiated.

a: Myelocytes are about half way down the differentiation steps in the granulocytopoiesis line.

c: Metamyelocytes are more differentiated than myelocytes.

d: Polychromatophilic normoblasts are about half way down the erythrocytopoiesis line of differentiation.

e: The reticulocyte or diffusely basophilic erythrocyte is one step short of being a fully formed RBC.

2. **Answer a:**

Given the choices from thrombocytopoiesis this is the correct sequence of events.

b: The platelet demarcation channels of SER form later in this list of events.

c: Thrombopoietin has to act on the stem cell before there can be endoreduplication and its resulting increase in ploidy in the differentiating magakaryocyte.

d: Rupturing of the filopods results in the release of platelets, and this is obviously very late in the sequence of events characterizing thrombocytopoiesis.

e: Choice 1 is first in this sequence but choice 5 is the last event in this series.

3. **Answer c:**

This is a description of the cell kinetic compartment at the mature end of hematopoiesis in which mature and not quite fully mature cells reside.

a: The stem cell compartment would be self-sustaining.

b: Cells in the DIM compartment are all in the process of differentiating. Therefore this compartment depends on influx of cells from the VIM or stem cell compartment.

d: The reverting post mitotic compartment is not a kinetic compartment of the bone marrow.

4. **Answer a:**

This is the correct series of events in the formation of a PMN or neutrophil and the exit of that cell from circulating blood to a CT area.

b: Nuclear indentation cannot come before the more undifferentiated step of a cell with 2 to 3 prominent nuclei (i.e., the myeloblast or promyelocyte stages).

c: The mature or almost mature cells are the ones, which after finishing most to all of the cytodifferentiation steps, exit the hematopoietic cord.

d, e: Specific granules, whether neutrophilic, basophilic, or eosinophilic, can-

not come before some of the more undifferentiated steps.

5. **Answer d:**

   The description best fits the promyelocyte and this would be promyelocytic
   leukemia.

   a: Lymphoblastic leukemia would be
   characterized by a large number of
   lymphoblasts, which do not have cytoplasm filled with azurophilic granules.
   b: Basophil leukemia is a rare leukemia in
   which various stages of undifferentiated
   basophils circulate, such as the basophil
   myelocyte, metamyelocyte, and band
   stages.
   c: Monoblastic leukemia would show a
   preponderance of monocytoblasts.
   e: Stem cell leukemia would show large
   numbers of very undifferentiated, immature cells, which would have prominent nucleoli but would not have differentiated far enough to show cytoplasmic granules.

Chapter 14: The Defense System

1. **Answer d:**

   The spleen filters blood by having the
   circulatory system dump blood directly
   into the cords of Billroth.

   a: The marginal zone is a region of T-B cell
   interaction and is not where worn-out
   RBCs are phagocytosed.
   b: The medulla of the thymus has nothing
   to do with the normal phagocytosis of
   RBCs.
   c: A hematopoietic cord in the bone
   marrow is where erythrocytopoiesis
   occurs, not erythrophagocytosis.
   e: The paratrabecular, subcapsular, and
   medullary sinuses in a lymph node have
   phagocytic cells bridging them, but
   these phagocytes are involved in filtering
   lymph, not blood, which is the job of the
   phagocytes in the cord of Billroth.

2. **Answer c:**

   This is the reverse order of the components of the blood-thymus barrier if an

antigen was moving from blood through
the barrier into the thymus. In this case
blood borne antigen would use the 3-2-
4-5-1 route.

   a: Thymocyte would be correct but the
   endothelium of a blood vessel would be
   the next to last component of the sequence, not second in the sequence.
   b: Thymocyte is correct, reticular cell is
   correct, perivascular space is correct, but
   thrombocyte or platelet cannot come
   before the endothelial lining of the blood
   vessel.
   d: Thymocyte is correct but the reticular
   cells would have to come between it and
   the perivascular space.
   e: Thymocyte is correct but the thrombocyte or platelet would have to be the very
   last structure in the sequence, not the
   second structure.

3. **Answer b:**

   The B effector cell is a plasma cell.

   a: Any lymphocyte seen in peripheral blood
   could be a T effector cell such as a Tk or
   T killer cell.
   c: Any lymphocyte seen in peripheral blood
   could be a T cell, which has yet to encounter the antigen it has been prepro-
   grammed against, and therefore it would
   be a "virgin" T cell.
   d: This is another way of describing a B
   memory cell. This is a cell which has had
   an encounter with an appropriate antigen and instead of differentiating into
   a plasma cell, it became a memory cell.
   Reexposure to the same antigen would
   activate the memory cells much faster
   (second set reaction) than a first set
   reaction.
   e: As is the case for explanation D, there are
   T memory cells too.

4. **Answer d:**

   The stromal reticular cells of the thymus,
   which are derived from the endoderm,
   not the mesoderm, produce thymosin,
   which is important for normal development of T cells in the thymus.

   a: Dendritic reticular cells in the germinal
   center of any lymph nodule is an antigen

trapping-presenting cell and not the source of thymosin.

   b: T helper cells make a lot of hormone-like substances, such as interleukins and cytokines, but they are not the cell source for thymosin.

   c: Tdth type cells make or may be involved in the production of MIF (migration inhibitory factor) and MAF (macrophage activating factor) but not thymosin.

   e: Hassall's corpuscles are remnants of the embryonic ectodermal grooves, which get "caught up" in the formation of the thymus and end up looking like little islands of keratin-producing cells in the thymus. They have no known function.

5. **Answer e:**

The CD8 cell is the same as the Ts cell, which can down-regulate antibody production by B cells, but it is not an antigen processing-presenting cell.

   a: Tissue macrophages or histiocytes are capable of antigen presentation after they have phagocytosed and processed foreign antigen.

   b: The Kupfer cell is basically a fixed macrophage and therefore can function as an antigen presenting cell.

   c: The dendritic reticular cell is a famous antigen trapper-presenter cell.

   d: Langerhans cells in the epidermis function as sort of the epidermal counterpart to the dendritic reticular cell found in the germinal centers of lymph nodules.

Chapter 15: The Digestive System

1. **Answer d:**

No matter where the muscularis mucosa is found it is composed only of smooth muscle. The muscularis externa can be either smooth or skeletal or both, depending on which part of the esophagus is involved.

   a: Meissner's autonomic ganglia/plexuses are a normal component of the submucosa.

   b: Antigen presenting cells, the M cells in the surface epithelium covering lymphoid tissue, are a normal component of the GI tract.

   c: The lamina propria is loose areolar connective tissue, which contains a diffuse lymphoid tissue infiltrate in response to all of the foreign antigens and bacteria ingested with the food.

   e: There is no region or component of the GI tract that does not have a proper blood and lymphatic as well as nervous component.

2. **Answer a:**

Stratified squamous wet epithelium abruptly changes to simple columnar epithelium at the gastroesophageal junction and again at the pectinate line in the anal canal.

   b: The lower anal canal-to-skin junction would be stratified squamous wet to stratified squamous dry epithelium.

   c: The lip contains the same junction described in B—only in reverse order.

   d: There would be no epithelial change between oropharynx and esophagus, both being lined by stratified squamous non-keratinized epithelium.

   e: There would be no epithelial change between the stomach and the duodenum, both being lined by simple columnar epithelium.

3. **Answer b:**

Every surface columnar epithelial cell in the stomach secretes a special kind of mucus, which is atypical in that it is insoluble.

   a: The esophagus is lined by stratified squamous wet type of epithelium, which does not manufacture mucus.

   c: The duodenum is lined by both simple columnar absorptive cells and goblet cells, which do produce mucus, but since they are intermingled with the absorptive cells (enterocytes), not all of the surface cells here produce mucus.

   d: Although the colon has a very high count of goblet cells in its surface epithelium, there are still enterocytes here absorbing water.

e: The lower anal canal is lined by stratified squamous wet type epithelium, which does not secrete mucus.

4. **Answer d:**

The lower anal canal is lined by stratified squamous wet epithelium, which has desmosomes attaching one cell to another but not zonula occludens or zonula adherens. All other cell types listed have classical junctional complexes at their apical lateral borders.

a: The simple columnar cells lining the gallbladder are actively involved in absorption and therefore have junctional complexes on their lateral sides at the apex of the cell.

b, c, e: The same explanation given for A applies to the duodenal, ilial, and jejunal lining epithelia.

5. **Answer e:**

The esophagus is lined by stratified squamous wet type epithelium, which functions as a "wear and tear" or protective type surface, not an absorptive surface.

a–d: All of these organs do absorb significant amounts of water and electrolytes.

CHAPTER 16: THE URINARY SYSTEM

1. **Answer a:**

ADH increases the permeability of the collecting tubules to water. This enables osmotic pressure to reabsorb water into the interstitium, increasing tonicity of urine.

b: It increases the reabsorption of water in the collecting tubules.

c: Since water is reabsorbed output is decreased.

d: The tonicity of the urine is increased.

2. **Answers b, b, a, a:**

b: Reabsorption of Na^+ is an active process in PCT.

b: Reabsorption of Na^+ is an active process in the thick ascending portion of the loop of Henle.

a: Noncarrier-mediated transport accounts for secretion of Na^+ into the thin segment.

a: Noncarrier-mediated transport accounts for reabsorption of water from the thin segment.

3. **Answers e, a, b, d:**

e: Extensive microvilli are found on the cells of the PCT.

a: Foot processes and pedicles are found on the cells of podocytes in the visceral layer of Bowman's capsule.

b: Cells with a large number of mitochondria are found in the thick ascending portion of the loop of Henle.

d: The endothelium of the glomerulus is fenestrated.

4. **Answers d, a, c, d:**

d: Angiotensin II causes vascular smooth muscle contraction.

a: Renin, an enzyme that causes conversion of angiotensinogen to Angiotensin I, is synthesized by JGA cells.

c: Angiotensinogen is synthesized in the liver.

d: Aldosterone, a hormone synthesized by the cells of the Z. glomerulosa, increases Na^+ resorption in the DCT.

5. (A) Na^+ ions in the afferent arteriole, appear in (B) glomerular filtratrate which proceeds to (C) the lumen of the PCT, to be absorbed into the (D) peritubular plexus that drains to the (E), arcuate vein.

CHAPTER 17: THE MALE REPRODUCTIVE SYSTEM

1. **Answer d:**

They have completed the reductional division at metaphase I and have only an X or a Y chromosome. Except for the results of crossing over, each chromosome is identical.

a: They have completed the reductional division at metaphase I and have only an X or a Y chromosome.

b: Except for the results of crossing over, each chromosome is identical.

c: Except for the results of crossing over, each chromosome is identical.

2. **Answer e:**

Having completed meiosis I, this is a haploid cell that demonstrates 2 chromatids per chromosome and contains the same amount of DNA as a G1 somatic cell.

a: The reductional meiosis I results in the haploid chromosome number.

b: Each chromosome contains 2 chromatids.

c: The cell contains the 2C amount of DNA.

d: The secondary spermatocyte having completed meiosis I contains 23 chromosomes, each having 2 chromatids (46 chromatids).

3. **Answer e:**

It takes about 62 days to go from the most mature spermatogonia to spermatozoan.

a: Spermatogonia labeled but not most advanced stage.

b: Primary spermatocytes labeled but not most advanced stage.

c: Secondary spermatocytes labeled but not most advanced stage.

d: Early spermatid labeled but not most advanced stage.

4. **Answers a, b, a, b:**

a: Spermatogonia are VIM cells and would be labeled.

b: Oocytes are in meiosis I and would not incorporate thymidine 3H.

a: Primary spermatocytes are in meiosis I and would not incorporate thymidine 3H, but 3H thymidine would be incorporated into spermatogonia, which would proceed to the primary spermatocyte phase within several hours.

b: Spermatids do not replicate DNA.

5. **Answers b, d, c, e:**

b: The acrosome is elaborated by the Golgi complex of the spermatid.

d: Enzymes involved in testosterone synthesis are found on the SER of the Leydig cell.

c: ABP is synthesized on the RER of the Sertoli cell.

e: The ZO of the Sertoli cell maintains the blood testis barrier.

Chapter 18: The Female Reproductive System

1. **Answer b:**

All of the oocytes are produced by mitotic events in the fetal ovary from the 5th to 7th month.

a: The follicular cells do undergo changes in shape and number during this cycle, e.g., the follicular cells begin as a single layer of squamous-like cells and end up stratified cuboidal.

c: During the ovarian cycle, an antrum does form in the stratified follicular cells.

d: The size of the nucleus of the oocyte increases as the cycle approaches ovulation.

e: The zona pellucida does form as the cycle progresses.

2. **Answer e:**

As the estrogen level decreases, which results in a rise of FSH-RF, this event does not occur before ovulation, but as the corpus luteum involutes.

a: Estrogen stimulates contraction in the smooth muscle of the uterine tube and in the myometrium.

b: The thickness of the vaginal epithelium is less during menses.

c: A drop in the level of LH as the corpus luteum ages will cause a drop in the amount of estrogen and progesterone produced by the corpus luteum. FSH stimulates a group of follicles to grow, and as they grow and increase the number of follicular cells, which are involved in the production of estrogen, the estrogen level will increase.

d: The estrogen level does not decrease and the FSH-RF does not increase immediately prior to ovulation.

3. **Answer e:**

This is the oocyte with the female pronucleus in it containing the gamete amount of DNA and a haploid number of chromosomes, each with only one chromatid.

a: This describes a prophase 1 situation.
b: This describes a regular G1 situation.
c: This is what a secondary oocyte would contain immediately before fertilization.
d: This is an erroneous situation that does not exist.

4. **Answer b:**

This is an example of an estrogen dominated epithelium, i.e., most differentiated state.

a, c, d: The cells that desquamate during the secretory phase, which would include the premenstrual phase and menses, are not as mature as those seen in the estrogen dominated epithelium.

5. **Answer d:**

The syncytiotrophoblast has the ultrastructural organelles consistent with the production of steroid and nonsteroid hormones.

a: The Hofbauer cell is a mesenchymally derived macrophage, not an endocrine cell.
b: No matter where the cytotrophoblast cells are found, they do not contain well-developed cytoplasmic organelles, which would be required to synthesize and release HCG.
c: Nitabuch's membrane is a fibrinoid area of interface between fetal tissue (outer cytotrophoblastic shell and the decidualized endometrium).

Chapter 19: The Endocrine System

1. **Answer c:**

The parenchyma of the adrenal medulla is directly innervated by preganglionic fibers of the sympathetic nervous system.

a: ACTH is the pituitary hormone that has a major influence on the zona fasciculata, not the medulla.
b: Corticotropin releasing factor is a hypothalamic hormone that stimulates a type of hypophyseal basophil to release ACTH.
d: Aldosterone is synthesized by the zona glomerulosa and is a mineralocorticoid that is not involved in the release of epinephrine or norepinephrine.
e: A decrease in the osmolarity of the blood does not cause the release of epinephrine or norepinephrine.

2. **Answer a:**

Since endocrine glands use their vascular supply as their functional duct system, all endocrine glands are highly vascularized.

b: The cell division rate is very low in endocrine glands.
c: Many endocrine glands depend on the pituitary gland for "instructions," but not all. For example, the parathyroid is directly influenced by the serum calcium levels, and the islets of Langerhans are directly influenced by the presence of glucose in the blood.
d: Most endocrine glands store relatively small amounts of their hormones in cytoplasmic granules. The thyroid gland is the only example of an endocrine gland that stores large amounts of hormone, and this storage is extracellular.
e: Most endocrine glands depend on an influence from the pituitary gland to control their secretion, not upon the autonomic nervous system. The adrenal medulla is directly influenced by direct innervation by the sympathetic division of the autonomic nervous system.

3. **Answers b, d, b, a, b, e:**

b: A type of pituitary basophil releases TSH.
d: A type of hypothalamic neuron releases TSH-RH.
b: A type of basophil releases ACTH.
a: A type of hypophyseal acidophil releases somatotrophin.
b: A third type of pituitary basophil releases FSH.
e: Glucagon is not released by any of the cells listed.

Chapter 20: The Eye and Ear

1. Answer a:

The optic disc is where the axons of the ganglion cells exit the eye forming the optic nerve. There is no photosensitive retina covering this disc; therefore, it is the blind spot.

b: The macula lutea is a yellowish spot in the retina lateral to the optic disc.

c: The fovea centralis is the special region of most acute vision. It is a small region in the center of the macula lutea. The fovea centralis has all of the innermost layers of the retina missing, allowing light to reach the outer nuclear layer unimpeded. This region is rod free with cones only.

2. Answer b:

Aqueous humor is formed by the ciliary processes; it then fills up the posterior chamber, flows through the pupil from posterior to anterior into the anterior chamber from which it is drained through the canal of Schlemm to episcleral veins.

a: Anterior chamber to pupil would be in reverse order.

c, d: Anterior chamber to the episcleral veins is in the correct order, but between these two choices the canal of Schlemm needs to be situated.

e: After formation by the ciliary processes the pupil and the anterior chamber would be next before reaching the canal of Schlemm.

3. Answer a:

First would be the sound waves in the air, which impact on the tympanic membrane, which transmits the vibrations over the ossicles to the oval window, then to the perilymph of the scala vestibuli, then to the endolymph of the cochlear duct, then to the perilymph of the scala tympani, and finally to the round window.

b: The foot plate of the stapes has to interact with the membrane in the oval window before the vibrations get transmitted to the perilymph of the scala vestibuli.

c: The endolymph of the cochlear duct cannot come before the perilymph of the scala vestibuli.

d: The oval window must come before the perilymph of the scala vestibuli.

e: The cochlear duct cannot come between the tympanic membrane and oval window. In the choices given the endolymph in the cochlear duct should be last.

4. Answer c:

These two chambers, which are filled with aqueous humor, communicate with each other or are connected to each other through the pupil.

a: The optic disc would have vitreous body anterior to it, but no aqueous humor.

b: Although the canal of Schlemm contains aqueous humor, it is not the region through which the anterior and posterior chambers are connected to each other.

d: The ora serrata is where the 10 layered photosensitive retina gives way anteriorly to the 2 layered, nonphotosensitive retina. It is not an opening through which the anterior and posterior chambers communicate with each other.

e: The ciliar zonules suspend the lens from the ciliary processes. They are little suspensory ligaments and not a chamber or opening through which aqueous humor moves.

5. Answer d:

The glands of Meibom in the eyelid secrete a substance that coats the edge of the eyelid, keeping the tear film posterior to it.

a: The stria vascularis is probably the vascular connective tissue area that produces the endolymph of the cochlear duct.

b: The olfactory mucosa is in the nose, not the eyelid.

c: The macula of the utricle is a sensory organ and has nothing to do with being a barrier to the movement of water (in this case, tears).

e: Ciliary processes are the site of formation of the aqueous humor and do not function as a barrier to water. They no doubt are involved in the movement of water from their stromal regions through the epithelium to the aqueous humor.

Index

Pages in italics indicate figures; pages with *t* indicate tables.

A

A band, 73
Acetylcholine, 76
Acquired immunological tolerance, 132
Acrosomal reaction, 186
Actin-containing microfilaments, 27, *28,* 74
Actinin, 28
Acute monocytic leukemia, 129
Acute myeloblastic leukemia, 128-129
Adenohypophysis, 200
Adherens junctions, 15, 48
Adipose cells, 53
   unilocular, 53
Adrenal gland, 207-208
Aganglionosis, 147
Agranulocytes, 114, 116
Air-blood barrier, 101-102, *102*
Alkaline phosphatase, 87
Allograft, 132
Alpha actinin, 75
Alpha cells, 208
Alveolar ducts, 98, 100
Alveolar macrophages, 102-103
Alveolar sacs, 98, 100, 101
Alveoli, 98, 101
Amacrine cells, 216
Amblyopia, 217
β-aminopropionitrile, 63
Anal canal, 152
Anaphase lagging, 42-43
Anchoring filaments, 110
Androstenedione, 186
Anemia, sickle cell, 114
Angiogenesis, 112
Angiogenic cell clusters, 121
Angiotensin II, formation of, 167-168
Angiotensinogen, 167-168
Ångstrom (Å), 1
Aniridia, 217
Ankyrin, 28
Annuli, 32
Anterograde degeneration, 67-68
Anterograde transport, 67
Antiangiogenesis factor, 86
Antibodies, 134
Antibody heterogeneity, 7

Antibody (humoral)-mediated immunological response, 134
Antigen-presenting cells, 134
Antigen trapping, 134
Antrum, 185
Apical dendrite, 221
Apocrine secretion, 47
Apocrine sweat glands, 83
Apoptosis, 184
Appendix, 152
Appositional deposition, 91
Appositional growth, 87, 88, 91
Aqueous humor, 213, 214
Arachnoid, 69
Arterial pressure, 107
Arteries, 105, 107
Arteriole, 107
Arteriosclerosis, 111
Arteriovenous anastomoses, 84, 105, 110
Articular cartilage, 91
Astrocytes, 68
Atresia, 184, 186
Atrial natriuretic hormone, 111
Atrial natriuretic peptide (ANP), 207
Atriopeptin, 207
Atrio-ventricular node, 111
Autograft, 132
Autolysis, 19
Autonomic nervous system, 65
Autophagic activity, 19
Autophagic vacuoles, 20
Autoradiography, *4,* 4-5
AV bundle of His, 111
Axon, 65-66
Axoneme, 26
Axoplasmic transport, 67

B

Barr body, 42
Basal cells, 221
Basal lamina, 62, 163
   composition of, 62, *62t*
Basement membrane, 62
Basophilic leukemia, 129
Basophilic normoblast, 127
Basophils, 116, 117, 126
B-cells, 134, 135
Beta cells, 208
Bimolecular layer, 9-10
Bipolar neurons, 66, 221

Mosby's Review Series
Copyright © 1996,
Mosby–Year Book, Inc.

How to install this program—Windows users

1. Place the disk in Drive A: (or B:)
2. From Program Manager, select File, then Run, then enter:
   A:SETUP (or B:SETUP if your disk drive is B:)
3. Follow the instructions on screen.

How to run this program—Windows users

Open the MOSBY Program Group and select the ACE program.

How to install this program—Macintosh users

1. Insert the disk into the disk drive. Double-click on the disk icon.
2. Double-click on the Install icon. The program will be saved to your hard drive.

How to run this program—Macintosh users

Open the MOSBY folder and select the ACE program.

For complete instructions on using the program, please read the "How to use this Program" file.

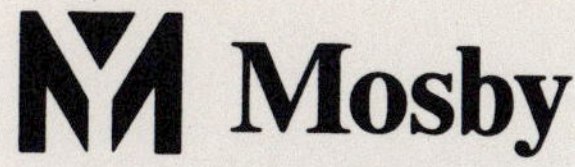

Mosby

Dedicated to Publishing Excellence

WE WANT TO HEAR FROM YOU!

To help us publish the most useful materials for students, we would appreciate your comments on this book. Please take a few moments to complete the form below, and then tear it out and mail to us. Thank you for your input.

Mosby's reviews: **HISTOLOGY & CELL BIOLOGY**

1. What courses are you using this book for?

___medical school   ___1st year
___pharmacy school   ___2nd year
___physician assistant program   ___3rd year
___nursing school   ___4th year
___dental school   ___other
___osteopathic school
___undergrad
___other _________________________

2. Was this book useful for your course? Why or why not?

___yes ___no____
____
____

3. What features of textbooks are important to you? (*check all that apply*)

___color figures
___summary tables and boxes
___summaries
___self-assessment questions
___price
___other ____
____

4. What influenced your decision to buy this text? (*check all that apply*)

___required/recommended by instructor
___recommendation by student
___bookstore display
___other ____

5. What other instructional materials did/would you find useful in this course?

___computer-assisted instruction
___lab time   ___slides
___case studies book
___other ____

Are you interested in doing in-depth reviews of our basic science textbooks? If so please fill out the information below.

NAME:_______________________________________

ADDRESS:____________________________________

____

TELEPHONE:__________________________________

THANK YOU!

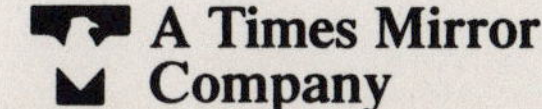
A Times Mirror Company

BUSINESS REPLY MAIL

FIRST CLASS MAIL   PERMIT No. 135   St. Louis, MO.

POSTAGE WILL BE PAID BY ADDRESSEE

CHRIS REID
MEDICAL EDITORIAL
MOSBY–YEAR BOOK, INC.
11830 WESTLINE INDUSTRIAL DRIVE
ST.LOUIS, MO 63146-9987